Musculoskeletal Pain, Myofascial Pain Syndrome, and the Fibromyalgia Syndrome

Musculoskeletal Pain, Myofascial Pain Syndrome, and the Fibromyalgia Syndrome

Søren Jacobsen, MD
Bente Danneskiold-Samsøe, MD, PhD
Birger Lund, MD, PhD
Editors

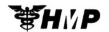

The Haworth Medical Press
An Imprint of
The Haworth Press, Inc.
New York • London • Norwood (Australia)

Published by

The Haworth Medical Press, 10 Alice Street, Binghamton, NY 13904-1580 USA

The Haworth Medical Press is an Imprint of The Haworth Press, Inc., 10 Alice Street, Binghamton, NY 13904-1580 USA.

Musculoskeletal Pain, Myofascial Pain Syndrome, and the Fibromyalgia Syndrome has also been published as *Journal of Musculoskeletal Pain,* Volume 1, Numbers 3/4 1993.

The development, preparation, and publication of this work has been undertaken with great care. However, the publisher, employees, editors, and agents of The Haworth Press and all imprints of The Haworth Press, Inc., including The Haworth Medical Press and Pharmaceutical Products Press, are not responsible for any errors contained herein or for consequences that may ensue from use of materials or information contained in this work. Opinions expressed by the author[s] are not necessarily those of The Haworth Press, Inc.

Library of Congress Cataloging-in-Publication Data

World Congress on Myofascial Pain and Fibromyalgia (2nd : 1992 : Copenhagen, Denmark)
Musculoskeletal pain, myofascial pain syndrome, and the fibromyalgia syndrome / Søren Jacobsen, Bente Danneskiold-Samsøe, Birger Lund, editors.
   p. cm.
Includes bibliographical references and index.
ISBN 1-56024-485-2 (alk. paper). – ISBN 1-56024-508-5 (pbk. : alk. paper)
   1. Myalgia–Congresses. 2. Fibrositis–Congresses. I. Jacobsen, Søren. II. Danneskiold-Samsøe, B. III. Lund, Birger. IV. Title.
   [DNLM: 1. Fibromyalgia–congresses. 2. Myofascial Pain Syndromes–congresses. WE 550 W927m 1992]
RC927.3.W67 1992
616.7–dc20
DNLM/DLC
for Library of Congress   93-30041
                                                                                                          CIP

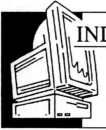

INDEXING & ABSTRACTING

Contributions to this publication are selectively indexed or abstracted in print, electronic, online, or CD-ROM version[s] of the reference tools and information services listed below. This list is current as of the copyright date of this publication. See the end of this section for additional notes.

- *Cambridge Scientific Abstracts*, *Health & Safety Science Abstracts*, Cambridge Information Group, 7200 Wisconsin Avenue #601, Bethesda, MD 20814

- *Dental Abstracts,* Mosby-Year Book, Inc., 200 N. LaSalle Street, Chicago, IL 60601-1080

- *Ergonomics Abstracts,* Taylor & Francis, Ltd., Rankine Road, Basingstoke, Hants RG24 0PR, England

- *Excerpta Medica/Electronic Publishing Division*, Elsevier Science Publishers, 655 Avenue of the Americas, New York, NY 10010

- *Pharmacist's Letter "Abstracts Section,"* Therapeutic Research Center, 8834 Hildreth Lane, Stockton, CA 95212

- *Physical Therapy "Abstracts Section,"* American Physical Therapy Association, 1111 North Fairfax Street, Alexandria, VA 22314-1488

- *Referativnyi Zhurnal [Abstracts Journal of the Institute of Scientific Information of the Republic of Russia],* The Institute of Scientific Information, Baltijskaja ul., 14, Moscow A-219, Republic of Russia

- *SilverPlatter Information, Inc.*, Information Resources Group, 101 West Walnut Street, Suite 200, Pasadena, CA 91103

- *Sport Database/Discus*, Sport Information Resource Center, 1600 James Naismith Drive, Suite 107, Gloucester, Ontario K1B 5N4, Canada

[continued]

SPECIAL BIBLIOGRAPHIC NOTES

related to indexing, abstracting, and library access services

☐ indexing/abstracting services in this list will also cover material in the "separate" that is co-published simultaneously with Haworth's special thematic journal issue or DocuSerial. Indexing/abstracting usually covers material at the article/chapter level.

☐ monographic co-editions are intended for either non-subscribers or libraries which intend to purchase a second copy for their circulating collections.

☐ monographic co-editions are reported to all jobbers/wholesalers/approval plans. The source journal is listed as the "series" to assist the prevention of duplicate purchasing in the same manner utilized for books-in-series.

☐ to facilitate user/access services all indexing/abstracting services are encouraged to utilize the co-indexing entry note indicated at the bottom of the first page of each article/chapter/contribution.

☐ this is intended to assist a library user of any reference tool [whether print, electronic, online, or CD-ROM] to locate the monographic version if the library has purchased this version but not a subscription to the source journal.

☐ individual articles/chapters in any Haworth publication are also available through the Haworth Document Delivery Services [HDDS].

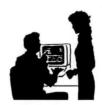

Musculoskeletal Pain, Myofascial Pain Syndrome, and the Fibromyalgia Syndrome

CONTENTS

PERIPHERAL AND CENTRAL MECHANISMS
IN MUSCLE PAIN

Preface:
MYOPAIN '92

Much has happened since MYOPAIN '89, including MYOPAIN '92. The latter was a wonderfully planned, international conference on musculoskeletal pain held during the month of August, 1992 in the beautiful environment of Copenhagen, Denmark. The success of that meeting was due to the vision of a multinational Program Committee and to the efficiency of local staff working under the direction of the conference president, Dr. Bente Danneskiold-Samsøe. More recently Dr. Danneskiold-Samsøe and Dr. Birger Lund have supervised the administrative efforts of Dr. Søren Jacobsen in editing for publication the proceedings of the main scientific presentations.

Drs. Lund and Danneskiold-Samsøe are well known to the international community for their work with rheumatic disease patients. This occasion, however, provides an opportunity to introduce a promising new investigator to the field of non-articular rheumatism. Dr. Søren Jacobsen's interest in fibromyalgia began in 1986 when he was a student at the Department of Rheumatology, Hvidovre Hospital. He was encouraged by the late Dr. Rasmus Bach Andersen and by Dr. Danneskiold-Samsøe to become involved in clinical research.

Some of the fruit of his labors is evidenced by the Denmark study examining the prevalence of fibromyalgia. Dr. Jacobsen is now a rheumatology fellow at the Copenhagen University Hospital. He already has 25 publications to his credit and there is good reason to expect many other valuable contributions from this gifted young colleague.

I. Jon Russell, MD, PhD

[Haworth co-indexing entry note]: "Preface: MYOPAIN '92." Russell, I. Jon. Co-published simultaneously in the *Journal of Musculoskeletal Pain* (The Haworth Press, Inc.) Vol. 1, No. 3/4, 1993, pp. xv-xvi; and: *Musculoskeletal Pain, Myofascial Pain Syndrome, and the Fibromyalgia Syndrome* (ed: Søren Jacobsen, Bente Danneskiold-Samsøe, and Birger Lund) The Haworth Press, Inc., 1993, p. xiii. Multiple copies of this article/chapter may be purchased from The Haworth Document Delivery Center [1-800-3-HAWORTH; 9:00 a.m. - 5:00 p.m. (EST)].

Introduction:
The Second World Congress on Myofascial Pain and Fibromyalgia, MYOPAIN '92, Copenhagen, August 17-20, 1992

Musculoskeletal pain is a common cause of both short- and long-term disability. Great efforts have been expended to categorize and describe the various types of musculoskeletal pain. Myofascial pain and fibromyalgia are two distinct syndromes which have been recognized and subjected to a large research effort as reflected by the First International Symposium on Myofascial Pain and Fibromyalgia, held in May of 1989 in Minneapolis (1). This successful meeting revealed much general interest in the field and a need for further research in specific disorders. The Second World Congress on Myofascial Pain and Fibromyalgia, held in August of 1992 in Copenhagen, was the follow-up meeting, in what hopefully will turn out to be a continuing series of conferences on these disorders. The Third World Congress on Myofascial Pain and Fibromyalgia is already scheduled for 1995 in San Antonio, Texas. Participants of MYOPAIN '92 will automatically receive information about that meeting.

At the opening of MYOPAIN '92 Drs. Janet Travell and David Simons were acknowledged for their pioneering efforts in revealing the mysteries of myofascial problems. They have published a most useful two volume manual on myofascial pain and dysfunction (2).

The Second World Congress on Myofascial Pain and Fibromyalgia was

[Haworth co-indexing entry note]: "Introduction: The Second World Congress on Myofascial Pain and Fibromyalgia, MYOPAIN '92, Copenhagen, August 17-20, 1992." Jacobsen, Søren, Bente Danneskiold-Samsøe, and Birger Lund. Co-published simultaneously in the *Journal of Musculoskeletal Pain* (The Haworth Press, Inc.) Vol. 1, No. 3/4, 1993, pp. 1-2; and: *Musculoskeletal Pain, Myofascial Pain Syndrome, and the Fibromyalgia Syndrome* (ed: Søren Jacobsen, Bente Danneskiold-Samsøe, and Birger Lund) The Haworth Press, Inc., 1993, pp. 1-2. Multiple copies of this article/chapter may be purchased from The Haworth Document Delivery Center [1-800-3-HAWORTH; 9:00 a.m. - 5:00 p.m. (EST)].

attended by participants from 34 countries and provided 177 podium or poster presentations. A full list of contributions is supplied in this volume and submitted abstracts are published in a supplementary issue of the *Scandinavian Journal of Rheumatology* (3). As editors, we appreciate the fact that most podium presenters have provided manuscripts detailing their work for these proceedings.

The congress was concluded by a consensus conference on fibromyalgia. This was the first attempt ever to reach international consensus on fibromyalgia. A written report entitled "Consensus Document on Fibromyalgia: The Copenhagen Declaration" was produced by a selected panel of experts in the field (4). It was refined by the panel from a preliminary consensus document available to all congress participants. This report now provides the current consensus on fibromyalgia by the world's most leading experts on fibromyalgia.

These proceedings provide the reader with the most updated information on both myofascial pain and fibromyalgia. It is our hope that they will benefit both researchers and patients suffering from painful musculoskeletal disorders.

Søren Jacobsen, MD
Bente Danneskiold-Samsøe, MD, PhD
Birger Lund, MD, PhD

REFERENCES

1. Myofascial Pain and Fibromyalgia. Fricton JR, Awad EA (eds.). Advances in Pain Research and Therapy Volume 17, Raven Press, New York, 1992.

2. Myofascial Pain and Dysfunction. The Trigger Point Manual. Volume I & II. Travell JG, Simons DG. Williams & Wilkins, Baltimore, 1983 & 1992.

3. MYOPAIN '92. Abstracts from the 2nd World Congress on Myofascial Pain and Fibromyalgia, Copenhagen, Denmark, August 17-20, 1992. Danneskiold-Samsøe B, Jacobsen S, Lund B (eds.). Scand J Rheumatology Supplement 94: 1-70, 1992.

4. Consensus Document on Fibromyalgia: The Copenhagen Declaration. J. Musculoskeletal Pain 1(3/4): 295-312, 1993. Also available from the Danish Rheumatism Association, Hauchsvej 14, 2000 Frederiksberg, Denmark.

REVIEW ARTICLES–MYOFASCIAL PAIN SYNDROMES AND FIBROMYALGIA

Pathogenesis of Fibromyalgia

Karl G. Henriksson

SUMMARY. The core symptoms and signs of the fibromyalgia [FM] syndrome are generalized chronic pain occurring mainly in muscles and hyperalgesia [tender points]. There is not one single cause to FM. The pathogeneses is a chain of events. Some links in the chain are still missing and some links are weak. The hypothesis presented is that FM is caused by a combination of peripheral factors mainly muscle and central factors. The central factors result in a decrease of pain inhibition.

KEYWORDS. Fibromyalgia, muscle pain

The patient with fibromyalgia [FM] is polysymptomatic. Symptoms that occur in 50% or more are generalized pain, sleep disturbance, fatigue,

Karl G. Henriksson, MD, PhD, is Associate Professor of Neurology, Neuromuscular Unit and Pain Clinic, University Hospital, S-581 85 Linköping, Sweden.

[Haworth co-indexing entry note]: "Pathogenesis of Fibromyalgia." Henriksson, Karl G. Co-published simultaneously in the *Journal of Musculoskeletal Pain* (The Haworth Press, Inc.) Vol. 1, No. 3/4, 1993, pp. 3-16; and: *Musculoskeletal Pain, Myofascial Pain Syndrome, and the Fibromyalgia Syndrome* (ed: Søren Jacobsen, Bente Danneskiold-Samsøe, and Birger Lund) The Haworth Press, Inc., 1993, pp. 3-16. Multiple copies of this article/chapter may be purchased from The Haworth Document Delivery Center [1-800-3-HAWORTH; 9:00 a.m. - 5:00 p.m. (EST)].

3

muscle stiffness, parasthesias and head ache (1). Muscular weakness and decreased muscular endurance are present in 50% or more of the patients (Bengtsson A et al., unpublished observation). Psychological distress is frequent. Social consequences for work, leisure time activities and for family relations are common. In one study, 90% of the FM patients state that fibromyalgia had markedly influenced their daily life (2).

There are two main ways to approach the fibromyalgia symptomatology. The first is to organize the symptoms in the following four groups.

1. Generalized chronic pain and tender points at 11 of 18 specified sites according to the classification criteria accepted by American College of Rheumatology (1).
2. Muscular weakness, decreased muscular endurance and increased perception of muscular effort. These symptoms may be a consequence of chronic muscular pain.
3. Typical symptoms that are common in FM but not specific for FM. The symptoms are, e.g., fatigue, sleep disturbance, stress symptoms and depressive symptoms.
4. Psychosocial consequences for work, leisure time activities, family relations etc.

The other way is to include all the symptoms described above in the concept of FM with the possible exception of symptoms that obviously are secondary to the pain. FM could then be regarded as a syndrome characterized by dysfunction of regulatory systems. In this overview the first approach will be followed and only the pathogenesis of chronic generalized muscular pain and of tender points will be discussed.

Morphological or biochemical or physiological changes have been found in a large number of studies in patients with FM. Changes are found both in peripheral tissues such as muscle and skin and in the central nervous system. There is no general agreement about the interpretation of these findings. With our present knowledge, it is difficult to know which findings are primary in the chain of events that result in FM and which changes are secondary to non-restorative sleep or chronic stress, which in turn could be secondary to the pain. Pain analyses of patients with FM support the notion that the pain is nociceptive, which means that at least part of pathogenesis is stimulation of nociceptors in muscles or other deep tissues. The pain disappears if the transmission of pain impulses is blocked by local anaesthesia (3). It also disappears after total blockade of sympathetic nerves (4). The pain diminishes on administration of opioids in a manner that is seen in nociceptive pain (3). The disappearance of pain on administration of local anaesthesia does not necessarily prove that the pain is peripheral.

MUSCULAR CHANGES

The muscle fibers themselves are not provided with pain receptors–nociceptors. Disorders with chronic muscle fiber degeneration like muscular dystrophies are usually pain-free. Muscle biopsy studies from different muscles in patients with FM do not show signs of ongoing muscle fiber degeneration (5).

The algogenic substances released in inflammation can excite pain neurones and also cause sensitization of pain receptors. Sensitization means that stimuli that normally do not evoke pain can elicit pain and that suprathreshold stimuli give rise to a more intensive pain than they normally do. Chronic inflammation in the muscle can be without pain. In a series of polymyositis and dermatomyositis comprising 107 patients, only 56% of the patients reported pain before treatment (6). Inflammation in the muscle may occur in FM but it is usually discreet and is found only in a minority of muscle biopsies (5).

During muscular contraction the intramuscular pressure increases. Resting values are, for example, around 4-6 mmHg in the anterior tibial muscle. At the pressure of 30-40 mmHg, the circulation is occluded. Even at a pressure of 15-18 mmHg, the microcirculation may be compromised, especially in the deeper part of the muscle (Fridén J, personal communication). At places where microcirculation is affected by increased intramuscular pressure, compensatory vasodilation may occur. This may minimize the risk of localized hypoxia. The disturbed microcirculation during contraction may, however, in any case lead to a decreased venous outflow. Algogenic substances may accumulate as long as the microcirculation is affected.

Ischemia or hypoxia alone does not necessarily give rise to muscular pain. Mense and Stahnke (7), in their animal studies, have found receptors in the muscles that are probably pain receptors which are excited by the combination of ischemia and muscle work. Ischemia can cause sensitization of pain receptors in the muscle, for example, through release of algogenic substances. Hypoxia interferes with ATP-production through oxidative metabolism. ATP is necessary for muscular work, muscle relaxation and for the integrity of the muscle fiber membrane. The storage of ATP in muscle is enough only for a few seconds of muscular work. Hypoxia, which may be localized, can mean that energy production in a certain population of the muscle fibers is inadequate for the energy demand. All situations where energy demand is greater than energy production are painful.

If the origin of the pain is in the muscle, signs of a disturbed microcirculation in combination with the presence of an energy-requiring process should be found. Pain in FM is present, not only during muscle work, but also at rest. Is there muscle tension also when there are no voluntary contractions in the painful muscle in FM? Or is the pain at rest a consequence of peripheral and/or central sensitization? Peripheral sensitization means a lowering of the threshold of nociceptors in the muscle. Central sensitization means increased excitation of second-order pain neurons in the CNS, or a changed processing in CNS of impulses in afferent nerves that are not nociceptive.

STUDIES ON MICROCIRCULATION
AND ENERGY METABOLISM IN PATIENTS WITH FM

1. Measurements of tissue oxygen pressure by an oxygen electrode placed directly on the surface of the trapezius and brachioradial muscles showed a distribution of pressure values which differed from normal controls. The distribution of the pressure values were similar to the one found in experimental ischemia. The results can be interpreted as a sign of a disturbed regulation of microcirculation (8).
2. Blockade of sympathetic efferent nerves increases microcirculation and relieves the pain and also the tender points (4,9).
3. Electronmicroscopical studies show that endothelial derangements occur more often in the trapezius muscle of patients with FM than in controls or in patients with localized shoulder pain (Rolf Lindman, unpublished observation).
4. In the descending part of the trapezius muscle, histochemical studies show that a proliferation, or accumulation, of mitochondria [the so called ragged red fibers–RR fibers] is found in patients with localized trapezius myalgia or fibromyalgia in 54%. The corresponding figure in patients with no pain is 31%. This difference in frequence is statistically significant [P < 0.02] (10). The RR fiber is a morphological sign of disturbed oxidative metabolism.
5. Energy rich phosphates are somewhat reduced in biopsies from the trapezius of patients with FM compared to controls (11). In a recent study (K Söderlund, unpublished observation), it has been found that the decrease in ATP is restricted to type 2 fibers [type 2 fibers are fast fibers].

6. That a slight change in energy metabolism is present in painful muscle is further supported by the discovery of a decreased relaxation rate (9).

Not all studies agree with the studies mentioned.

Simms et al. (12) and Blécourt et al. (13) found no differences in energy metabolism between FM patients and controls in their study using P-magnetic resonance spectroscopy.

The discrepancy between the results of different studies can have many causes. Different methods have different resolutions. The pathological findings may be localized and difficult to detect. The changes of importance for pathogenesis may differ from one muscle to another. The changes may be confined to certain motor units or a small population of muscle fibers. Findings may be different if the tests are performed at a time when the patients are pain-free compared with tests performed at intensive pain.

At present, we cannot rule out the fact that microcirculation and oxidative energy metabolism are affected in FM. It is important to observe that the studies referred to above, with the exception of the relaxation rate studies, have been performed in resting muscles. What causes the changes in microcirculation which are present in muscles at rest? We don't know. Static work and deficient relaxation over long periods of time are possible factors. Some motor units may be active more or less continuously both during static and dynamic muscular contractions. Postischemic damage is another possibility. Hypoxia or ischemia alone do not necessarily give pain, as mentioned above. The finding of RR fibers, for example, is an unspecific sign of any disorder or pathophysiological state that affects oxidative metabolism. RR fibers are often found in conditions where there is no pain.

ARE THERE ANY SIGNS OF AN ENERGY REQUIRING PROCESS IN PAINFUL MUSCLES WHEN THERE IS NO VOLUNTARY MUSCLE CONTRACTION?

In one study with surface EMG we did not find any signs of muscle tension at rest in painful muscles in FM (14). In a recent study by Elert et al. (15), it was shown that the relaxation between contractions were less efficient in patients with FM and in patients with localized trapezius myalgia than in persons with no pain. The relaxation was studied in several shoulder muscles. The insufficient relaxation could mean that the microcirculation could be affected also at rest between contractions in patients with chronic muscular pain. The difference between FM and localized trapezius pain was that in localized pain the insufficient relaxation was confined to the trapezius muscle. In FM the insufficient relaxation was found in all tested shoulder muscles. Another important observation was that the patient's perception of muscle tension correlated to the objectively demonstrated insufficient relaxation (16).

Muscle tension caused by reflex mechanisms involving the gamma system has also been proposed as a possible cause of muscle tension in pain conditions (17).

The muscle tension that occurs in relation to mental stress situations could be another possible cause of an energy requiring process present even when there are no voluntary contractions.

The muscular pain in FM often starts as a localized pain. The most common sites are the shoulder muscles and the lumbal back muscles. Pain from the muscle is generally more diffuse than pain from the skin. The spreading of the pain is probably due to central mechanisms. The tendency to spreading is greater if the pain is intensive. The generalized pain in FM may be triggered from a few muscle groups, and muscle pathology and pathophysiology may, as mentioned above, be restricted to a few muscles or muscle groups.

REFERRED PAIN

The pain that the patients localize to the muscle may be referred to the muscle from other deep structures. Such structures could be joint capsules, ligaments, skeleton and joints. Of special interest in this context are changes in the vertebral joints or ligaments, preferably in the lumbar spine and cervical spine. Inflammation or stretching that occurs in the joint capsules or ligaments may also give rise to reflexogenic muscular tension in the muscle in the same segment. This muscle tension may then, in addition to the changes in microcirculation described above, be of importance for the pathogenesis and the muscular pain (17). Before damage in other deep structures than the muscle is accepted as a cause of a chronic muscular pain it is required that a structural or physiological pathology is diagnosed and that the symptoms diminish after treatment.

CHANGES IN PAIN MODULATION

The generalized pain in FM can hardly be explained only by peripheral mechanisms. The acute peripheral pain caused by tissue damage induces changes at the dorsal horn levels. Clifford Wolf has summarized the central effect as follows (18):

1. Reduction in threshold–that could give alodynia [alodynia is present when non-nocious stimuli evoke pain]; amplication of responses [that could give hyperalgesia]; expanded receptive field [that could cause the spread of sensitization]; and, finally, after-discharges that could cause persistent pain.

In animal experiments it has been shown that activity in central nociceptive neurons receiving input mainly from the muscle are under more central inhibitory control than central nociceptive neurons receiving inputs mainly from the skin (19). An important inhibitory transmittor substance is serotonin. Changes in serotonin levels could influence pain inhibition.

There are, at present, a fairly large number of studies that indicate that FM patients have either a disturbance of pain modulation or a disturbed function of regulatory systems. These pathological findings have recently been reviewed by Boissevain and McCain (20) and by Zimmerman (21) and by Yunus (22). In summary, deviation from controls have been found with respect to

a. serotonin metabolism: the findings indicate a serotonin deficiency in the central nervous system (23,24,25,26).
b. norepinephrine, epinephrin and dopamine metabolism: no conclusive statement can be made about these transmittor substances in FM (23).
c. levels of substance P: substance P is increased in CSF in FM patients compared to controls (27).
d. function of the autonomus nervous system: the baseline sympathetic activity is probably not increased in patients with FM (28). Værøy et al. (29) found a decreased vasoconstrictor response to auditive and cold pressor tests in FM patients. vanDenderen et al. (30) tested the physiological effects of exhaustive physical exercise and measured also cortisol epinephrin and norepinephrine levels. The levels were lower than in controls. These findings together with lower heart rates were interpreted as signs of a disturbed reactivity of the sympathetic nervous system.
e. the function of the hypothalamus–pituitary-adrenal axis (30,31) and finally
f. the function of the immune system: there are few reports of immunological disturbance. Hader et al., for example, found a defect in the interleukin-2 pathway in patients with FM (32). Bengtsson et al.

determined the titres of different autoantibodies in serum from patients with FM. They found that the occurrence of antibodies did not differ from the reference values (33).

The findings indicating serotonin deficiency or increased values of substance P in CSF fit very well with the assumption that there is a decreased pain inhibition in patients with FM. However, it is difficult to evaluate whether the findings referred to above are primary or secondary to sleep disturbance, for example, or secondary to chronic stress or secondary to chronic pain at large.

SLEEP DISTURBANCE

Sleep disturbance characterized by increased occurrence of alpha-delta sleep in the EEG and clinically by non-restorative sleep is common in FM. The question as to whether sleep disturbance is a primary or a secondary event in FM is not settled (34,35). Low levels of somatomedine-C have been found in patients with FM. Somatomedine levels reflect growth hormone secretion. Growth hormone is produced during deep sleep, and low levels may effect protein metabolism in the muscle (36).

PSYCHOLOGY

FM patients suffer more often from depression and psychological illness than controls and, for example, patients with RA (37,38). Quality of life is related to the degree of psychological distress. The majority of FM patients have, however, no psychiatric or psychological disorder and there is no basis for the statement that the pain and tenderness in FM are primarily caused by emotional stress, depression or anxiety. These factors may, however, increase the intensity of the pain (39).

MUSCULAR FUNCTION

In a study by Bennet et al. (40), aerobic fitness was reduced in 80% of FM patients compared with controls. Bennet and co-workers have proposed that the "detraining phenomenon" and mechanical microlesions in disused muscle could be of importance for the pathogenesis of muscle pain in FM (41). However, in a Scandinavian study no difference in aerobic capacity was found between FM patients and healthy matched controls (42).

Muscular weakness and reduced muscular endurance have been found in several studies (42,43 and Bengtsson A, unpublished observation). In one study, where the muscle strength during electrical stimulation of the muscle nerve was compared with maximal voluntary contraction strength, the results indicated that the muscular weakness was of central origin (9). Clinically, one common complaint from FM patients is an increased perceptions of effort. That the FM patients have an increased perception of effort compared both with patients with localized trapezius myalgia and with persons with no pain has been shown (44). There are no indications in studies of muscle function that the results can be explained only by decreased motivation. However, it cannot be totally ruled out that motivation plays a role. Central effects of chronic pain could also contribute to the difficulty for patients with FM to activate their motor units in voluntary muscular contractions.

SKIN CHANGES

Increased extravasation of IgG was found in a series comprising 25 consecutive FM patients. The results do not indicate an immunological disorder, but suggest that the attachment of IgG was unspecific. The IgG attachment to collagen in the dermis could possibly be caused either by a defect of collagen or a damage to vessels by anoxia, for example. An increased number of connective tissue mastcells was found (45). Whether this has anything to do with the finding by Littlejohn et al. (46) of an increased tendency towards neurogenic inflammation in the skin is not known. The diagnostic importance of a skin biopsy has so far not been further investigated.

THE PATHOGENESIS OF TENDER POINTS

The presence of tender points at 11 of 18 specified sites is one of the requirements for the diagnosis for FM according to the ACR criteria (1). The tender point represents an area with mechanical hyperalgesia. The localization of the tender point may simply reflect the point or areas that are most densely provided with receptors for noxious and non-noxious stimuli. Two possible pathogenetic mechanisms for tender points will be discussed. The first is that tender points represent an area with neurogenic inflammation. Impulses in primary pain neurons from the skin can give rise to neurogenic inflammation. The neurogenic inflammation is caused by the release of substance P and other neuropeptides. There is some evidence that neurogenic inflammation in the skin is present in fibromyalgia (46). Whether or not neurogenic inflammation also occurs in the muscle has not been established and consequently we do not know if neurogenic inflammation can explain tender points in the muscle. Tender points that are not localized to the muscle could possibly be explained by neurogenic inflammation.

The second explanation of the tender points is that they represent areas of primary and secondary hyperalgesia. In the skin, primary hyperalgesia can be produced experimentally by injecting capsaicin, which gives rise to a C-fiber mediated primary hyperalgesia. Around the area of primary hyperalgesia, a larger area of secondary hyperalgesia develops. In experiments in humans with the use of microneurography and neuro-microstimulation. Torebjörk et al. (47) have shown that secondary hyperalgesia is caused by activity in low threshold mechanoreceptive group A afferents, and that secondary hyperalgesia is the result of a changed signal processing in the spinal cord. The pain can thus be caused by activity in afferent neurons that do not normally convey the sensation of pain. The presence of same type of sensitization and secondary hyperalgesia in the muscle in FM, for example, has not been shown. There is a possibility that the hyperalgesia in the muscle that has been called tender point is a result of both peripheral and central sensitization. Peripheral sensitization can be caused by ischemia.

The presence or absence of tenderness at a specific point may be due to the presence or absence of a disturbed microcirculation at the time of examination.

CONCLUSIONS AND HYPOTHESES

The morphological, physiological and biochemical changes found in the muscle are localized and comparatively discrete and, regarding some changes, there is more of a quantitative than a qualitative difference between findings in FM patients and controls. Localized disturbed microcirculation is a possible cause of some of the pathological findings. Mechanical microlesions could possibly explain other findings. It has not been proven that disturbed microcirculation alone can cause pain. In animals, the muscles contain pain receptors that are activated by the combination of ischemia and an energy requiring muscle tension. The pain in FM is a pain also at rest. Discrete muscle tension caused by reflexes possibly via the gamma-system or a discrete muscle tension caused by emotional or mental stress, or an insufficient relaxation between contractions together with disturbed microcirculation, could possibly cause muscular pain. Changes in the periphery, for example, in muscle could not, however, explain the generalized pain at rest in FM patients. It is hypothesized that the key to the problem of FM is a combination of peripheral factors and a disturbed pain modulation in CNS. Studies indicating a serotonin deficiency and an increase of the neuropeptide substance P indicate that there really is a disturbed pain modulation in CNS. The changed pain modulation could occur alone or as a part of a more generalized syndrome characterized by a disturbance in the regulatory systems. Chronic fatigue syndrome, for example, could be such a syndrome.

There is no single cause for a pain condition like FM. The pathogenesis is a chain of events. Some links in this chain are still missing, and some links are weak. Further studies are obviously needed. FM could very well be the key to the puzzle of chronic pain as suggested by Reilly and Littlejohn (48).

REFERENCES

1. Wolfe F, Smythe HA, Yunus MB, Bennett RM, Bombardier C, Goldenberg DL, Tugwell P, Campbell SM, Abeles M, Clark P, Fam AG, Farb er SJ, Fiechtner JJ, Franklin CM, Gatter RA, Hamaty D, Lessard J, Lichtbroun AS, Masi AT, McCain GA, Reynolds WJ, Tomano TJ, Russel IJ, Sheon RP: The American College of Rheumatology 1990 Criteria for the Classification of Fibromyalgia. Report of the Multicenter Criteria Committee. Arthritis Rheum 33:2: 160-172, 1990.

2. Henriksson C, Gundmark I, Bengtsson A, Ek A-C: Living with Fibromyalgia. Consequences for Everyday Life. Clin J Pain 8: 138-144, 1992.

3. Bengtsson M, Bengtsson A, Jorfeldt L: Diagnostic epidural opioid blockade in primary fibromyalgia at rest and during exercise: Pain 39: 171-180, 1989.

4. Bengtsson A, Bengtsson M: Regional sympathetic blockade in primary fibromyalgia. Pain 33: 161-167, 1988.

5. Bengtsson A, Henriksson KG, Larsson J: Muscle Biopsy in Primary Fibromyalgia. Scand J Rheumatol 15: 1-6, 1986.

6. Henriksson KG, Sandstedt P: Polymyositis–treatment and prognosis. A study of 107 patients. Acta Neurol Scand 65: 280-300, 1982.

7. Mense S, Stahnke M: Contraction–Sensitive Fine Muscle Afferents. J Physiol (Lond) 342: 383-397, 1983.

8. Lund N, Bengtsson A, Thorborg P: Muscle Tissue Oxygen Pressure in Primary Fibromyalgia. Scand J Rheum 15: 165-173, 1986.

9. Bäckman E, Bengtsson A, Bengtsson M, Lennmarken C, Henriksson KG: Skeletal muscle function in primary fibromyalgia. Effect of regional sympathetic blockade with guanethidine. Acta Neurol Scand 77: 187-191, 1988.

10. Henriksson KG, Bengtsson A, Lindman R, Thornell LE: Morphological changes in muscle in fibromyalgia and chronic shoulder myalgia. In: Progress in Fibromyalgia and Myofascial Pain. Eds.: Merskey H, Værøy H. Elsevier Science Publishers.

11. Bengtsson A, Henriksson KG, Larsson J: Reduced high-energy phosphate levels in the painful muscles of patients with primary fibromyalgia. Arthritis Rheum 29: 7, 817-821, 1986.

12. Simms RW, Roy S, Hrovat M, Anderson JJ, Skrinar G, LePoole SR, Zerbini CF, DeLuca C, Jolesz F: Fibromyalgia syndrome (FMS) is not associated with abnormalities in muscle energy metabolism. Scand J Rheumatol (suppl 94): 19, 1992.

13. de Blécourt, Wolf RF, van Rijswijk MH, Kamman RL, Knipping AA, Mooyaart EL: In vivo 31P magnetic resonance spectroscopy (MRS) of tender points in patients with primary fibromyalgia syndrome. Rheumatol Int 11: 51-54, 1991.

14. Zidar J, Bäckman E, Bengtsson A, Henriksson KG: Quantitative EMG and muscle tension in painful muscles in fibromyalgia. Pain 40: 249-254, 1990.

15. Elert JE, Rantapää-Dahlqvist SB, Henriksson-Larsén K, Lorentzon R, Gerdle BUC: Muscle Performance, Electronmyography and Fibre Type composition in Fibromyalgia and Work-related Myalgia. Scand J Rheumatol 21: 28-34, 1992.

16. Elert J, Rantapää-Dahlqvist, Almay B, Eisemann M: Muscle endurance, muscle tension and personality traits in patients with muscle or joint pain. A pilot study. Scand J Rheumatol (suppl 94): 31, 1992.

17. Johansson H, Sojka P: Pathophysiological mechanisms involved in genesis and spread of muscular tension in occupational muscle pain and in chronic musculoskeletal pain syndromes. A hypothesis: Med Hypotheses 35: 196-203, 1991.

18. Woolf CJ: Central mechanisms of acute pain. In: MR Bond, JE Charlton, CJ Woolf (Eds). Proceedings of the Vth World Congress on Pain, Elsevier Science Publishers BV: 3, 25-34, 1991.

19. Mense S: Physiology of Nociception in Muscles. In: JR Fricton, E Awad (Eds) "Advances in Pain Research and Therapy," Raven Press Ltd, New York 17: 67-85, 1990.

20. Boissevain MD, McCain GA: Clinical Section, Review Article. Toward an integrated understanding of fibromyalgia syndrome. I. Medical and pathophysiological aspects. Pain 45: 227-238, 1990.

21. Zimmerman M: Pathophysiological Mechanisms of Fibromyalgia. Clinical J Pain (Suppl 1): 8-15, 1991.

22. Yunus M: Towards a model of pathophysiology of fibromyalgia: Aberrant central pain mechanisms with peripheral modulation. J Rheumatol 19:6: 846-850, 1992.

23. Russell IJ, Værøy H, Javors M, Nyberg F: Cerebrospinal fluid biogenic amine metabolites in fibromyaglia/fibrositis syndrome and rheumatoid arthritis. Arthritis Rheum 35:5: 550-556, 1992.

24. Russell IJ, Michalek JE, Vipraio GA, Fletcher EM, Javors MA, Bowden CL: Serum serotonin and platelet ^{3}H-imipramine binding receptor density in patients with fibromyalgia/fibrositis syndrome. J Rheumatol 19: 104-109, 1992.

25. Russell IJ, Michalek JE, Vipraio GA, Fletcher EM, Wal K: Serum amino acids in fibrositis/fibromyalgia syndrome. J Rheumatol 16: 158-163, 1989.

26. Yunus MB, Dailey JW, Aldag JC, Masi AT, Jobe PC: Plasma tryptophan and other amino acids in primary fibromyalgia: a controlled study. J Rheumatol 19: 90-94, 1992.

27. Værøy H, Helle R, Øystein F, Kåss E, Terenius L: Elevated CSF levels of substance P and high incidence of Raynaud phenomenon in patients with fibromyalgia: new features for diagnosis. Pain 32: 21-26, 1988.

28. Elam M, Johansson G, Wallin BG: Do patients with primary fibromyalgia have an altered muscle sympathetic nerve activity?. Pain 48: 371-375, 1992.

29. Værøy H, Qiao ZG, Mørkrid L, Øystein F: Altered Sympathetic nervous system response in patients with fibromyalgia (fibrositis syndrome). J Rheumatol: 16:11: 1460-1465, 1989.

30. van Denderen JC, Boersma JW, Zeinstra P, Hollander AP, van Neerbos BR: Physiological effects of exhaustive physical exercise in primary fibromyalgia syndrome (PFS): Is PFS a disorder of neuroendocrine reactivity? Scand J Rheumatol 21: 35-37, 1992.

31. McCain GA, Tilbe KS: Diurnal hormone variation in fibromyalgia syndrome: A comparison with rheumatoid arthritis. J Rheumatol (suppl 19) 16: 154-157, 1989.

32. Hader N, Rimon D, Kinarty A, Lahat N: Altered interleukin-2 secretion in patients with primary fibromyalgia syndrome. Arthritis and Rheumatism 34:7: 866-872, 1991.

33. Bengtsson A, Ernerudh J, Vrethem M, Skogh T: Absence of autoantibodies in primary fibromyalgia. J Rheumatol 17: 1682-1683, 1990.

34. Moldofsky H: The contribution of Sleep-Wake physiology to fibromyalgia. In: JR Fricton, E. Awad (Eds) "Advances in Pain Research and Therapy," Raven Press Ltd, New York 17: 227-240, 1990.

35. Anch AM, Lue FA, MacLean AW, Moldofsky H: Sleep physiology aspects of the fibrositis (fibromyalgia) syndrome. Can J Psychol 45:2: 179-184, 1991.

36. Bennett RM, Clark SR, Campbell SM, Burckhardft CS: Low levels of somatomedin-C in fibromyalgia: A neuro-endocrine defect involving the sleep related secretion of growth hormone. Scand J of Rheumatol (suppl 94): 35, 1992.

37. Goldenberg DL: An overview of psychologic studies in fibromyalgia. J Rheumatol (suppl 19) 16: 12-14, 1989.

38. Boissevain MD, McCain GA: Review Article. Toward an integrated understanding of fibromyalgia syndrome. II. Psychological and phenomenological aspects. Pain 45: 239-248, 1991.

39. Yunus MB, Ahles TA, Aldag JC, Masi AT: Relationship of clinical features with psychological status in primary fibromyalgia. Arthritis & Rheumatism 34:1: 15-21, 1991.

40. Bennett RM, Clark SR, Goldberg L, Nelson D, Bonafede RP, Porter J, Specht D: Aerobic fitness in patients with fibrositis. A controlled study of respiratory gas exchange and [133] Xenon clearance from exercising muscle. Arthritis & Rheumatism 32:4: 454-460, 1989.

41. Bennett RM: Beyond fibromyalgia: Ideas on etiology and treatment. J Rheumatol (suppl 19) 16: 185-191, 1989.

42. Mengshoel AM, Førre Ø, Komnæs HB: Muscle strength and aerobic capacity in primary fibromyalgia. Clin Exp Rheumatol 8: 475-479, 1990.

43. Jacobsen S, Danneskiold-Samsøe B: Isometric and isokinetic muscle strength in patients with fibrositis syndrome. Scand J Rheumatol 16: 61-65, 1987.

44. Elert JE, Rantapää Dahlqvist SB, Henriksson-Larsén K, Gerdle: Increased EMG activity during short pauses in patients with primary fibromyalgia. Scand J Rheumatol 18: 321-323, 1989.

45. Eneström S, Bengtsson A, Lindström F, Johan K: Attachment of IgG to dermal extracellular matrix in patients with fibromyalgia. Clin Exp Rheumatol 8: 127-135, 1990.

46. Littlejohn GO, Weinstein C, Helme RD: Increased neurogenic inflammation in fibrositis syndrome. J Rheumatol 14: 1022-1025, 1987.

47. Torebjörk HE, Lundberg LER, Lamotte RH: Central changes in processing of mechanoreceptive input in capsaicin-induced secondary hyperalgesia in humans. J Physiol 448: 765-780, 1992.

48. Reilly PA, Littlejohn GO: Fibrositis/fibromyalgia syndrome: the key to the puzzle of chronic pain. Med J Aust 152: 226-228, 1990.

Fibromyalgia:
On Diagnosis and Certainty

Frederick Wolfe

SUMMARY. Objectives: To review the construct of fibromyalgia in light of current methods of diagnosis and classification.

Results: Although current criteria satisfactorily identify most persons with fibromyalgia and have added much to our ability to perform fibromyalgia research, problems are still present. Clinical and classification criteria are different and identify different sets of patients. Tenderness can occur with limited pain, and pain and symptoms without tenderness. "Mild" fibromyalgia and "early" fibromyalgia are not well captured by current criteria. Fibromyalgia and fibromyalgia criteria application can be influenced by psychological factors and the settings of compensation and litigation.

Conclusion: ACR classification criteria work well in studies [for which they were designed], but clinical as well as classification criteria may be useful in the clinic where uncertainty can not be dealt with by exclusion. More research is required to classify and conceptualize patients who intermittently meet criteria, and those with

---

Frederick Wolfe, MD, is affiliated with the Arthritis Research Center [St. Francis Research Institute] and is Clinical Professor of Internal Medicine and Family and Community Medicine, University of Kansas School of Medicine, Wichita, KS.

Address correspondence and reprint requests to: Frederick Wolfe, MD, Arthritis Research Center, 1035 N. Emporia, STE 230, Wichita, KS 67214.

Supported in part from a grant from the Los Angeles Chapter, Arthritis Foundation.

[Haworth co-indexing entry note]: "Fibromyalgia: On Diagnosis and Certainty." Wolfe, Frederick. Co-published simultaneously in the *Journal of Musculoskeletal Pain* (The Haworth Press, Inc.) Vol. 1, No. 3/4, 1993, pp. 17-35; and: *Musculoskeletal Pain, Myofascial Pain Syndrome, and the Fibromyalgia Syndrome* (ed: Søren Jacobsen, Bente Danneskiold-Samsøe, and Birger Lund) The Haworth Press, Inc., 1993, pp. 17-35. Multiple copies of this article/chapter may be purchased from The Haworth Document Delivery Center [1-800-3-HAWORTH; 9:00 a.m. - 5:00 p.m. (EST)].

17

remittent or mild symptoms. The certainty requested by the compensation and legal system conflicts with the uncertainty of fibromyalgia diagnosis and prognosis in that setting.

KEYWORDS. Fibromyalgia, diagnosis, criteria

During the decade of the 1980s, and following on ideas of Smythe and Moldofsky (1), a small, rump group of clinicians and investigators turned a foggy and somewhat disreputable concept into a widely recognized and generally accepted syndrome. The success has been almost complete. In the academic world grants for fibromyalgia are increasingly awarded. Fibromyalgia is routinely a subject in prestigious journals. Primary care physicians recognize, diagnose, and treat the disorder; and referrals to specialists are routine. Yet there are some days where I, as a clinician and investigator, have stood there and thought, "what have we created." In this paper which is about criteria, I want to discuss some of these problems [Table 1].

In the United States, in a major turn-around, disability benefits are being awarded for fibromyalgia. Litigation within the workplace is increasing and many very large judgments have been awarded. The questions that we have been asked by the courts have not been easy. Diagnosis of fibromyalgia is not always easy. I have been involved in cases where rheumatologists have testified on opposing sides as to whether the plaintiff had the disorder. If a plaintiff injures a shoulder and later seems to have developed more generalized pain and fibromyalgia tenderness, but in whom the shoulder is the major problem, does the plaintiff have fibromy-

TABLE 1. Problems associated with diagnosis in fibromyalgia.

1. Diagnostis is uncertain.

2. Diagnosis is correct, but main problem is not fibromyalgia.

3. Diagnosis is correct, but contra-productive.

4. Diagnostic criteria are satisfied, but clinically fibromyalgia is not present.

5. Diagnosis seems correct, but criteria are not satisfied.

6. Diagnosis is correct, but patient improves and does not satisfy criteria at all
   follow-up visits.

7. Diagnosis is correct, but psychological factors are predominant.

algia which is often then considered to be a life-long disorder [with the help of many of us] and worthy of life long compensation, or is it a shoulder disorder which might be expected to heal? I have also been involved in cases where the plaintiff was malingering [or at least exaggerating]. In one instance the plaintiff and attorney had read the literature of fibromyalgia and knew the symptoms and where tenderness was supposed to be. None of us planned this when we performed our studies of *patients* with the syndrome.

Next, I see patients who meet our various criteria, but surely are not benefited by a diagnosis of fibromyalgia; young people, often under stress, and having psychological difficulties. When diagnosed and referred by primary care physicians, I often have to try to talk the patient out of the diagnosis.

Then there are those who have widespread tenderness, but with pain that is partially or completely explained by other conditions. They have the tenderness of fibromyalgia but not the usual concomitants of irritable bowel syndrome, sleep disturbance, and the qualitative diffuse pain. And some patients are tender all over but have a single, limited complaint.

There are those patients who have met most of our criteria but not enough to be called fibromyalgia. But they have it. There are those patients who have met our criteria, have fibromyalgia, but when they return for re-visits have limited tenderness but most of the fibromyalgia symptoms.

Finally, there are those patients with overwhelming psychological distress who have the symptoms and meet the criteria, but whose primary difficulty is not musculoskeletal.

FIBROMYALGIA AND ITS CRITERIA

With problems like these in mind I would like to discuss the nature of fibromyalgia and its criteria. The concept of fibromyalgia with which I think few would disagree is that it is a syndrome of generally wide spread pain, decreased pain threshold as manifested by tender points, most often associated with fatigue, stiffness, disturbed or poor sleep, and associated with a usual and common set of signs and symptoms including mild soft tissue swelling, irritable bowel syndrome, paresthesias, headache, anxiety, depression, and modulation of symptoms by weather, activity, etc. Patients who fit this picture are easily recognized in the clinic. Indeed it is that they are so easily recognized that forms the basis for our claim to fibromyalgia as a syndrome.

There are, I believe, 4 characteristics that need to be considered in understanding fibromyalgia: pain, tenderness, characteristic signs and symptoms, and psychological distress [Table 2]. In grouping fibromyalgia in this way I have removed anxiety and depression from the "signs and symptoms" and placed them into the category of psychological distress.

Smythe and Moldofsky (1) and some others before them (2,3) called our attention to pain and tenderness and to some of the signs and symptoms [sleep disturbance, morning stiffness, and fatigue] of the syndrome. The 3 symptoms differed in many ways from those that Yunus was later to suggest (4). They all were representations of the fibromyalgia "sleep disturbance," and I want to omit them at this moment and concentrate on pain and tenderness. One way of looking at this original construct is to assume that almost everyone who has the syndrome has all of these features [Figure 1]. In fact, the Smythe and Moldofsky criteria, by making all criteria items mandatory, enforced this assumption.

In 1981 Mohammed Yunus and his colleagues wrote a very important paper in which they suggested certain criteria for the diagnosis of fibromyalgia [Table 3] (4). The Yunus et al. paper pointed out and stressed a series of physical findings and symptoms. These included the Smythe and Moldofsky "3" [fatigue, morning stiffness, and disturbed sleep], and expanded them by adding irritable bowel syndrome, subjective swelling, headache, and exacerbation and amelioration by a series of factors including rest, heat cold, stress, poor sleep, anxiety, weather change, and vacation. Not only did they emphasize symptoms, but they down-played pain location. Only three regions were needed. As for tenderness, as few as 3 or 4 points would satisfy the criteria. In fact, Professor Yunus once told me that he thought you could have fibromyalgia without any tender points. Kind of a heresy, I guess, to those of us that have measured tenderness and pain with a series of dolorimeters and pain assessment instruments. I hope Dr.

TABLE 2. Features of the fibromyalgia symptom complex.

1. *Pain:* location, intensity, tolerability.

2. *Tenderness* [decreased pain threshold].

3. *Signs and Symptoms:* fatigue, morning stiffness, disturbed sleep, irritable bowel syndrome, subjective swelling headache; exacerbation and amelioration by a series of factors including rest, heat cold, stress, poor sleep, anxiety, weather change, and vacation.

4. *Psychological distress.*

FIGURE 1. Smythe and Moldofsky (1) conjunction of pain, tenderness [At least 12 of 14 tender points], and symptoms [Sleep disturbance, morning stiffness, and fatigue]. Note that criteria definition requires all features to be present simultaneously.

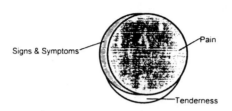

Yunus will not take it amiss if I characterize what I think the older Yunus criteria mean. It is, I believe, a view of fibromyalgia which says that it is the symptoms of the syndrome rather than the tenderness or the locations of the pain that are most important. In our clinics we have all seen patients with every one of the Yunus "minor criteria" but with little or no tenderness and with regional pain. Let us then set aside for a moment this third view of fibromyalgia and take up the 4th factor, psychological distress.

Although there is "controversy" concerning psychological abnormality in fibromyalgia, almost all of the data supports the notion of psychological distress. That concept is supported by > 38,000 psychological tests administered to more than 6,600 rheumatic disease patients [Table 4] (5). By any measure fibromyalgia patients have higher depression scores than all of the other disease groups. More than that, they have higher divorce rates (6), and a higher non-participant rate in studies.

These 4 features, then, constitute the base of fibromyalgia *as it is known in the clinic*. As we consider the nature of the syndrome and its validity let us rethink it all in light of all of the available evidence. In this discussion I am not concerned about criteria, but concepts.

Fibromyalgia Pain

In fibromyalgia one of the most important aspects of pain is its location. The 1990 American College of Rheumatology criteria study noted that 67.0% of those with fibromyalgia described "pain all over" (7). Of 30 body regions described on a pain diagram, 55.6% with fibromyalgia had at least 15 painful sites. Among the most characteristic sites were the neck [85.3%], the posterior thorax [72.3%], and the low back [78.8%]. If one defined "wide spread pain" as pain involving the axial skeleton, the upper

TABLE 3. The Yunus et al. 1981 criteria (4).

1. *Obligatory Criteria*

A] Aching and pain or prominent stiffness of 3 anatomical areas for 3 months.

B] Absence of secondary causes.

2. *Major criteria*

A] 5 tender points

3. *Minor criteria*

A] Modulation of symptoms by physical activity.

B] Modulation of symptoms by weather factors.

C] Aggravation of symptoms by anxiety or stress.

D] Poor sleep.

E] General fatigue or tiredness.

F] Anxiety.

G] Chronic headache.

H] Irritable bowel syndrome.

I] Subjective Swelling.

J] Numbness.

Must meet obligatory criteria plus 1 major criterion and 3 minor criteria; if 3-4

tender points then 5 minor criteria.

half of the body, and the lower half of the body, then 97.6% of fibromyalgia patients met that definition.

Figure 2 shows typical pain diagrams from 4 patients with fibromyalgia. There are certain characteristic features in these diagrams. First, there is a sense of distress that no statistical parameter can convey. Pain is drawn with broad strokes, and is everywhere. There are additional factors that are important. Pain is contiguous. It also has a quality suggesting radiation, as if from central sources [e.g., low back or cervical spine].

Beyond location, fibromyalgia pain is characterized by severity, unpleasantness, and unendurability. In the 1990 ACR study (7), fibromyalgia subjects had a visual analog scale pain rating of 6.6 on a 10 point scale. This is a high pain score. Control subjects from rheumatic disease clinics had a score of 4.5. In our clinic the pain scores of 248 fibromyalgia

TABLE 4. Depression and depressive symptoms in fibromyalgia.

	Number of Subjects	Percent Depressed *†	Aims Depression Scores †
Fibromyalgia	762	49.6/29.3	3.3
Clinic Controls	5,840	32.9/17.9	2.6

* Refers to AIMS depression scores | 3.0 / | 4.0

† Differences between Fibromyalgia and control subjects are significant at
 p <0.001.

FIGURE 2. Pain diagrams from 4 patients with fibromyalgia. Note the widespread and contiguous nature of the pain complaint.

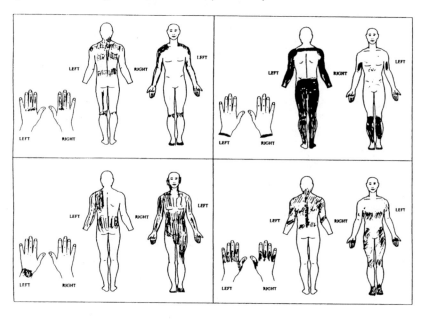

patients was 6.1 (8), quite similar to that noted in the ACR study. Studies using the McGill pain scale and other instruments have underscored the components of suffering in fibromyalgia pain. Leavitt et al. found fibromyalgia subjects tended to use more affective and sensory words than controls with RA (9), and Scudds et al. noted that the pain and other characteristics of fibromyalgia patients allowed them to be separated diagnostically from other pain patients (10).

Clinicians can usually suspect fibromyalgia on the basis of pain description and location and often by its interaction with severity. The more "characteristic" the description and location, the more likely it is for the patient to have fibromyalgia.

Let us now examine 3 important questions:

> *Can you have widespread tenderness with local or regional pain?*
> *If you have limited pain can you have fibromyalgia?*
> *Do you have to have pain to have tenderness?*

Figures 3, 4, and 5 reflect 3 different views of fibromyalgia. Figure 3 indicates that widespread pain, tenderness, and symptoms are merely chance overlaps. We will come back to this below. Figure 4 is, I believe, a contemporary view of fibromyalgia *in the clinic* and as reflected by the 1990 ACR criteria. First, the figure reflects the ubiquity of widespread pain in the clinic. Few patients have ACR tenderness [at least 11 of 18

FIGURE 3. Overlap of pain, tenderness, and signs and symptoms of fibromyalgia assuming these factors are "chance" conjunctions. This model suggests that fibromyalgia is part of a continuum rather than a distinct syndrome.

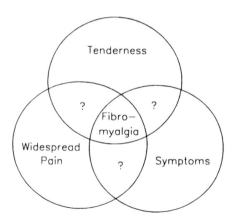

FIGURE 4. A model of fibromyalgia in the clinic. In this model ACR tenderness [at least 11 of 18 tender points] is almost always found in conjunction with widespread pain and fibromyalgia signs and symptoms. Symptoms alone may be found with non-widespread pain and with no pain. This model reflects the prevalence of fibromyalgia in the clinic and the relative relationship between tenderness, pain, and symptoms found in the clinic.

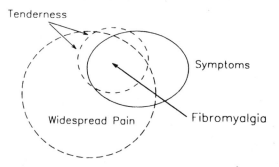

FIGURE 5. A model of fibromyalgia in the clinic that goes beyond the Figure 4 model by introducing the concept of distressful, contiguous, and often generalized and "all over" pain [hatched area].

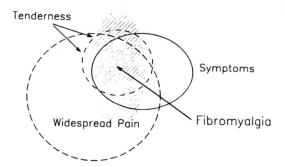

tender points] without widespread pain, reflecting the selection bias toward more severely afflicted persons in the clinic. For example, if the prevalence of fibromyalgia is 3% in the community, it is greater than 10% in the clinic. Note that ACR tenderness is generally found with widespread pain and with the characteristic fibromyalgia symptom complex. Fibromyalgia symptoms, however, may be found in a small number of subjects without the requisite widespread pain and in many subjects without ACR tenderness.

Figure 5 takes this model one step further, introducing the kind of distressful, contiguous, and often generalized and often "all over" pain typically found in the syndrome. It is this qualitative feature of fibromyalgia pain, that has not been captured well in any criteria set, that provides one of the most important "proofs" of the fibromyalgia construct in the clinic. It is of interest that it is generally easy to measure pain severity in the clinic, but measures of pain quality and location [found in instruments such as the McGill Pain Questionnaire (11)] are difficult to impossible to use in routine clinic practice.

Can You Have Widespread Tenderness with Local or Regional Pain? If You Have Limited Pain Can You Have Fibromyalgia?

Figures 4 and 5 do not set specific boundaries for fibromyalgia, but suggest that "characteristic" fibromyalgia is found at the point of the arrow from which it spreads outward. At this juncture, as we consider the nature of fibromyalgia and fibromyalgia diagnosis, it is well to remember that there is a difference between "diagnostic" and "classification" criteria. Classification criteria, designed to identify patients for studies *works on a set of patients already diagnosed.* Just because a subject meets classification criteria doesn't mean that he must have fibromyalgia. A person with widespread burns, for example, would meet classification criteria for fibromyalgia, but would not be diagnosed as having the syndrome. Classification criteria tend to be exclusive, aiming at specificity rather than sensitivity, but depend on a previous diagnosis. The "classification area" in the figures is subsumed by the intersection of the widespread pain and ACR tenderness sets [circles].

Figures 4 and 5 suggest, particularly when the qualitative aspects of pain are considered, that ACR widespread pain might not always be necessary. Conceptually, a patient with extensive upper torso pain, ACR tenderness, and fibromyalgia symptoms might reasonably be considered to have fibromyalgia. Another factor, usually considered in the clinic, but not considered in any criteria sets, is past pain. Fibromyalgia patients often have a history of significant, long-lived pain in multiple regions that clinicians use in making a diagnosis of fibromyalgia, although some of those regions might not be painful at the time of the current clinic visit.

In the community and in subsets of patients designated as having the myofascial pain syndrome the above outline is not as clear. Reports from Raspe (12), and others indicate that ACR tenderness often occurs in the community in the absence of ACR widespread pain. As shown in Figure 6, from our ongoing community survey, 24.1% of subjects have chronic regional pain, and about 3% of those of have at least 18 tender points. Of interest, we recently studied fibromyalgia and myofascial pain syndrome patients in a blinded protocol (13). We expected limited tenderness in the MFP group, but found a great deal of tenderness. In some ways the MFP patients in their symptoms and tenderness resembled those with fibromyalgia. Dworkin found more tenderness than expected in patients with the TMJ syndrome (14), as did Scudds (15). Would such community and MFP patients have the same contiguity of pain and distress that might lead us to label them as fibromyalgia? Would we be wrong?

Do You Have to Have Pain to Have Tenderness?

In the clinic this is most certainly true. For why else do patients come to us except for pain? In the community, though, this may not be true. Professor Dr. Heiner Raspe (personal communication) reported that in community surveys he has found subjects with multiple tender points, but no pain! Although we have not yet found such a patient in our surveys [we have one with 7 tender points], such data suggest that tenderness represents a continuum. Although tenderness is critical to clinical fibromyalgia, pain

FIGURE 6. Tender point counts in 84 community subjects. Ten percent of subject with widespread pain have at least 11 of 18 tender points. Three percent of those with regional or local pain have at least 11 tender points.

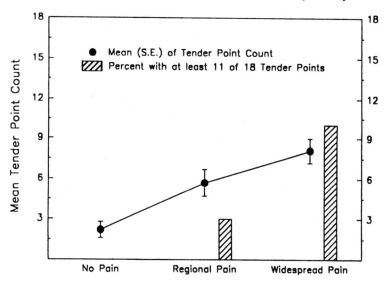

Tender Point Counts in 84 Community Subjects

pressure threshold [tenderness] has meaning beyond and separate from fibromyalgia. Buskila, Smythe and coworkers have found differences in pain threshold by dolorimetry in specific disease states (16). Patients with systemic lupus erythematosus, for example, have lower thresholds while those with psoriatic arthritis have higher thresholds. Finally, Lyddell reports that many subjects in a community survey who had ACR level tenderness had no pain (17).

Are Symptoms Most Important?

There is something more to having fibromyalgia than just pain and tenderness as Yunus et al. were trying to tell us in their [older] 1981 criteria (4). The symptoms of fibromyalgia are fatigue, morning stiffness, disturbed sleep, irritable bowel syndrome, subjective swelling, headache, exacerbation and amelioration by a series of factors including rest, heat, cold, stress, poor sleep, anxiety, weather change, and vacation [after Yunus et al.] (4). Most of us would be very uncomfortable diagnosing fibromyalgia without a few of these features. Such features have [at least] two meanings. The first is obviously psychological. The second is that they reflect pain: often deep, radiating pain; and autonomic contributions. Many of the same features are seen in low back pain syndromes, sympathetic dystrophy syndromes, and osteoarthritis. Thus one measure of the symptoms is that they reflect pain, important pain, often referred pain as suggested in the contiguity of pain on the pain diagrams. As we will note later, there are some problems with a strong reliance on symptom criteria. But they have a special importance in evaluating patients with limited distribution of pain and less than the usual tenderness.

What Is the Role of Psychological Factors?

It has always been known that psychological factors play a major role in fibromyalgia. As noted above, fibromyalgia patients have higher levels of depression than all other clinic disease groups (5,18). By essentially any psychological test or type of observation those with fibromyalgia score highest (5). It has been argued that the issue is complex and that the severe pain and/or disability of fibromyalgia causes rather than is the consequence of psychological distress. My own view is that is true in some patients, but not in others; and that, taken as a whole, psychological factors are more often causative rather than the consequence of fibromyalgia. The psychological arguments go around and around, and will not be solved here. But we should examine some newer evidence concerning the relationship between psychological factors and pain, pain location, and tenderness. Important, insightful work has come from Heiner Raspe of Lübeck who pointed out (personal communication), and we later confirmed, that in the community there is an important association between psychological factors and every feature we consider common to fibromyalgia, and that this interaction is not dependent on clinical diagnosis. In our community survey we studied a sample without pain, those with chronic but non-widespread pain, and those with chronic widespread pain, according to the ACR definitions. Dolorimetry scores had Spearman correlations in excess of 0.35 with depression. Depression was correlated with the pain grouping at about 0.25, and with pain scores at about 0.40. I want to suggest one meaning to these data, harkening back to Yunus's observation: fibromyalgia is often exacerbated by factors such as "stress" and "anxiety." One mechanism or model suggests that psychological factors enlarge the circles of tenderness, pain and symptoms noted in Figures 4 and 5. This has important consequences in a number of areas, including diagnosis which will be discussed below. First, it is possible to see how fibromyalgia might be a "psychological" disorder since as psychological factors enlarge the circles more patients will meet diagnostic and classification criteria for the syndrome. Remembering that the model we have proposed here is only a model, one might speculate on whether a patient whose fibromyalgia is determined by psychological factors does or does not have fibromyalgia? One further consequence of this model is, of course, that psychological factors are not necessary for the fibromyalgia construct.

THE DIAGNOSIS OF FIBROMYALGIA

What is it that makes fibromyalgia or allows us to diagnose it? It is first the unexpected nature of the pain and the unexpected tenderness that suggests fibromyalgia. The 30 year old with pain in the arms, legs and back, and has all of the tender points, certainly has fibromyalgia. We are surprised and have no other explanation. But what if the regions of pain are only somewhat more than expected or if the patient is older and has other potential reasons for pain. We are not so surprised. Should we diagnosis cervical and/or lumbar degenerative disease and perhaps osteoarthritis of the hand or knees or should we call this fibromyalgia. It is here that we examine the factors described to us by Yunus and added to by others. Is there irritable bowel syndrome, disturbed sleep, paresthesias, fatigue, etc? If these factors are present we tend to diagnose fibromyalgia, and if they are not we stay with local pathology or are uncertain. In fact, if the signs and symptoms of fibromyalgia are so characteristic [to those of us sitting in the clinic] then we might consider fibromyalgia with lesser tender points or, as suggested by Yunus, consider it when there is scant or no tenderness.

Both the diagnostic and classification criteria for fibromyalgia suggests that one either has or does not have the syndrome. More realistic is the appreciation that beyond those who clearly do or do not have fibromyalgia are a group of patients who have some of the features of the syndrome and "possibly or probably have" fibromyalgia. The terms "possible" and "probable" have important echoes for rheumatologists since they bring to mind the older [1958] ACR criteria for the diagnosis of rheumatoid arthritis (19). The most important thing about these criteria was that they didn't work. Almost everyone had "possible RA," and many other disorders easily fit into "probable RA." With signs and symptoms in fibromyalgia being somewhat "softer" than in RA, it would seem hazardous to introduce similar terms to this syndrome. Yet it is probably necessary, and probably can be done effectively if the differences between diagnostic and classification criteria are kept in mind.

Table 5 suggests an outline of features that are associated with fibromyalgia at differing degrees of certainty. I want to suggest the following as diagnostic criteria definition:

Definite fibromyalgia: All of the definite fibromyalgia features.
Probable fibromyalgia: Two of the three definite fibromyalgia features.
Possible fibromyalgia: One of the three definite fibromyalgia features and two of the three possible fibromyalgia features.

TABLE 5. Diagnostic criteria for fibromyalgia.

	Non Fibromyalgia Features	Possible Fibromyalgia Features	Definite Fibromyalgia Features
Pain	None or limited Pain	Regional to extensive, often with contiguity, but not widespread	Widespread
Tenderness	0-5	6-10	11 or >
[Tender Points]	0-20%	20-55%	> 60%
Symptoms	None or rare	Few to many	Many

These "Copenhagen Diagnostic Criteria" are clinical criteria, and they are vague as to how many symptoms factors are required since the list of symptoms associated with fibromyalgia is large. But they should aid in the clinic since they allow us to deal with the continuum of signs and symptoms that we find in the real world of the clinic. They may be an aid in a number of other settings as well. First, they may allow us to better describe patients with fibromyalgia type symptoms. Next, they may help in understanding the patient with recent onset of symptoms whose future course in not known. Here they may document the passage from one grouping to another with time. Remember this passage may go in both directions. They can also express the uncertainty that is present, but ignored by the ACR classification criteria.

Do we need still another set of criteria? Let us first examine fibromyalgia in light of the 1990 American College of Rheumatology classification criteria. The classification criteria simply represent the best [most accurate and best sensitivity/specificity tradeoff] method to choose between those with and those without fibromyalgia [in the setting of the ACR study population]. The criteria committee, as noted in their paper (7), examined a number of other possible criteria sets. As might be expected from Figure 4, it was possible to put together criteria which stressed symptoms and performed almost as well as adopted criteria. When we looked at the patients identified by these two potential criteria sets, although sensitivities, specificities, and accuracies were generally similar, certain patients were identified by one potential set of criteria and other patients by the remaining set. This too might be suspected by examining Figure 4. For example, we might fail to identify the patient with symptoms, widespread pain, and only 10 tender points by the ACR criteria. When we try to use such criteria in the clinic, we are perplexed. The call is for yes or no, black or white when the true shading is gray. I often find myself writing to a referring physician: "While the patient does not quite meet current criteria, he almost certainly has the disorder." The true value of classification criteria is in studies and as a model.

How do our classification criteria perform? All criteria sets were developed in the clinic. This means they should work best in the clinic. All authors in proposing their criteria had some notion of how the criteria might work in the community, but were, like those in Plato's cave, influenced by spectrum bias. It seemed likely that the original Yunus et al. criteria (4) might not work as well in the community since their heavy reliance on symptoms might identify others in the community with those symptoms. It was also likely that psychological factors might influence the

Yunus symptom criteria more than they would influence the tender point criterion. Studies presented in this symposium, in fact, indicate that the Yunus criteria identify subjects in the community more than 3 times more frequently than the ACR criteria (12).

Table 6, modified from the ACR 1990 criteria study, describes sensitivity, specificity, and accuracy of a number of criteria sets that have been used in fibromyalgia studies. It is likely that the proportion of persons in the community who are identified as having fibromyalgia will be inversely related to the specificity of the criteria set used in identification. Criteria that are highly specific [> 95%] will miss too many persons with fibromyalgia to be useful in community surveys. Similarly, it is likely that criteria that rely on the presence of some symptom criteria, regardless of their apparent specificity in the clinic, will not perform well in the community. Given the difference between clinic and community, the ACR criteria will probably yield the best approximation of fibromyalgia when applied to the community based upon what fibromyalgia looks like in the clinic.

TABLE 6. Comparison of sensitivity, specificity, and accuracy of the 1990 criteria for the classification of fibromyalgia with previous criteria sets.

Criteria Set	Year	Fibromyalgia Syndrome [n=558]		
		Sens.	Spec.	Accuracy
Criteria committee	**1990**	**88.4**	**81.1**	**84.9**
Wolfe et al	1985	95.8	73.8	85.6
Yunus et al	1988	86.3	80.7	83.7
Goldenberg et al	1986	78.8	82.3	80.4
Yunus et al	1981	83.6	76.6	80.3
Campbell, Bennett, Clark	1983	45.8	95.0	68.2
Smythe & Moldofsky	1977	39.2	95.5	64.6

* Tender point sites and historical data items may differ slightly in current study compared with previous criteria sets. Therefore sensitivity, specificity, and accuracy data for previous criteria sets should be considered close approximations.

FUTURE TRENDS

Clinical diagnostic criteria and classification criteria. It may well be that the compromise of using *clinical diagnostic criteria* as well as *classification criteria* will prove useful since the classification criteria have an appropriate level of specificity and the clinical criteria often some additional usefulness. In fact, the suggested clinical criteria do not preclude the simultaneous use of the classification criteria since the data contained in the diagnostic assessment are sufficient for classification.

The impact of psychological factors. The problem with the "creation or causation" of fibromyalgia by psychological factors is likely to remain since there are no easily applicable rules or instrumentation to screen out those with *inordinate* psychological contribution to the diagnosis of fibromyalgia. Thus the *omnia et sempre* patient that Heiner Raspe feels does not have fibromyalgia and the slightly less affected subject with positive control points will continue to remain problems.

Permanency of the fibromyalgia diagnosis. Current criteria do not address the issue of "once fibromyalgia always fibromyalgia" versus "only fibromyalgia when you meet criteria." In illnesses such as rheumatoid arthritis, for example, patients in remission or with just minor disease activity are still considered to have rheumatoid arthritis. When one treats fibromyalgia a major goal is to reduce pain and tender points, but succeeding in this goal may mean that the patient no longer meets criteria! Longitudinal studies of the course of fibromyalgia are needed since little is known about what happens to fibromyalgia patients except when they appear with symptoms in the clinic.

When does fibromyalgia begin? Patients with fibromyalgia often have a long history of musculoskeletal problems before they are diagnosed as having fibromyalgia. By history, at least, some of these complaints appear discrete. Cervical pain [10 years ago], shoulder "bursitis" [7 years ago], foot pain [6 years ago], carpal tunnel syndrome [3 years ago], but generalized pain and increase in severity within the last six months. It is not known if such patients had many tender points or characteristic fibromyalgia symptoms during the many bouts of musculoskeletal problems, but it is certainly possible. Even without tender points, did such a patient have fibromyalgia when the first complaint began or perhaps somewhere along the time course of the illness? Or was it only during the last 6 months? Was fibromyalgia developing during this period? How could it have been identified?

Reliability of the fibromyalgia diagnosis in the courts and in the clinic. Physician discussion and informational materials about fibromyalgia tell patients about the symptoms of fibromyalgia, about tender points, and about diagnosis. Fibromyalgia, like chronic fatigue syndrome and "lupus" is an "in" diagnosis. Its diagnosis depends on patient reporting. Can a patient "learn" to have fibromyalgia? Sophisticated persons participating in legal and quasi-legal disability and compensation hearings may be able to mislead the examiner. How often this occurs is unknown. But with increasing compensation for "traumatic" fibromyalgia, issues of diagnostic reliability need to be addressed. If psychological factors can exacerbate fibromyalgia, why should not the compensation setting also drive the system? It is probably useful to reemphasize that what we know about this difficult and distressful syndrome derives from the clinic, and that no data regarding the reliability of the fibromyalgia diagnosis and prognosis exists out of that setting. Here, as in the areas previously discussed, more research will be required.

REFERENCES

1. Smythe HA and Moldofsky H: Two contributions to understanding of the "fibrositis" syndrome. Bull Rheum Dis:28:928-931, 1977.

2. Graham W: The fibrositis syndrome. Bull Rheum Dis:3:33-34, 1953.

3. Traut EF: Fibrositis. J Am Geriatr Soc:16:531-538, 1968.

4. Yunus MB, Masi AT, Calabro JJ, Miller KA and Feigenbaum SL: Primary fibromyalgia (fibrositis): clinical study of 50 patients with matched normal controls. Semin Arthritis Rheum:11:151-171, 1981.

5. Hawley DJ and Wolfe F: Depression is not more common in rheumatoid arthritis: a 10 year longitudinal study of 6,608 rheumatic disease patients. J Rheumatol:1993 (In Press).

6. Hawley DJ, Wolfe F, Cathey MA and Roberts FK: Marital status in rheumatoid arthritis and other rheumatic disorders: a study of 7,293 patients. J Rheumatol:18:654-660, 1991.

7. Wolfe F, Smythe HA, Yunus MB, et al.: The American College of Rheumatology 1990 Criteria for the Classification of Fibromyalgia: Report of the Multicenter Criteria Committee. Arthritis Rheum:33:160-172, 1990.

8. Hawley DJ and Wolfe F: Pain, disability, and pain/disability relationships in seven rheumatic disorders: a study of 1522 patients. J Rheumatol:18:1552-1557, 1991.

9. Leavitt F, Katz RS, Golden HE, Glickman PB and Layfer LF: Comparison of pain properties in fibromyalgia patients and rheumatoid arthritis patients. Arthritis Rheum:29:775-781, 1986.

10. Scudds RA, Rollman GB, Harth M and McCain GA: Pain perception and personality measures as discriminators in the classification of fibrositis. J Rheumatol:14:563-569, 1987.

11. Melzack R: The McGill pain questionnaire: major properties and scoring methods. Pain:1:277-299, 1975.

12. Raspe H, Baumgartner, Ch: The Epidemiology of the fibromyalgia syndrome in a German town (Abstract). Scand J Rheumatol (Suppl):94:S8, 1992.

13. Wolfe F, Simons DG, Fricton JR, et al.: The fibromyalgia and myofascial pain syndromes: a study of tender points and trigger points in persons with fibromyalgia, myofascial pain syndrome, and no disease. J Rheumatol:19:944-951, 1992.

14. Dworkin SF, Huggins KH, LeResche L, et al.: Epidemiology of signs and symptoms in temporomandibular disorders: clinical signs in cases and controls. JADA:10:11-23, 1990.

15. Scudds RA, Trachsel LC, Luckhurst BJ and Percy JS: A comparative study of pain, sleep quality and pain responsiveness in fibrositis and myofascial pain syndrome. J Rheumatol Suppl:19:120-126, 1989.

16. Buskila D, Langevitz P, Gladman D, Urowitz S and Smythe HA: Patients with rheumatoid arthritis are more tender than those with psoriatic arthritis. J Rheumatol:19:1115-1119, 1992.

17. Lyddell C: The prevalence of fibromyalgia in a South African community (Abstract). Scand J Rheumatol (Suppl):94:S8, 1992.

18. Hawley DJ and Wolfe F: Depression in fibromyalgia: a comparative study of 1522 rheumatic disease patients. Scand J Rheumatol (Suppl):94:S14, 1992.

19. Ropes MW, Bennett GA, Cobb S, Jacox R and Jessar RA: 1958 Revision of diagnostic criteria for rheumatoid arthritis. Arthritis Rheum:2:16-20, 1959.

Myofascial Pain:
Clinical Characteristics
and Diagnostic Criteria

James R. Fricton

SUMMARY. Myofascial pain [MFP] is a common cause of persistent regional pain characterized by local pain, associated muscle tenderness, and slight decrease in range of motion. Although many definitions exist for MFP, little research has been done on the reliability and validity of proposed diagnostic criteria for this disorder. In this series of studies, operational definitions were developed for the most common signs of MFP and then tested for inter- and intra-rater reliability. This standardized examination was then applied to 30 MFP patients and 30 normal subjects by an examiner blinded to the status of the subject. Discriminant analysis was then used to evaluate the relative predictive value of each individual item and to generate diagnostic criteria. The scope of tenderness [percent of specific muscles sites tender] was the most predictive sign with adequate reliability. The sensitivity and specificity was 93.5% and 80.6%, respectively with diagnostic criteria at 28% or more muscle sites tender.

James R. Fricton, DDS, MS, is affiliated with the Department of Diagnostic and Surgical Sciences, University of Minnesota School of Dentistry, Minneapolis, MN 55455.

Address correspondence to: James R. Fricton, DDS, MS, 6-320 Moos Tower, Division of TMD and Orofacial Pain, University of Minnesota School of Dentistry, Minneapolis, MN 55455.

[Haworth co-indexing entry note]: "Myofascial Pain: Clinical Characteristics and Diagnostic Criteria." Fricton, James R. Co-published simultaneously in the *Journal of Musculoskeletal Pain* (The Haworth Press, Inc.) Vol. 1, No. 3/4, 1993, pp. 37-47; and: *Musculoskeletal Pain, Myofascial Pain Syndrome, and the Fibromyalgia Syndrome* (ed: Søren Jacobsen, Bente Danneskiold-Samsøe, and Birger Lund) The Haworth Press, Inc., 1993, pp. 37-47. Multiple copies of this article/chapter may be purchased from The Haworth Document Delivery Center [1-800-3-HAWORTH; 9:00 a.m. - 5:00 p.m. (EST)].

37

KEYWORDS. Myofascial pain, muscles, pain, diagnostic criteria

Myofascial pain is a common muscular pain disorder characterized by regional pain and associated localized muscle tenderness. In clinical studies, it has been reported as the most common diagnosis responsible for chronic pain syndromes and related disability (1-4). However, it often is regarded by some as a wastebasket term for soft-tissue complaints and by others as a psychological problem. Part of this confusion stems from high variability in case definitions and the lack of diagnostic criteria or objective methods for assessment.

This situation creates both clinical and research dilemmas that have hindered adequate diagnosis and management of MFP. For example, in disability determination, cases involving chronic benign pain had been so often neglected in the United States Social Security Administration and litigation so common that the U.S. Congress had to pass legislation to ensure that these patients were dealt with fairly (5). In the clinic, many clinicians have a tendency to recognize and treat only disorders that are diagnosed with objective tests. As a result, patients with MFP are often poorly recognized and inadequately treated perpetuating the chronic pain syndrome. In addition, the epidemiology of MFP including prevalence, incidence, progression, and etiology is unclear because of the lack of tested case definitions sufficiently accurate to predict the presence and severity of MFP. For example, in a study by Le Resche and associates, there were considerable differences among clinicians in comparing diagnoses in the masticatory system for the same cases (6).

For these reasons, the development of diagnostic criteria for MFP is a critical next step in improving our understanding of MFP. In developing these criteria, only items that characterize myofascial pain with sufficient reliability and validity can be used. In addition, they need to rely on the subjective appraisal of the subject as little as possible. Since MFP can occur in muscles throughout the body, its criteria also need to be broad enough to allow potential application to different regional muscle groups and to distinguish MFP from systemic disorders affecting the muscles such as fibromyalgia. For each regional MFP syndrome such as in the low back or neck, discussion among experts need to occur to obtain consensus on the definition of MFP and ensure construct validity of the clinical items that are potentially used to diagnose MFP.

Once these are established, studies can be accomplished with these items using discriminate analysis between various populations and disorders to determine which items best predict MFP of each region. In establishing these diagnostic criteria, care must be taken to minimize false positives and false negatives so that the sensitivity and specificity are acceptable and repeatable by the same and different investigators. The purpose of this paper is to discuss research studying the clinical characteristics of myofascial pain in one region of the body, the muscles of mastication, and how they have been used to begin the process of developing diagnostic criteria for masticatory MFP [MMFP].

SELECTION OF ITEMS CHARACTERIZING MASTICATORY MYOFASCIAL PAIN

The most common characteristics of myofascial pain include regional pain complaints, localized muscle tenderness in a taut band of muscle [termed trigger point], slightly limited range of motion, local and referred pain, and reproducible alteration of the pain complaints with specific palpation of the associated tender muscle (7-10). Clinical techniques that have been proposed and tested to objectively characterize MFP include pressure algometry to document tenderness, measurement of tissue consistency, electromyography to document muscle activity, thermography to detect temperature differences, and injections of the trigger point to alleviate pain (11-19).

Tenderness is the most common sign and, although still based on patient reports, has been tested the most extensively for reliability and validity (11-12,14-15). Tenderness parameters include scope or number of muscles tender, absolute pressure pain threshold with a pressure algometer, relative pressure pain threshold [compared to a control point], localization of tenderness, presence of a taut band with tenderness, radiation of pain with palpation of tenderness, and presence of a twitch response with palpation of tenderness. Other tests that have been studied for diagnosis of MFP have been electromyography and surface thermography. However, both have produced mixed results in showing adequate reliability and validity in preliminary studies of their efficacy (17,20). Thus, in this study, tenderness parameters warranted further study as potential criteria.

STUDIES OF TENDERNESS IN MASTICATORY MYOFASCIAL PAIN [MMFP]

The inter- and intra-rater reliability of the scope of tenderness for MFP, the reliability, validity, and norms for pressure pain threshold using a precision pressure algometer in the diagnosis of MFP, and studies to help establish content validity of diagnostic criteria for MFP have been completed. Table 1 presents the correlation coefficients for reliability of the scope of tenderness of MMFP [muscle index] (21). Although intraoral palpation was less reliable, reliability of all of these were within acceptable range.

Despite these findings, muscle palpation in MFP has been criticized for poor reliability (11). For example, in a study of signs of temporomandibular disorders, Dworkin and colleagues found that palpation of individual muscle sites by untrained examiners was unreliable (22). However, training of examiners did improve reliability almost to the level of more objective items that were measured with a device such as a millimeter rule. This supports the importance of training and calibrating of examiners to a standard as well as the need for developing objective devices to measure tenderness.

A pressure algometer or dolorimeter is a device that has been designed to improve reliability of muscle and joint palpation and requires further research. This device allows accurate measurement of the degree of pressure being placed over a standardized surface area (23). In one study, a precision strain gauge pressure algometer for muscle palpation [PAMP] was developed at the University of Minnesota and tested for inter-rater reliability [two raters in one day] as compared to the manual palpation technique (15). This algometer, which incorporates a precision strain gauge, will not warp over time and has high clinical agility.

The palpation technique with PAMP consisted of locating the distinct muscle band or part of joint with gentle index finger pressure and then using the tip of PAMP to place pressure on the band at the specific muscle location. An "ascending method of limits" technique was used to determine the pain threshold. The pain threshold was the first level at which the patient reports even the slightest pain due to ascending pressure from palpation with PAMP. The ascending pressure is timed in order to standardize the slope of increasing pressure. The threshold was recorded and repeated in five seconds to determine mean pain threshold for each muscle location. All patients were given the following instructions: "Please raise your hand when the pressure first becomes even the slightest bit painful." If no pain was reported at the

Table 1. Reliability of the scope of tenderness in different groups of masticatory muscles

	Intra-rater reliability(n=40)	Inter-rater reliability(n=19)
	Intraclass correlation	Intraclass correlation
Extra- oral muscle palpation	0.86	0.81
Intra-oral muscle palpation	0.68	0.58
Neck muscle palpation	0.85	0.84

highest level, then that level was recorded as the pain threshold. The second rater, blind to the first rater's determinations repeated the evaluation after a fifteen minute rest to minimize aggravation of the trigger point.

The mean values at each site for the 45 comparisons for both the PAMP technique and manual technique were then compared using the KAPPA statistic for inter-rater agreement [Table 2]. This statistic was used in order to provide a standardized comparison of both the PAMP and manual technique that takes into consideration the factor of random agreement. The PAMP scores were digitized [converted to 0 to 1] by using the mean as the threshold value. The results demonstrated that moderate to good reliability was demonstratable for 13 to 15 sites with PAMP and in only 2 of 15 sites with manual palpation. A corollary to the study was that experienced raters were more reliable than inexperienced raters suggesting that palpation is technique sensitive and calibration of examiners is needed. As a result of this study and the use of the muscle index and PAMP in other studies, a calibration procedure for muscle palpation has been developed and tested with numerous other raters here and other institutions (24). A video tape of the examination procedures has been made to allow for standardization at other sites.

CONTENT VALIDITY OF DIAGNOSTIC CRITERIA FOR MASTICATORY MYOFASCIAL PAIN

With these and other studies, sufficient evidence of reliability and validity of individual items associated with tenderness have been shown and

Table 2. Reliability, validity , and norms for pressure algometer for masticatory muscles

Muscles	Inter-rater rel. K- value	Mean Pain Thresholds		
		males w/ MFP	females w/ MFP	Normals
Ant. temporalis	0.55*	0.50	0.33**	0.79***
Mid. temporalis	0.49*	0.66	0.43**	0.84***
post. temporalis	0.38	0.51	0.36**	0.81***
Deep masseter	0.36	0.63	0.32**	0.78***
Ant. masseter	0.63*	0.51	0.30**	0.68***
Inf. masseter	0.68*	0.51	0.27**	0.65***
Post. digastric	0.40*	0.36	0.23**	0.46***
Medial pterygoid	0.51*	0.35	0.21**	0.38***
Vertex	0.69*	0.68	0.61**	0.84***

*Moderate to good reliability.

** Significance(p<.05) when comparing males and females with MFP.

***Significance(p<.05) when comparing normals to combined male-female scores.

development of diagnostic criteria has proceeded. Regional and national committees in the past year were organized independently of each other to determine which items should be included in diagnostic criteria for masticatory myofascial pain and other temporomandibular disorders. Each item was reviewed with the experts on the different committees to determine which items have the highest potential to be representative of MMFP and have adequate reliability. These untested criteria are compared in Table 3. The first committee, consisting of faculty at the University of Minnesota, developed diagnostic criteria which were later tested for sensitivity and specificity against normals (20). The second committee consisted of the members of the White Paper Committee of the American Academy of Orofacial Pain [formerly American Academy of Craniomandibular Disorders] (25). This committee developed diagnostic criteria that were clinically relevant using both research results on diagnostic criteria and objective clinical tests, but did not develop operational definitions to be used for clinical research. The third committee was an NIDR sponsored Research Diagnostic Criteria Study and included a national group of experts to develop research criteria and operational definitions for them (26). Each of these committees contained experts in the field to ensure that any items included in criteria exhibited adequate content validity and reliability.

Table 3. Content validity for diagnostic criteria for MMFP: results of 3 committees

University of Minnesota Criteria(3 of 4 criteria need to be met)

1. presence of taut bands of skeletal muscles, tendons and ligaments.

2. presence of tenderness to specific palpation in a taut band (jump sign).

3. radiation to or replication of a present pain problem after specific palpation of a tender spot.

4. The presence of four or more trigger points of 18 sites(22%) on a masticatory muscle index.

Academy of Orofacial Pain Clinical Criteria

1. Continuous pain, usually dull in one or more muscles.

2. localized tenderness in firm bands of muscle

3. can have reproducible alteration of pain complaints with palpation of specific trigger points.

4. may be associated with parafunction, postural hypertonicity, or secondary to trauma

NIDR Research Diagnostic Criteria for masticatory MFP with and without limitation

1. Report of orofacial pain at rest.

2. Pain reported by the subject in response of palpation of four or more of 18(22%) muscle sites

3a. With limitation: Unassisted mandibular opening of less than 40 mm and passive stretch opening of 4 or more mm greater than than unassisted opening.

3b. Without limitation: Unassisted mandibular opening of 40 mm or more than.

Although each of these committees worked independently of each other, there were similarities in the results and also produced criteria that could be tested through research.

TESTING OF DIAGNOSTIC CRITERIA FOR MMFP

We then completed a study of these criteria using discriminate analysis to determine which items best predict the diagnosis of MMFP (20). The sensitivity and specificity of these items as diagnostic criteria were determined as compared to normals. In essence, this study was designed to confirm or refute the diagnostic criteria of the committees. Thirty one patients with MMFP and 31 subjects who met criteria for being normal were each examined by a rater who was blind to their status. Measures included a muscle index of 44 extraoral, intraoral and cervical muscle sites to assess the scope of tenderness in the muscles involved in masticatory function; pressure algometry to measure the absolute and relative pressure pain thresholds of the muscles, the presence of taut bands, twitch response, and pain radiation with palpation. The techniques used for examination were identical to those discussed earlier for the Craniomandibular Index and the pressure algometer. Validity of the original MMFP diagnosis or the normal status of the subjects was determined based on all relevant clinical data and another independent examiner different than the first rater.

The results shown in Table 4 confirmed what the committees had suggested; that the scope of tenderness [% of muscle sites tender] is a valid predictor of the presence of MMFP. Other items including pressure algometry to measure the absolute pressure pain thresholds of the muscles, the twitch response and pain radiation with palpation were predictive but not to the same extent as scope of tenderness. Items that showed no difference between the groups included taut bands and relative pain thresholds. With scope, different cutoff levels were analyzed to determine which one provide the best sensitivity and specificity to arrive at the 28th percentile. This is similar to diagnostic criteria that were developed for fibromyalgia

Table 4. Final tested diagnostic criteria for masticatory myofascial pain and it's sensitivity and specificity with and without including subjective reports of temple or jaw pain

	12 of 44 sites	12 of 44 sites plus pain in temples/jaw
Sensitivity	93.5%	93.5%
Specificity	80.6%	100%
% Agreement	87.1%	97%

[where 11 of 18 sites need to be tender] (27) in order to have a diagnosis of MMFP.

DISCUSSION

This paper presents results of a number of studies that have examined the reliability and validity of characteristics of myofascial pain and led to the development and testing of diagnostic criteria for masticatory myofascial pain. In this series of studies, the scope of tenderness in muscles, i.e., the percentage of muscle sites tender, appears to the most reliable and valid predictor of MMFP confirming expert opinions. Although, one committee suggested that tenderness in 22% of muscle sites would be adequate for diagnosis, this study suggests that patients with 28% or more of their masticatory muscles being tender is a better predictor of a diagnosis of masticatory myofascial pain in this study population. Although these figures are close enough to be comparable, future larger multicenter studies are needed to determine which percentage would be the best cutoff for epidemiological purposes.

Other items that were different between the two populations could also be included in future studies as minor criteria including pressure algometry to measure the absolute pressure pain thresholds of the muscles, the twitch response and pain radiation with palpation. Items that showed no difference between the groups included taut bands and relative pain thresholds may be insignificant as single criteria in diagnosing MMFP. However, taut bands are useful in determining the presence of the muscle prior to palpation but seem to occur in both normals and patients.

Certain methodological problems found in completing this study should be addressed in future studies. For example, the gold standard in this case was an independent expert clinician using common definitions and all available data on patients to arrive at a diagnosis of MMFP. Since the definition of MMFP is based upon subjective pain and related tenderness, it is not surprising that tenderness is a key diagnostic feature. However, as pointed out earlier, there are many different methods of measuring tenderness and each was factored into the statistical analysis.

Tenderness can be measured using finger pressure to determine whether a site is tender or not. Finger pressure techniques have borderline reliability and require a standardized method combined with a calibration process to enhance reliability between raters. In addition, the sites must be carefully chosen and identified as well known trigger point sites since many sites have localized tenderness of less than 5 mm in diameter. The scope of tenderness may be calculated as the mean pressure pain threshold of all trigger point sites or as the percentage of sites that were tender using a standardized pressure. This latter measure appears to be the most predictive item.

A pressure algometer can also be used to determine the pressure pain threshold of a site alone or as compared to adjacent sites for relative measurements. We found that a pressure algometer does increase reliability of the measurements and should be used whenever possible. An algometer that includes a strain gauge with a standardized surface that is small, agile and allows for standardizing of the rate of pressure increase improves the potential reliability. In addition, other factors such as twitch response, taut bands, and radiation of pain were considered and found to be less significant criteria. Future studies need to examine other criteria which may be as significant as the scope of tenderness including range of motion, surface skin changes, electromyograghic recordings of the twitch response, skin conductivity, thermography, and other regional measurements.

It is interesting to note that these conclusions are similar to the criteria developed for fibromyalgia, a systemic muscle disorder (27). For myofascial pain, the cutoff for confirming the diagnosis was 28% of the muscle sites being tender, whereas fibromyalgia requires 61%. It is interesting to note that of the 18 palpation sites proposed for a fibromyalgia diagnosis, 16 of them are well known myofascial trigger point sites (7). This finding suggests that fibromyalgia may be a physical disorder closely related to myofascial pain with regard to peripheral pain mechanisms. However, they may be distinguished from each other by different contributing factors that cause the widespread pain and tenderness in fibromyalgia versus the regional characteristics of myofascial pain. The most common contributing factors cited in fibromyalgia are systemic or central in nature such as sleep disorders, inactivity, or depression whereas the most commonly cited contributing factors to myofascial pain are regional in nature such as poor posture, repetitive strain, and local trauma (8).

The scope of tenderness as a diagnostic criteria for masticatory myofascial pain also has implications for diagnosing myofascial pain in other parts of the body such as the low back, upper back or torso, the neck, and the extremities. In each of these areas there are well known trigger point sites which may be examined for tenderness using a similar standardized technique for patients presenting with regional pain in those areas. Studies need to be performed in a similar fashion to determine if the scope of tenderness is the best predictor of the diagnosis in these other regions. Confounding factors in all of these studies may be the frequent presence of muscular pain in other pain disorders such as joint disorders, neuralgias, and sympathetic dystrophies. Cases of multiple diagnoses frequently complicate the diagnostic process in determining which disorder is causing which pain and contribute to the neglect of the myofascial component.

In summary, although the scope of the tenderness appeared to be the most reliable and valid criteria for masticatory myofascial pain in this series of studies, it is important to realize that the gold standard for diagnosis of MMFP in a clinical setting is an expert clinician's analysis of all available data to render a decision on diagnosis. In addition, there continues to be a need for further research to test criteria for myofascial pain in different samples, with different criteria, for other chronic pains, and against other chronic pain disorders. In particular, there is a need for more objective measures of myofascial pain that do not depend upon the patient's subjective reports. This is a critical step is the process of establishing myofascial pain as a common, universally accepted and eminently treatable disease.

REFERENCES

1. Fricton JR, Kroening R, Haley D, Siegert R: Myofascial pain and dysfunction of the head and neck: a review of clinical characteristics of 164 patients. Oral Surg Oral Med Oral Path 60:615-623, 1985.

2. Fishbain DA, Goldberg M, Meagher BR, Steele R, Rosomoff H: Male and female chronic pain patients categorized by DSM III. Psychiatric Diagnostic Criteria. Pain 26:181-197, 1986.

3. Skootsky SA, Jaeger B, Oye RK: Prevalence of myofascial pain in general internal medicine practice. West J Med 151:157-160, 1989.

4. Rosomoff, et al.: Physical findings in patients with chronic intractable benign pain of the neck and or back. Pain 26:181-197, 1988.

5. Foley, K. *The Report of the Commission on the Evaluation of Pain.* DHHS, SSA, Office of Disability, SSA Pub. No. 64-031.

6. LeResche L, Dworkin S, Von-korff M, Truelove E, Sommers, E: Epidemiologic evaluation of two diagnostic classifications schemes for TMD. J Dent Res 68(supp):258, 1989.

7. Simons D: Muscle pain syndromes. In Fricton J, Awad E, (eds) Myofascial Pain and Fibromyalgia, Raven Press, pp 1-41, 1990.

8. Bennett R: Myofascial pain syndromes and the fibromyalgia syndrome: A comparative analysis. In Fricton J, Awad E, (eds), Myofascial Pain and Fibromyalgia. Raven Press, pp 43-66, 1990.

9. Travell J, Simons DG: Myofascial pain and dysfunction: The trigger point manual. Baltimore, Williams and Wilkins, 17-25, 1983.

10. Simons DG: Muscle Pain Syndromes (I and II). Am J Phys Med 54 (6): 288-311 and 55(1):15-42, 1975.

11. Fisher AA: Documentation of Myofascial Trigger Points. Arch Phys Med Rehab 69:286-291, 1988.

12. Reeves JL, Jaeger B, Graff-Radford SB: Reliability of the pressure algometer as a measure of myofascial trigger point sensitivity. Pain 24:313-321, 1986.

13. Jaeger B, Reeves LJ: Quantification of changes in myofascial trigger point sensitivity with the pressure algometer following passive stretch. Pain 27:203-210, 1986.

14. Ohrbach R, Gale EN: Pressure pain thresholds, clinical assessment, and differential diagnosis: reliability and validity in patients with myogenic pain. Pain 39(2):157-170, 1989.

15. Schiffman E, Fricton J, Haley D, Tylka D: A pressure algometer for myofascial pain syndrome: Reliability and validity testing in Dubner R, Gebhart GF, and Bond MR, (eds). Proceedings of the Vth World Congress on Pain, Elsevier Science Publishers, BV. Chpt 46, pp. 407-413, 1988.

16. Fischer AA, Chang CH: Temperature and pressure threshold measurements in trigger points. Thermology 1:212-15, 1986.

17. Mohl ND (b), Ohrbach RK, Crow HC and Gross AJ: Devices for the diagnosis and treatment of temporomandibular disorders. Part III: Thermography, ultrasound, electrical stimulation, and electromyographic biofeedback. J Prosthet Dent 63:472-77, 1990.

18. Fischer AA: Pressure threshold measurement for diagnosis of myofascial pain and evaluation of treatment results. Clin J Pain 2:207-14, 1987.

19. Lewit K: The needle effect in relief of myofascial pain. Pain 6:83-90, 1979.

20. Meister T: Thermography in diagnosis of Myofascial pain (M.S.Thesis). University of Minnesota, 1990.

21. Fricton JR, Schiffman, EL: Reliability of a craniomandibular index. J Dent Res 65:1359-64, 1986.

22. Dworkin SF, LeResche L, DeRoven T: Reliability of clinical measurement in temporomandibular disorders. Clin J Pain 4:89-100, 1988.

23. Jensen K: Pressure Algometry. In Fricton J, Awad E, (eds), Myofascial Pain and Fibromyalgia, Raven Press, pp 165-182, 1990.

24. Dahlstrom L, Keeling S, Fricton J, Helsenbeck S, Clark G, and Rugh J: Evaluation of a Training Program Intended to Calibrate Raters of Temporomandibular Disorders. J of Cranio Dis Oral and Facial Pain (submitted) 1993.

25. McNeil C, (ed): Craniomandibular Disorders: Guidelines for Evaluation, Diagnosis, and Management (American Academy of Craniomandibular Disorders). Chicago, Quintessence Books, 1990.

26. Dworkin S, (ed): Research Diagnostic Criteria for Temporomandibular Disorders: J of Craniomandibular Disorders, Oral and Facial Pain, 6:301-354, 1992.

27. Wolfe F, Smythe HA, Yunus MB, Bennett RM, et al.: Criteria for fibromyalgia. Arth Rheum 33:160-172, 1990.

A Chronobiologic Theory of Fibromyalgia

Harvey Moldofsky

SUMMARY. Objectives: The paper reviews the evidence in favour of a chronobiologic theoretical model of fibromyalgia.

Findings: The physiology and behaviour of sleep and wakefulness are important components of the features of fibromyalgia. Detailed analyses of recurrent changes over time in the patterns of these fundamental brain functions and symptoms provide evidence for central nervous system mechanisms that underlie the disorder. Consistent with the chronobiologic theory, the constellation of diffuse pain, nonrestorative sleep, fatigue and depression is shown to be the result of altered biologic rhythms that involve diurnal physiologic functions, seasonal environmental influences, and social-behavioural disturbances.

Conclusions: The chronobiologic theory stresses the importance of temporal variation and the factors that influence and govern recurrent patterns of biologic functions and behaviour that determine health and the evolution of the illness. Finally, the chronobiologic theory of fibromyalgia allows for an integrated study of brain, behaviour and somatic functions over time and emphasizes that such a comprehensive approach is core to any therapeutic intervention.

KEYWORDS. Chronobiology, sleep, fibromyalgia

Harvey Moldofsky, MD, is Professor of Psychiatry and Medicine, University of Toronto.

Address reprint requests to: Dr. H. Moldofsky, Centre for Sleep and Chronobiology, Toronto Western Division, the Toronto Hospital, 399 Bathurst Street, EC 3D-022, Toronto, Ontario, Canada M5T 2S8.

[Haworth co-indexing entry note]: "A Chronobiologic Theory of Fibromyalgia." Moldofsky, Harvey. Co-published simultaneously in the *Journal of Musculoskeletal Pain* (The Haworth Press, Inc.) Vol. 1, No. 3/4, 1993, pp. 49-59; and: *Musculoskeletal Pain, Myofascial Pain Syndrome, and the Fibromyalgia Syndrome* (ed: Søren Jacobsen, Bente Danneskiold-Samsøe, and Birger Lund) The Haworth Press, Inc., 1993, pp. 49-59. Multiple copies of this article/chapter may be purchased from The Haworth Document Delivery Center [1-800-3-HAWORTH; 9:00 a.m. - 5:00 p.m. (EST)].

49

INTRODUCTION

While considerable interest has focussed upon the characteristic distribution of pain and tenderness in fibromyalgia (1), unrefreshing sleep, chronic fatigue and emotional distress are common to patients with this disorder. A review of the evidence from clinical, sleep physiologic and treatment studies in patients with fibromyalgia show that disordered sleep physiology, e.g., the alpha [7.5-11 Hz] electroencephalographic [EEG] sleep anomaly, reflects a state of vigilance during sleep which accompanies the experience of unrefreshing sleep, generalized aching, fatigue and emotional distress (2). The amalgam of disordered sleep physiology and symptoms comprise a nonrestorative sleep syndrome that is a common feature of patients with fibromyalgia (3). Such sleep and somatic symptoms also characterize patients who are especially distressed by fatigue and cognitive difficulties following a febrile illness [chronic fatigue syndrome] or by functional bowel symptoms [irritable bowel syndrome]. Indeed, these disorders appear variably or commonly coexist in patients with fibromyalgia (4,5,6).

The research shows that the nonrestorative sleep syndrome is a final common pathway that emerges from heterogeneous disturbances of the central nervous system. Metabolic dysfunctions that have been found to affect fibromyalgia involve the sleeping-waking brain. These altered metabolic functions include neurotransmitters such as serotonin and substance P, immune and neuroendocrine substances, such as interleukin-1, growth hormone and cortisol (7). Secondly, environmental disturbances have been shown to affect brain functions and the somatic symptoms. The experimental disruption of slow wave [deep] sleep by noise has been shown to be accompanied by myalgia, fatigue and emotional distress in a vulnerable group of sedentary people (8). Thirdly, the altered sleep physiology, somatic and psychological symptoms have been shown to follow acute social and behavioural disturbances such as those following a motor vehicle or industrial accidents (9).

Since the physiology and behaviour of sleep and wakefulness are important components of the features of fibromyalgia, the detailed study of recurrent changes over time in the patterns of these brain functions and symptoms should provide for further understanding of the central nervous system mechanisms that underlie the disorder. The paper reviews the evidence in favour of a chronobiologic theoretical model of fibromyalgia. According to this theory, the constellation of diffuse pain, nonrestorative sleep, fatigue and depression is the result of disturbed biologic rhythms that involve diurnal physiologic functions, seasonal environmental influences, and social-behavioural disturbances.

DIURNAL SYMPTOMS AND PHYSIOLOGIC FUNCTIONS

Various research studies on the 24 hour pattern of changes in sleep and wakefulness show increased sleep tendency, negative mood, diminished capacity for intellectual functions, and reduced performance skills from approximately 0200 h to 0700 h. To a lesser degree, the sleepiness and behavioural changes occur during the afternoon from 1300 h to 1600 h. After a suitable duration of restful nocturnal sleep there is increased wakefulness and optimal behavioural functioning during the morning, then again, at around 1900 h until before evening bedtime (10). That is, normal healthy adults experience reduced well being during two distinct periods over the course of the daily cycle: a nocturnal period and a lesser afternoon period. Figure one provides an illustration of the double peak pattern of well-being that has been shown in a variety of studies of changes in sleep tendency and human performance over the 24-hour day (10,11). On the other hand, patients with fibromyalgia and chronic fatigue syndrome report increased lethargy, emotional distress, cognitive and performance difficulties that accompany the diffuse pain and stiffness in the morning after awakening from unrefreshing sleep (2,8,12,13). As the morning progresses, often the symptoms recede. Optimal levels of energy, mood, and performance along with improved tolerance to discomfort or least pain occur during an interval from approximately 1000 h to 1400 or 1500 h. Typically, the symptoms gradually increase during the latter half of the afternoon so that often the individual is obliged to rest. The symptoms do not improve in the evening, but continue without respite until the evening bedtime. In contrast to healthy subjects, fibromyalgia subjects feel at their relative best during the midday time interval when normally healthy people may be beginning to experience a decline in alertness, mood, cognitive and performance capabilities [see Figure 1]. In this figure, the hypothetical inverse bimodel curve illustrates the changes in symptoms of fibromyalgia during the period of wakefulness. The curve in well-being is extrapolated from self-ratings of pain, fatigue and sleepiness before and after sleep physiologic studies and unpublished self-ratings of time of day for least symptoms and overall well being. These diurnal changes in symptoms are similar to the curve that describes the circadian variation in chest pain of patients admitted to a coronary care unit following a myocardial infarction (14).

Whereas healthy subjects have least pain sensitivity in the morning (15), patients with fibromyalgia show increased tenderness upon awakening in the morning or no overnight improvement in dolorimeter ratings (16). Furthermore, decreased pain threshold toward the end of the menstrual cycle (15) is consistent with the clinical observation of increased fibromyalgia symptoms during the premenstrual time interval.

FIGURE 1. Hypothetical curves that describe diurnal changes in well being for healthy subjects [top] and for fibromyalgia patients [bottom]. Double plot of 24 hr. day is used to show overnight sleep-related changes.

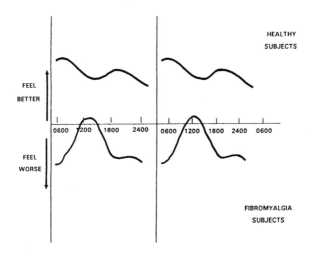

The significance of sleep physiology to the diurnal changes in pain is evident in the findings of increased overnight tenderness and subjective pain measures in normals when their slow wave sleep was disrupted by noise. Such diurnal changes did not occur with REM sleep deprivation. Furthermore, on the night following the resumption of undisturbed sleep, the normal subjects experienced an overnight decline in tenderness measures with the dolorimeter (8). In an experimental longitudinal study of a comparison of the use of 100 mgm chlorpromazine to 5 G of L-tryptophan at bedtime, EEG sleep measures were found to be related to the overnight change in symptoms of fibromyalgia. That is, the mean percent time per minute or mean percent power per minute of the alpha EEG frequency during sleep correlated with overnight increase in tenderness, increased hostility and decreased energy. On the other hand, mean percent time per minute of slow wave [delta] sleep was related to overnight decrease in tenderness. The mean percent delta power per minute was associated with decreased anxiety and hostility, and increased energy (17).

The overnight chronobiologic pattern of the alpha EEG sleep frequency of fibromyalgia patients differs from that found in normal subjects. Not only is the overall amount of the alpha EEG frequency greater during sleep, but fibromyalgia patients also show that the amount of alpha EEG is highest during the first few hours of sleep (18). The alpha EEG sleep declines over the course of the night to the same low level that persists unchanged throughout the sleep of normal subjects. On the other hand, the exponential decline in slow wave sleep after sleep onset that characterizes normals also occurs in patients with fibromyalgia. The overnight pattern of decline in slow wave sleep is identical to a previously determined mathematical formula (19). The normal amount of EEG slow wave sleep in fibromyalgia differs from the reduced slow wave sleep found in patients with major depressive disorder (20). These observations, together with the absence of an abbreviated onset to REM sleep that is often found in patients with major depressive disorder, provide chronobiologic evidence that does not support the notion that fibromyalgia is a variant of major depressive disorder (21). Furthermore, the decline to normal levels of alpha EEG sleep in the few hours before morning awakening is consistent with the subjective experience of fibromyalgia patients who report that their best sleep occurs just prior to arising in the morning.

Animal and human studies have demonstrated linkages among neurotransmitters [e.g., serotonin], certain cytokines, aspects of the immune, neuroendocrine, and sleep-wake systems. Slow wave sleep of animals is promoted by serotonin, interleukin-1 [IL-1], and certain immunologically-active peptides including Factor S, muramyl dipeptide [a product of bacterial cell walls], vasoactive intestinal peptide, prostaglandin D-2, α2-interferon; tumour necrosis factor (22) and IL-2 (23). Human studies show that maximum plasma IL-1 and IL-2-like activities, reduced natural killer cell activity, maximum growth hormone secretion and least cortisol secretion occur during nocturnal [slow wave] sleep (24,25). Krueger and colleagues suggest that various immunologically active peptides interact in a complex fashion with hypothalamic pituitary hormones in regulating the delicate balance of sleep-wake functions (22). We showed that sleep deprivation with 40 hours of wakefulness produced dramatic changes in aspects of immune, endocrine and behavioural functions. Plasma IL-1 and IL-2 activities were higher during the early hours of the night of sleep deprivation than during baseline and resumed sleep (26). As previously shown by other researchers, the normal nocturnal rise in growth hormone secretion did not occur, but was increased over the baseline on the following night of resumed sleep. The average 24 hour cortisol levels were not altered by a single night of sleep deprivation, but the late nocturnal cortisol rise occurred one hour earlier suggesting that sleep provides an inhibitory influence on cortisol secretion which is otherwise not dependent on sleep (25). Serial behavioural and performance assessments showed that negative mood, sleepiness and fatigue were related to responses of lymphocytes to stimulation by pokeweed mitogen. Reaction time and logical reasoning were related to the cellular response to phytohemagglutinin mitogen and to plasma IL-1 activity. These observations in animal and human studies are consistent with the notion that sleep-related immune and neuroendocrine functions are related to the physiological restorative function of sleep. Interference with sleep by sustained wakefulness is accompanied by alteration in these functions and with nonrestorative sleep symptoms.

The limited data on alteration of serotonin metabolism, neuroendocrine and immune functions are consistent with the theory that relates disordered biologic rhythmic functions to the clinical features of fibromyalgia. The initial observation of an inverse relationship of plasma-free tryptophan to the pain of patients with fibromyalgia (27) and recent metabolic studies by Russell et al. (28) and Yunus et al. (29) of reduced serotonin metabolism are consistent with the hypothesis of disordered brain serotonin metabolism in fibromyalgia patients (27). The finding of reduced somatomedin-C, that is considered to reflect reduced growth hormone secretion, is thought to be related to the disturbances in the nocturnal sleep of fibromyalgia patients (30). McCain et al. (31) showed an absence of the expected decline between morning and late afternoon levels of serum cortisol in fibromyalgia patients. Serum IL-2 levels are increased in patients with chronic fatigue disorder (22). IL-2 used in the treatment of cancer produces decreased energy, fatigue, malaise, depression, sleep disturbances and diffuse musculoskeletal pain symptoms similar to those of fibromyalgia (33,34). Most of these studies involve single or post hoc observations so that the temporal relationships of the sleep-wake system with behaviour and biologic measures are not well defined. Future studies will require time series analyses of measures of the circadian pattern of the sleep-wake system neurotransmitters, neuroendocrine and immune functions. The effect of behaviour and environment on this dynamic system will further our understanding of the disorder. Recent research on the effects of fitness (35) or exercise suggest dysfunction of the hypothalamic-pituitary axis and peripheral autonomic activity in fibromyalgia (36).

SEASONAL-ENVIRONMENTAL INFLUENCES AND FIBROMYALGIA

Environmental stimuli [e.g., climate] and mood [e.g., depression] may modulate the symptoms of patients with fibromyalgia. Numerous studies have shown that depression may be subject to seasonal variation. In particular, considerable interest has focussed upon the periodic recurrence of depression during the fall and winter months with remission in the summer. Such people have been identified as having a seasonal affective disorder (37). Because of the possibility that seasonal variation may influence the mood and symptoms of fibromyalgia, we hypothesized that fibromyalgia patients would show seasonal changes in mood, pain, energy and sleep. Furthermore, in order to evaluate the role of inflammatory disease pain, we hypothesized that patients with fibromyalgia would differ from those with rheumatoid arthritis [RA] in the seasonality of their symptoms. In a study that compared such patients and normal controls, the Seasonal Pattern Assessment Questionnaire (38) which has been used to rate seasonal mood changes showed that fibromyalgia patients had a higher rating than RA and controls. Indeed, 43 percent of fibromyalgia patients in the Toronto region rated mood impairment equivalent to seasonal affective disorder compared to 25% of controls and 16% RA patients. An analogous questionnaire that addressed seasonal fluctuations in pain, energy and restful sleep revealed that seasonal variation of pain was greater in fibromyalgia vs. RA. Furthermore, monthly evaluation of symptoms showed that fibromyalgia patients claimed most pain, worst mood, least energy and least restful sleep from November to March. They reported least symptoms from May to August. RA patients did not describe consistent monthly pattern of symptoms. While the method depends upon peoples' beliefs about climatic effects on health, nevertheless the study indicated that seasonal environmental influences appear to be important for mood and symptoms of patients with fibromyalgia (39). These findings may account for the opposing claims for the primacy of depression in the etiology of fibromyalgia (40,41,42,43). As shown by the study, depressive symptoms vary with the seasons. Moreover, the observations have treatment implications. That is, seasonal changes in symptoms may mask treatment trials so that time of year for scheduling treatments need to be considered. Finally, given the beneficial effects of light therapy on seasonal affective disorder, such treatment may prove useful for the management of fibromyalgia during the fall-winter season in northern latitudes. A pilot study carried out in Toronto during the winter of 1991-92 suggests that some patients who are sensitive to seasonal variation in light may benefit from this treatment. These preliminary results justify further research on the role of light and seasonal influences on biologic rhythms and symptoms of fibromyalgia.

TIME, SOCIAL-BEHAVIOURAL FUNCTIONS AND SYMPTOMS

Studies have shown that the altered sleep physiology and symptoms of fibromyalgia may follow upon a nonphysically injurious motor vehicle or industrial accident (9,16). We speculated that the disordered sleep physiology induced by the emotional distress of the accident mediated the subsequent nonrestorative sleep, musculoskeletal pain, and fatigue symptoms (9). Our current research findings, in a longitudinal prospective study of post accident pain in 150 workers following an industrial accident, are consistent with this hypothesis. The data show that at the point of entry into the study at 3 months following a work-related soft-tissue strain, sprain injury, all subjects had comparable ratings of pain severity, number of tender points, and threshold tenderness. All subjects were quite similar with regard to the severity of their sleep disturbances and their fatigue. However, after repeated measures at 9, 15 and 21 months, subjects who failed to return to work showed more painful regions, more behavioural pain dysfunction, and greater emotional distress. Even though there was a progressive decline in the number of tender points and improvement in threshold tenderness, after 9 months post accident, those who failed to return to work showed progressive increase in sleep disturbance, fatigue ratings, and emotional distress. Conversely, those who returned to work showed a progressive decline in pain severity and pain behaviour. They did not show any changes in sleep, fatigue, or emotional distress over the 21 months. Those who failed to return to work rated themselves as persistently physically disabled and socially handicapped. They indicated that they were experiencing progressively increasing physical and psychological impairment. On the other hand, those who returned to work claimed a decline in disability and handicap. They did not indicate any change in scores of impairment (Crook and Moldofsky, unpublished data). Therefore, study of the evolution of pain symptoms and the ability to return to work are related to psychologic distress, sleep disturbance and fatigue. The temporal patterns are consistent with the chronobiologic theoretical model for understanding the evolution of persistent pain, fatigue and nonrestorative sleep. Furthermore, the theory allows for an analysis of those factors that discriminate those workers with post accident pain who will return to work from those who will not be able to work. The theory would appear to have practical implications for designing rehabilitation and social assistance programmes for injured workers with hitherto poorly understood chronic pain problems.

CONCLUSION

A review of the evidence from diurnal physiologic, seasonal environmental and prospective studies of social-behavioural functions suggest that a chronobiologic theoretical model provides a comprehensive basis to the dynamics of central nervous system mechanisms, the assessment and management of patients with fibromyalgia. The chronobiologic model stresses the importance of temporal variation and the factors that influence and govern recurrent patterns of biologic functions and behaviour that determine health and illness. Finally, the theory allows for an integrated study of brain, behaviour and somatic functions over time and emphasizes that such a comprehensive approach is core to any therapeutic intervention.

REFERENCES

1. Wolfe F, Smythe HA, Yunus MB, Bennett RM, Bombardier C, Goldenberg DL, Tugwell P, Campbell SM, Abeles M, Clark P, Fam AG, Farber SJ, Fiechtner JJ, Franklin CM, Gatter RA, Hamaty D, Lessard J, Lichtbroun AS, Masi AT, McCain GA, Reynolds WJ, Romano TJ, Russell IJ, Sheon RP: The American College of Rheumatology 1990 criteria for the classification of fibromyalgia: Report of the multicenter criteria committee. Arthritis Rheum 33: 160-172, 1990.

2. Anch AM, Lue FA, MacLean AW, Moldofsky H: Sleep physiology and psychological aspects of fibrositis (fibromyalgia). Can J Psychol 45:179-184, 1992.

3. Moldofsky H: Sleep and musculoskeletal pain; Progress in Fibromyalgia & Myofascial Pain, a volume in the series, Pain Research and Clinical Management. Edited by H Vaeroy, H Merskey. Elsevier Science Publishers BV, Amsterdam (in press).

4. Yunus MB, Masi AT, Aldag JC: A controlled study of primary fibromyalgia syndrome: clinical features and association with other functional syndromes. J Rheumatol 16 (suppl 19): 62-71, 1989.

5. Goldenberg DL: Fibromyalgia and its relation to chronic fatigue syndrome, viral illness and immune abnormalities. J Rheumatol 16 (suppl 19): 91-93, 1989

6. Moldofsky H, Lue FA: Disordered sleep, fatigue and gastrointestinal symptoms in fibromyalgia, chronic fatigue and irritable bowel syndromes; Pain Research and Clinical Management Series. Edited by HE Raybould, EA Mayer. Elsevier Science Publishers BV, Amsterdam (in press).

7. Moldofsky H: Fibromyalgia, sleep disorder and chronic fatigue syndrome, Ciba Foundation Symposia. John Wiley & Sons Ltd, Sussex, U.K. (in press).

8. Moldofsky H, Scarisbrick P: Induction of neurasthenic musculoskeletal pain syndrome by selective sleep stage deprivation. Psychosom Med 38: 35-44, 1976.

9. Saskin P, Moldofsky H, Lue FA: Sleep and post-traumatic rheumatic pain modulation disorder (fibrositis syndrome). Psychosom Med 48: 319-323, 1986.

10. Mitler MM, Carskadon MA, Czeisler CA, Dement WC, Dinges DF, Graeber RC: Catastrophes, sleep, and public policy: Consensus report. Sleep 11: 100-109, 1988.

11. Mitler MM: The realpolitik of narcolepsy and other disorders of impaired alertness. Psychosocial Aspects of Narcolepsy. Edited by M Goswami, CP Pol-

lock, FL Cohen, MJ Thorpy, NB Kavey. Haworth Press, Binghamton, NY, 1992, pp. 129-146.

12. Whelton CL, Salit I, Moldofsky H: Sleep, Epstein-Barr virus infection, musculoskeletal pain, and depressive symptoms in chronic fatigue syndrome. J Rheumatol 19: 939-943, 1992.

13. Moldofsky H, Lue FA: Sleep and symptoms in 205 fibromyalgia patients vs. 876 patients with various sleep disorders. Sleep Research 21: 303, 1992.

14. Thompson DR, Sutton TW, Jowett NI, Pohl JEF. Circadian variation in the frequency of onset of chest pain in acute myocardial infarction. Br Heart J 65: 177-178, 1991.

15. Procacci P: Methods for the study of pain threshold in man; Advances in Pain Research and Therapy. Vol 3. Edited by JJ Bonica et al. Raven Press, New York, 1979, pp. 781-790.

16. Moldofsky H, Scarisbrick P, England R, Smythe HA: Musculoskeletal symptoms and nonREM sleep disturbance in patients with "fibrositis syndrome" and healthy subjects. Psychosom Med 34: 341-351, 1975.

17. Moldofsky H, Lue FA: The relationship of alpha and delta EEG frequencies to pain and mood in fibrositis patients treated with chlorpromazine and L-tryptophan. EEG Clin Neurophysiol 50: 71-80, 1980.

18. Shahal B, Moldofsky H: Process S and alpha EEG sleep in fibrositis and controls. Sleep Res 20: 137, (abstract) 1991.

19. Daan S, Beersma GDM, Borbély AA: Timing of human sleep recovery process gated by a circadian pacemaker. Am J Physiol 246: R161-R183, 1984.

20. Borbély AA: The S-deficiency hypothesis of depression and the two process model of sleep regulation. Pharmacopsychiat 20: 23-29, 1987.

21. Hudson JI, Pope HG: Fibromyalgia and psychopathology: Is fibromyalgia a form of "Affective Spectrum Disorder"? J Rheum 16 (suppl 19): 15-24, 1989.

22. Krueger JM, Johannsen L: Bacterial products, cytokines and sleep, Molecular mimicry in health and disease. Edited by A Lenmark, T Dyrberg, L Terenius, B Hokfelt. Elsevier Science Publ, Amsterdam, 1988, pp. 35-46.

23. Nistico G, De Sarro G: Is interleukin-2 a neuromodulator in the brain? Trends Neurosci 14: 146-151, 1991.

24. Moldofsky H, Lue FA, Eisen J, Keystone E, Gorczynski: The relationship of interleukin-1 and immune functions to sleep in humans. Psychosom Med 48: 309-318, 1986.

25. Davidson JR, Moldofsky H, Lue FA: Growth hormone and cortisol secretion in relation to sleep and wakefulness. J Psychiatr Neurosci 16: 96-102, 1991.

26. Moldofsky H, Lue FA, Davidson JR, Gorczynski RM: Effects of sleep deprivation on human immune functions. FASEB J 3: 1972-1977, 1989.

27. Moldofsky H, Warsh JJ: Plasma tryptophan and musculoskeletal pain in nonarticular rheumatism (fibrositis syndrome). Pain 5: 65-71, 1978.

28. Russell IJ, Michalek JE, Vipraio GA, Fletcher EM, Javors MA, Bowden CA: Platelet ^{3}H-imipramine uptake receptor density and serum serotonin levels in patients with fibromyalgia/fibrositis syndrome. J Rheumatol 19: 104-109, 1992.

29. Yunus MB, Dailey JW, Aldag JC, Masi AT, Jobe PC: Plasma tryptophan and other amino acids in primary fibromyalgia: A controlled study. J Rheumatol 19: 90-94, 1992.

30. Bennett RM, Clark SR, Campbell SM, Burckhardt CS: Low somatomedin-C levels in fibromyalgia. Arthritis Rheum 34 (suppl 3): S188 (abstract), 1991.

31. McCain GA, Tilbe KS: Diurnal hormone variation in fibromyalgia syndrome: A comparison with rheumatoid arthritis. J Rheumatol 16 (suppl 19): 154-157, 1989.

32. Cheney PR, Dorman SE, Bell DS: Interleukin-2 and the chronic fatigue syndrome. Ann Intern Med 110: 321, 1989.

33. Denicoff KD, Rubinow DR, Papa MZ, Simpson C, Seipp CA, Lotze MT, Chang AE, Rosenstein D, Rosenberg SA: The neuropsychiatric effects of treatment with interleukin-2 and lymphokine activated killer cells. Ann Intern Med 107: 293-300, 1987.

34. Wallace DJ, Peter JB, Bowman RL, Wormsley SB, Silverman S: Fibromyalgia, cytokines, fatigue syndromes and immune regulation. Adv Pain Res Therapy 17: 277-287, 1990.

35. Bennett RM: Beyond fibromyalgia: Ideas on etiology and treatment. J Rheumatol 16 (suppl 19): 185-191, 1989.

36. Van Dendern JC, Boersma JW, Zeinstra P, Hollander AP, van Neerbos BR: Physiological effects of exhaustive physical exercise in primary fibromyalgia syndrome (PFS): Is PFS a disorder of neuroendocrine reactivity? Scand J Rheumatol 21: 35-37, 1992.

37. Rosenthal NE, Sack DR, Gillin JC, Lewy AJ, Goodwin FK, Mueller PS, Newsome DA, Wehr TA: Seasonal affective disorder: A description of the syndrome and preliminary findings with light therapy. Arch Gen Psychiat 41: 72-80, 1984.

38. Rosenthal NE, Bradt GH, Wehr TA: Seasonal Pattern Assessment Questionnaire; National Institute of Mental Health. Bethesda, MD, 1984.

39. Moldofsky H, Lue FA, Natarajan MN, Reynolds WJ: Seasonality of pain, mood, energy and sleep in fibromyalgia. Arthritis Rheum 35 (suppl): R40, (abstract) 1992.

40. Hudson JI, Hudson MS, Pliner LF, Goldenberg DL, Pope HG: Fibromyalgia and major affective disorder: A controlled phenomenology and family history study. Am J Psychiatr 142: 441-446, 1985.

41. Tariot PN, Yocum D, Kalin NH: Psychiatric disorders in fibromyalgia. Am J Psychiatr 143: 812-813, (letter) 1986.

42. Kirmayer LJ, Robbins JM, Kapusta MA: Somatization and depression in fibromyalgia syndrome. Am Psychiatr 145: 950-954, 1988.

43. Ahles TA, Khan SA, Yunus MB, Spiegel DA, Masi AT: Psychiatric status of patients with primary fibromyalgia, patients with rheumatoid arthritis, and subjects without pain: A blind comparison of DSM-III diagnoses. Am J Psychiatr 148: 1721-1726, 1991.

Chronic Muscular Pain–
A Life Stress Syndrome?

H. Merskey

SUMMARY. Objective: To examine the relationship between emotional factors, muscle activity, psychological stress and the occurrence of myofascial pain and fibromyalgia.

Findings: Pain may be associated with anxious arousal or with muscle tension but psychological evidence does not relate anxiety to the amount of muscle tension. Psychological illness is common in cases of severe chronic pain but is often only temporary and does not explain persistent pain. Psychological changes commonly follow chronic pain from physical illness. Patients with fibromyalgia often are free from psychological illness, although they show more than patients with rheumatoid arthritis. A close relationship between stress and muscle pain has not been shown.

Conclusions: Chronic muscular pain is not a life stress syndrome and has to be understood in terms of organic disorders made worse by psychological factors. Psychological change which occurs in consequence of muscle pain needs appropriate psychiatric treatment.

KEYWORDS. Fibromyalgia, myofascial pain and psychological illness

---

H. Merskey, MD, is affiliated with the London Psychiatric Hospital, 850 Highbury Avenue, P.O. Box 2532, London, Ontario, Canada N6A 4H1.

Address correspondence to: Dr. H. Merskey, Department of Research, London Psychiatric Hospital, 850 Highbury Avenue, P.O. Box 2532, London, Ontario, Canada N6A 4H1.

[Haworth co-indexing entry note]: "Chronic Muscular Pain–A Life Stress Syndrome?" Merskey, H. Co-published simultaneously in the *Journal of Musculoskeletal Pain* (The Haworth Press, Inc.) Vol. 1, No. 3/4, 1993, pp. 61-69; and: *Musculoskeletal Pain, Myofascial Pain Syndrome, and the Fibromyalgia Syndrome* (ed: Søren Jacobsen, Bente Danneskiold-Samsøe, and Birger Lund) The Haworth Press, Inc., 1993, pp. 61-69. Multiple copies of this article/chapter may be purchased from The Haworth Document Delivery Center [1-800-3-HAWORTH; 9:00 a.m. - 5:00 p.m. (EST)].

61

PAIN AND AROUSAL

It has long been supposed that pain may follow from emotional stress and there is a well accredited relationship between pain, anxiety and arousal. Montaigne (1) was not the first to observe it but perhaps the most economical when he said "We feel one cut from the surgeon's scalpel more than ten blows of the sword in the heat of battle" ["Nous sentons plus un coup de rasoir du chirurgien que dix coups d'espée en la chaleur du combat."]. A relationship between pain and anxiety is well established in the literature (2) both clinically and experimentally. At the same time very high arousal, e.g., in combat may be associated with relative neglect of wounds, at least initially. Thus, men injured in battle or sportsmen in the heat of a game may continue with activity without pain when we would expect that the injury would cause them to withdraw. This may be explained as resulting from an overwhelming degree of arousal, suggesting a curvilinear relationship between anxiety, fear and pain. It may also be the case that some initial injuries are not particularly painful for physical reasons since as many as one-third of individuals with significant physical trauma do not complain of pain at first (3). In any event the relationship between pain and anxiety in clinical practice has been repeatedly confirmed. Hence, we might expect that emotional stress could be an important cause of painful syndromes including muscle syndromes even if the mechanism of muscle contraction pain has not been adequately confirmed.

TENSION AND MUSCLE PAIN

The literature of this century is replete with the concept of tension headache, muscle contraction headache, back pain and pain in the limbs which may be attributed among other favourite causes, to muscle contraction (2,4). It is probably true to say that, in the absence of clear cut alternative explanations, muscle contraction became the preferred explanation for pain.

This approach was probably undermined first in the field of headache. Early workers (5) who used quantitative EMG, showed a modest relationship between pain and anxiety and muscle contraction. But the most influential series of studies was probably the one initiated by Pozniak-Patewicz (6) who demonstrated that muscle contraction was greater in patients with migraine between attacks than in patients with so called tension or muscle contraction headache. In general it has been hard to establish that any relationship found accounts for more than 10% of the variance. However, muscle tension may still play a role. Clark and Sakai (7) reviewing the dental literature, suggest that the assumption that masticatory muscle hyperactivity leads to pain and dysfunction cannot be discarded since evidence does exist for elevated masticatory muscle hyperactivity during sleep. Some habitual muscle over-activity in the jaw has also been demonstrated with EMG monitoring. In the low back, Arena et al. (8) have shown recently that a relationship exists between the quantitative EMG and symptoms, provided that measurements are made under the appropriate condition of activation rather than relaxation. In those circumstances patients with back pain have increased muscle action potentials compared with controls. This does, however, tend to discount the psychological explanation of the origin of much back pain. With respect to fibromyalgia, Zidar et al. (9) have shown that spontaneous and involuntary activity, in patients with fibromyalgia display no difference in motor unit potentials compared with normal controls. Thus, it seems likely both for fibromyalgia and muscle pain in general that muscle contraction may contribute to pain but is far from being a sufficient explanation for it, and also that the links with states of mind are often tenuous. With respect to fibromyalgia, there is an additional consideration, namely that, to the extent that muscle pain is based upon local tenderness, this would be hard to link with certain important locations in fibromyalgia, such as the insertions of tendons and the medial fat pad at the knee.

THE FREQUENCY OF PSYCHOLOGICAL ILLNESS IN CHRONIC PAIN

In physical states which are promoted by anxiety the psychological illnesses which are marked by anxiety should be prominent. The usual frequency for psychological illness is associated with chronic pain is some 30%, depending upon the population studied. Anxiety and depression, often linked with each other, are common psychiatric conditions. Specific evidence on depression and pain has been well reviewed by Romano and Turner (10). They note that in populations with pain, as few as 10% and as many as 83%, were found to have a depressive syndrome of some type. A survey of musculoskeletal pain in the general population showed that using the depression scale of the Centre for Epidemiological Studies [CES-D] 18% of people with chronic pain were found to have depression, in contrast to 8% of those who did not have chronic pain (11). An increase in depression and other psychological symptoms may also be expected in individuals who attend hospital compared with those who remain in the community (12). In addition, a series of studies (13,14,15) using the General Health Questionnaire 28-item version (16) revealed that psychiatric illness at one point in time ranged from 30% of patients in an oral medicine facial pain clinic to 51% in a psychiatrist's service for the assessment and treatment of patients with pain. Thus, patients with pain are not constantly subject to psychiatric illness, although on retrospective examination in the psychiatric sample mentioned above, a DSM-III diagnosis could be made for 84% at some point during their painful illness.

These findings indicate that in muscle pain and in other types of pain, psychiatric illness may be relevant in many during the time in which the patient is in pain, but is usually only present in a minority on a long term basis. The explanation of this psychiatric illness remains to be considered. It may be causal and responsible for the illness; it may be a coincidental finding; it may be a factor which has led the patient with chronic pain to seek hospital care, thus biasing selection; or it may be a consequence of pain. From the population study of Magni et al. quoted above, we can calculate that more than 40% of subjects with chronic pain in the community who also had depression might have had their depression for coincidental reasons.

There are, also, a number of studies which indicate the importance of painful illness in causing emotional change. Woodforde and Merskey (17) showed that psychological illness was as severe in patients with physical complaints of pain as in those without, suggesting that the presence of a painful lesion had caused emotional changes; Atkinson et al. (18) demonstrated that patients with back pain had depression twice as often after the onset of their back pain as before; Sternbach et al. (19) and Kukull et al. (20) showed similarly that among out patients in a general medical clinic, depression appeared to result most often from physical illness. Those who were not depressed initially, but became depressed, had more new physical illness. Radanov et al. (21) have shown that in patients with cervical sprain injury, the initial intensity of neck pain, the initial cognitive impairment related to injury, and age were the significant factors which predicted the presence of continuing symptoms at six months. Psychosocial factors have little power to explain the course of recovery from "Common Whiplash." Patients who improved and those who did not improve did not differ at baseline in respect of personality features. Thus, a variety of sources support the view that, in clinical practice, depression or other psychological changes frequently result from the presence of chronic pain.

A better estimate of the relevant contribution of different factors may only emerge from prospective studies of populations with and without chronic pain and depression, which are not easy to undertake.

PSYCHOLOGICAL ASPECTS OF FIBROMYALGIA

A review of the psychological findings in fibromyalgia leads to the conclusion that fibromyalgia is probably an independent physical illness. Usually only some of the patients with fibromyalgia can be identified as having recognizable psychological illness (22,23,24,25). Hudson et al. (26) did report that most of their patients with fibromyalgia had evidence of anxiety and depression, either past or present, but not all the patients had contemporary psychiatric diagnoses with their illness. Kirmayer et al. (27), using a diagnostic interview schedule, could find only seven cases with a lifetime diagnosis of a psychiatric disorder among 20 patients with fibromyalgia, and seven among 23 patients with rheumatoid arthritis. In general, the proportions resemble those found in studies in family practice, e.g., Shepherd et al. (28). This leads to the conclusion that while depression and other psychological problems may complicate muscle pain and fibromyalgia, and may occasionally promote such illnesses, they are not likely to be the principal cause of more than a minority of cases.

STRESS AND MUSCLE PAIN

It is theoretically possible that stressful circumstances might give rise to muscle pain including fibromyalgia, that the disorder might persist independently even after the stress subsided, and that there might be no signs of psychological illness [except those secondary to pain] after some weeks or months, even though such a disturbance might have been present initially. Such a sequence is not likely, but the possibility that fibromyalgia is sometimes promoted by stress, and more often exacerbated by it, and that the same applies to muscle pain, is much more plausible. Good evidence is hard to obtain because the task is very time-consuming. The popular check lists for stress are not efficient or satisfactory and an adequate measure usually requires a lengthy interview to determine prior life events. The methodology is difficult (29). Jensen (30) compared patients with low back pain, with and without nerve root compression, and two groups of headache patients. Comparison of the frequency of single life events within the previous twelve months revealed no statistically significant differences among the diagnostic groups. The same applied to the total number of life events and the number of life events with transient distress or enduring distress. A number of life events with transient distress were found to show a significant negative association with the persistence of pain in patients with headache, but not in other groups, but even this finding does not appear to be significant after correction from multiple tests.

The Nuprin Study (31) showed that individuals in the community would report a strong association between stress and pain, in that minor ongoing stresses and strains of daily living–"hassles"–were related to pain in different locations including headache and back ache. However, the contribution did not appear large. Marbach et al. (32) undertook a thorough study of life events in patients with temporomandibular pain and dysfunction syndrome. They found no preponderance of life events in the patients with facial pain compared with controls, except after the onset of the symptom. The occurrence of other physical illness was more common in the patients. This may suggest an association of types of musculoskeletal change but it does not suggest an effect of stress in producing the illnesses originally. Most studies have not shown, either, that stressful life events will precipitate or increase headache or low back pain, and life events have not been used for predicting the results of treatment. Moldofsky (33) has demonstrated clearly that similar phenomena may occur both in response to stress and in fibromyalgia. The symptoms of widespread aching and stiffness, tender points at specific anatomical sites, chronic fatigue and non-restorative sleep have been shown to occur in some people after an emotionally stressful but physical non-injurious experience. The symptoms are disruption of electroencephalographic non-REM slow wave sleep by noise. Such exogenous noxious events produce an arousal disturbance in sleep indicated by the alpha EEG non-REM sleep anomaly [Alpha delta sleep] and could be part of an arousal disturbance which is responsible for the symptoms of fibromyalgia. Thus, the possibility exists that fibromyalgia may be produced by sleep disturbance, or at least some type of sleep disturbance. At this point, however, we lack the evidence which would indicate that such a sequence occurs in preference to the possibility that fibromyalgia is a diffuse syndrome which appears first, and that the EEG change develops in consequence. Moldofsky (33) may be able to indicate the extent to which stress might provoke fibromyalgia. To date, however, it appears to be more a contributory factor than a principal cause.

Taking into account also the indications of ill effects arising from the experience of pain in muscle disorders, the only reasonable conclusion at the moment appears to be that while some muscle conditions may be exacerbated, or even initiated, by psychological factors, the evidence that psychological factors are the main cause or the principal sustaining cause of most muscle conditions is rather poor. Psychological change does occur with muscle pains of a variety of types and it is important to treat it when present.

REFERENCES

1. Montaigne ME de: Essais. Book I, Chap. 40: 374-375. J.-V. Le Clerc (ed.). Paris: Garnier Freres, 1865. (1580. Essais. Book I, Chap. 14. Trans. EJ Trechmann. Oxford University Press, London, 1927. (N.B. In some editions Chaps. 14 and 40 are transposed.).

2. Merskey H, Spear FG: Pain: Psychological and Psychiatric Aspects. Bailliere, Tindall & Cassell, 1967, London.

3. Melzack R, Wall PD, Ty TC: Acute pain in an emergency clinic: Latency of onset and descriptor patterns related to different injuries. Pain 14: 33-43, 1982.

4. Merskey H: Psychological aspects of pain. Postgrad Med J 44: 297-306, 1968.

5. Sainsbury P, Gibson JG: Symptoms of anxiety and tension and the accompanying physiological changes in the muscular system. Psychosom Med 17: 216-224, 1954.

6. Pozniak-Patewicz E. "Cephalgic" spasm of head and neck muscles. Headache 15: 161-166, 1976.

7. Clark GT, Sakai S: Masticatory muscle hyperactivity and muscle pain. Advances in Pain Research and Therapy. Edited by JR Fricton, E Awad. Raven Press, New York, 1990, pp. 201-212.

8. Arena JG, Sherman RA, Bruno GM, Young TR: Electromyographic recordings of 5 types of low back pain subjects and non-pain controls in different positions. Pain 37: 57-65, 1989.

9. Zidar J, Backman E, Bengtsson A, Henriksson KF: Quantitative EMG and muscle tension in painful muscles in fibromyalgia. Pain 40: 249-254, 1990.

10. Romano JM, Turner JA: Chronic pain and depression: Does the evidence support a relationship? Psych Bull 97: 18-34, 1985

11. Magni G, Caldieron C, Rigatti-Luchini S, Merskey H: Chronic musculoskeletal pain and depressive symptoms in the general population. An analysis of the 1st national health and nutrition examination survey data. Pain 43: 299-307, 1990.

12. Crook J, Weir R, Tunks E: An epidemiological follow-up survey of persistent pain sufferers in a group family practice and specialty pain clinic. Pain 36: 49-61, 1989.

13. Salter M, Brooke RI, Merskey H: Is the temporomandibular pain and dysfunction syndrome a disorder of the mind? Pain 17: 151-166, 1983.

14. Merskey H, Brown A, Brown J, Malhotra L, Morrison D, Ripley C: Psychological normality and abnormality in persistent headache patients. Pain 23, 1: 35-47, 1985.

15. Merskey H, Lau CL, Russell ES, Brooke RI, James M, Lappano S, Nielsen J, Tlsworth RH: Screening for psychiatric morbidity. The pattern of psychological illness and premorbid characteristics in four chronic pain populations. Pain 30: 41-157, 1987.

16. Goldberg DP: Manual of the General Health Questionnaire. NFER Publications, Windsor, 1978.

17. Woodforde JM, Merskey H: Personality traits of patients with chronic pain. J Psychosom Res 16: 167-172, 1972.

18. Atkinson JH, Slater MA, Grant I, Patterson TL, Garfin SR: Depressed mood in chronic low back pain: Relationship with stressful life events. Pain 35: 47-55, 1988.

19. Sternbach RA, Wolf SR, Murphy RW, Akeson WH: Traits of pain patients: The low-back "loser." Psychosomatics 13: 226-229, 1973.

20. Kukull WA, Koepsell TD, Inui TS, Borson S, Okimoto J, Raskind MA, Gale JL: Depression and physical illness among elderly general medical clinic patients. J Affect Dis 10: 153-162, 1986.

21. Radanov, Bogdan P, Stefano G, Schnidrig A, Ballinari P: Role of psychosocial stress in recovery from common whiplash. Lancet 338: 712-715, 1991.

22. Payne TC, Leavitt F, Garron DC, Katz RS, Colden HE, Glickman PB, Vanderplate C: Fibrositis and psychologic disturbance. Arthritis Rheum 25: 213-217, 1982.

23. Ahles TA, Yunus MB, Riley SD, Bradley JM, Masi AT: Psychological factors associated with primary fibromyalgia syndrome. Arthritis Rheum 27: 1101-1106, 1984.

24. Wolfe F, Cathey MA, Kleinheksel SM, Amos SD, Hoffman RS, Young DY, Hawley DJ: Psychological status in primary fibrositis and fibrositis associated with rheumatoid arthritis. J Rheumatol 11: 500-506, 1985.

25. Clark S, Campbell SM, Forehand ME, Tindall EA, Bennett RM: Clinical characteristics of fibrositis. II: A "blinded" controlled study using standard psychological tests. Arthritis Rheum 28: 132-137, 1985.

26. Hudson JI, Hudson MS, Pliner LF, Goldenberg DL, Pope HG: Fibromyalgia and major affective disorder: A controlled phenomenology and family history study. Am J Psychiatry 142: 441-446, 1985.

27. Kirmayer LJ, Robbins MJ, Kapusta MA: Somatization and depression in fibromyalgia syndrome. Am J Psychiat 145: 950-954, 1988.

28. Shepherd M, Cooper B, Brown MC, Kalton G: Psychiatric Illness in General Practice. Oxford University Press, London, 1966.

29. Brown GW, Sklair F, Harris TO, Birley JLT: Life events and psychiatric disorders. Part I: Some methodological issues. Psychol Med 3: 74-87, 1973.

30. Jensen J. Life events in neurological patients with headache and low back pain (in relation to diagnosis and persistence of pain). Pain 32: 47-53, 1988.

31. Sternbach RA. Survey of pain in the United States: The Nuprin Pain Report. Clin J Pain 2: 49-53, 1986.

32. Marbach JJ, Lennon MC, Dohrenwend BP: Candidate risk factors for temporomandibular pain and dysfunction syndrome: psychosocial, health behavior, physical illness and injury. Pain 34: 139-151, 1988.

33. Moldofsky H: The contribution of sleep-wake physiology to fibromyalgia. Advances in Pain Research and Therapy. Edited by JR Fricton, E Awad. Raven Press, New York, 1990, pp. 227-240.

Fibromyalgia:
Treatment Programs

Don L. Goldenberg

SUMMARY. **Objective:** To provide a concise overview of current treatment approaches in fibromyalgia.

Findings: This review first discusses methodologic problems in prior fibromyalgia therapeutic trials. Then, controlled medication and non-medication studies are reviewed, with emphasis on the largest and most important reports. Finally, a discussion of multidisciplinary treatment of fibromyalgia is provided.

Conclusions: No single therapeutic modality has been highly effective in patients with fibromyalgia. Judicious use of medications that decrease pain and promote better sleep, in conjunction with physical and psychosocial management, is currently the best approach to treatment.

KEYWORDS. Fibromyalgia, treatment, medication

One of the more challenging therapeutic dilemmas in medicine involves the treatment of chronic pain syndromes. Idiopathic low back pain syndrome, migraine or tension headaches and chest wall pain disorders are examples of common painful conditions that defy usual therapeutic ap-

Don L. Goldenberg, MD, is Chief of Rheumatology, Newton-Wellesley Hospital, and also Professor of Medicine, Tufts University School of Medicine.

Address reprint requests to: Don L. Goldenberg, MD, Arthritis-Fibromyalgia Center, Newton-Wellesley Hospital, 2014 Washington Street, Newton, MA 02162.

[Haworth co-indexing entry note]: "Fibromyalgia: Treatment Programs." Goldenberg, Don L. Co-published simultaneously in the *Journal of Musculoskeletal Pain* (The Haworth Press, Inc.) Vol. 1, No. 3/4, 1993, pp. 71-81; and: *Musculoskeletal Pain, Myofascial Pain Syndrome, and the Fibromyalgia Syndrome* (ed: Søren Jacobsen, Bente Danneskiold-Samsøe, and Birger Lund) The Haworth Press, Inc., 1993, pp. 71-81. Multiple copies of this article/chapter may be purchased from The Haworth Document Delivery Center [1-800-3-HAWORTH; 9:00 a.m. - 5:00 p.m. (EST)].

proaches. Fibromyalgia is now recognized as one of the more common chronic pain syndromes, and its treatment has proven to be equally frustrating (1). Since no specific cause or pathophysiologic abnormalities have been identified, treatment has been largely empirical. Initial therapeutic trials employed antiinflammatory medications and central nervous system active medications. These trials as well as newer approches to the treatment of fibromyalgia will be reviewed below.

METHODOLOGIC PROBLEMS
IN FIBROMYALGIA CLINICAL TRIALS

Before 1986, most clinical trials in fibromyalgia were uncontrolled. More recently, there have been a number of controlled therapeutic trials. However, most of these studies have had major methodologic problems. Until the recent generally accepted American College of Rheumatology fibromyalgia diagnostic criteria were published, investigators did not use a uniform case definition for fibromyalgia. Most clinical trials have been reported from tertiary medical centers with a specific interest in fibromyalgia, which may select out patients with more "severe" illness than community cases. Such a selection referral bias is a common criticism of many rheumatic disease trials, and future trials in fibromyalgia should attempt to enroll a broad-based patient population. No standard outcome variables have been measured in clinical trials and rarely has mood or function been assessed. Most studies have been of short duration, usually 6-12 weeks, whereas fibromyalgia is a chronic illness.

In evaluating prior and future therapeutic trials in fibromyalgia, appropriate methodology should include the random assignment of patients to treatment or control groups and such groups should be comparable in regard to variables as sex, age, duration of illness and the severity of symptoms [Table 1]. An adequate number of patients should be included in both control and intervention groups to assure statistical power to detect group differences. All patients should have met the 1990 American College of Rheumatology criteria for the classification of fibromyalgia (2). Clinically relevant, standardized measures should be used to evaluate change in fibromyalgia symptoms. Examples of such measures include selfadministered anchored Likert scales or visual analog scales that ask patients to rate current levels of pain, fatigue, or sleep disturbances. Psychological status, either using simple self-administered questionnaires such as the Hamilton or Beck depression surveys, or structured interviews should be assessed. Functional assessment, either using instruments validated in other rheumatic diseases, such as the Arthritis Impact Measure-

TABLE 1. Methodologic issues in fibromyalgia clinical trials

Study Design:
Random assignment
Comparable intervention and control groups
Adequate number of patients, including after drop-out
All patients should meet ACR fibromyalgia diagnostic criteria
Patient and evaluator should be "blinded"

Standardized Measures of Disease Activity:
Symptoms, such as pain, sleep, mood
Psycholgical evaluation
Tender point scores
Evaluation of function

ment Scale [AIMS] or the Stanford Health Assessment Questionnaire [HAQ] or alternatively an instrument designed to evaluate the functional impact of fibromyalgia, such as the Fibromyalgia Impact Questionnaire [FIQ] (3), should be measured. A tender point examination, either performed manually or with a dolorimeter, should also be evaluated. Patients and evaluators should be blinded as to whether the patient is receiving intervention or is a control.

A set of preliminary criteria for response to treatment in fibromyalgia was recently developed (4). Outcome measures from a prior clinical trial which best distinguished patients with effective medications from those treated with ineffective medication or placebo were identified using stepwise logistric regression analysis. The combination of outcome variables providing the best ability to distinguish effective treatment were physician global assessment of less than 4 of 10 [with 10 = doing extremely poorly], patient sleep score of less than 6 of 10, and a tender point score of less than 14 of maximum 20. Such methodology can be used by others to develop their own set of criteria for treatment response.

MEDICATIONS

Randomized, controlled, clinical therapeutic trials have demonstrated that low doses of tricyclic medications are more effective than placebo in the treatment of fibromyalgia [Table 2]. The largest controlled studies have been with amitriptyline (5-8) and cyclobenzaprine(9,10). Although there are some minor variations in the chemical structure of these two tricyclic compounds, their efficacy and adverse side effects have been very

TABLE 2. Medications tested in controlled therapeutic trials in fibromyalgia

Medication	Dose(mg/day)	Better than placebo
Amitriptyline	10-50	Yes
Cyclobenzaprine	10-30	Yes
Dothiepin	75	Yes
Alprazolam	0.5-3	Yes
Carisoprodol	1200	Yes
5-Hydoxytryptophan	1000	Yes
S-Adenosylmethionine	800	Yes
Prednisone	15	No
Naproxen	1000	No
Ibuprofen	2400	No

comparable in fibromyalgia clinical trials. Generally, a clinical response in pain and quality of sleep was seen by 2 weeks, and within 6 weeks these medications were significantiy better than placebo in most outcomes. Our study (6) demonstrated improvement in tender point scores with amitriptyline but Carette's report (5) did not find such improved tender point scores. The effective doses of amitriptyline have varied from 10-50 mg/day and of cyclobenzaprine from 10-30 mg/day. In most of these trials the tricyclic medications were administered in a single dose at bedtime although the trials with cyclobenzaprine have used divided doses. Our study (6) also found amitriptyline to be more effective in fibromyalgia than 1000 mg of naproxen per day. This is the only study directly that compared a central nervous system acting medication to a non-steroidal anti-inflammatory medication [NSAIDS] in the treatment of fibromyalgia. Naproxen alone was no more effective than placebo treatment. Such a lack of response to NSAIDS was also noted with ibuprofen in the treatment of fibromyalgia (11). We did find that the combination of 25 mg of amitriptyline at bedtime and 500 mg of naproxen twice daily was slighlly more effective than the amitriptyline alone (6). A possible synergism of NSAIDS with a central-nervous system-active medication was also demonstrated by Russell with the combination of alprazolam and ibuprofen (12). There have been no controlled studies using doses of tricyclic antidepressants that are usually employed in the treatment of depression. For example, the highest dose used in a clinical trial was 75 mg/day of dothiepin (13). However, adverse side effects, such as grogginess, constipation, fluid retention, and weight gain, even at these low doses, have been very common. In short-term clinical trials of 4-10 weeks, there has been approximately a 35% drop-out rate. Even more sobering, a clinically meaningful response has been noted in only about one-third of patients.

Uncontrolled longitudinal observations have suggested that patients perceive the efficacy of tricyclics wanes over time (14). Preliminary results from the first long-term clinical trial of tricyclic medication also demonstrated that the short-term effectiveness of these medications appears to regress to the mean over time (15). Carette et al. enrolled 208 fibromyalgia patients in a six month, double-blind, controlled trial of amitriptyline, 10-50 mg/day, cyclobenzaprine, 10-30 mg/day, and placebo (15). A total of 13 outcome measures were evaluated at one, three and six months. Patients on either medication reported significant improvement from baseline on all measures except the tender point and HAQ scores. Patients on placebo improved only on one measure at month one but improved on 9 of the 13 measures at month 6. Significant improvement was more often found in the medication treated patients at one month but at six months there was no significant difference in the percentage of patients in each of the three groups who satisfied the authors' criteria for significant improvement [Table 3]. Thus, although this study confirms the short-term efficacy of amitriptyline and cyclobenzaprine in fibromyalgia, long term efficacy could not be demonstrated because of a significant placebo response over time. In this study, approximately 30% of patients had a meaningful response to the two tricyclic medications, which is similar to results of prior reports.

There are a number of potential mechanisms of action of tricyclic medications in fibromyalgia. Obviously, they are capable of treating depression, however the doses used in these trials were much lower than generally employed in the treatment of depression. Furthermore, the response was quicker than generally noted in depression and we found no correlation of levels of improvement with preexisting psychopathology. Most patients report sleeping better with these medications, but we have

TABLE 3. Results of a six month controlled trial amitriptyline, cyclobenzaprine, and placebo in fibromyalgia*

	Percent of Patients with Significant Improvement		
	Amitriptyline n=84	Cyclobenzaprine n=82	Placebo n=42
Month 1	20.7**	11.7**	0.00
Month 3	18.4	19.4	13.5
Month 6	35.9	32.9	19.4

*From Carette, et al; Arthritis Rheum 1992;35:S112
**$p<0.05$

not found a consistent correlation of response with sleep disturbances (6) and cyclobenzaprine was not found to improve the slow-wave sleep anomaly during a recent clinical trial (16). The tricyclic antidepressants also have an analgesic effect, at least partially mediated by potentiating the action of endogenous opioids. They also cause muscle relaxation, by reducing motor neuron efferent activity at a supraspinal level, and they may even produce modest anti-inflammatory effects. Amitriptyline, in particular, has a wide range of pharmacological actions that include inhibition of serotonin and norepinephrine reuptake, blocking alpha-adrenergic receptors and antagonism of muscarinic, cholinergic and histamine receptors. Scudds reported that the improvement in pain with amitriptyline was related to changes in pain threshold, implying that the mode of action was related to the effect of amitriptyline on peripheral pain sensation (7).

Other central nervous system [CNS] active medications that have been reported to be effective in controlled clinical trials include alprazolam (12) and temazepam [Hench, unpublished observations]. The efficacy of alprazolam was difficult to assess because it was studied in combination with ibuprofen (12). Medications that may also have a number of different actions promoting analgesia in fibromyalgia include SOMA which contains 1200 mg of carisoprodol, 960 mg of acetaminophen, and 192 mg of caffeine (17), S-hydroxytryptophan (18), and S-adenosylmethionine (19), which has analgesic and anti-inflammatory, as well as analgesic properties. The nonbenzodiazepine hypnotic, zopiclone, was found to improve sleep complaints, but not sleep structure, pain, or stiffness (20). Uncontrolled reports have described that fluoxetine, which blocks serotonin uptake, has not been effective in treating the pain in fibromyalgia, although it may help mood and energy. Desipramine, a relatively selective blocker of norepinephrine reuptake was as effective as amitriptyline in relieving the pain of diabetic neuropathy whereas fluoxetine was no better than placebo (21). The only controlled trial of corticosteroids in fibromyalgia demonstrated that 15 mg/day of prednisone was not better than placebo (22).

NON-MEDICINAL THERAPY

Non-medicinal approaches to fibromyalgia therapy have included exercise, physical therapy, various physical and mechanical modalities, and relaxation techniques. It is much more difficult to perform controlled therapeutic trials of such forms of intervention. However, controlled trials have demonstrated improvement in fibromyalgia patients who underwent cardiovascular fitness training (23), EMG-biofeedback (24), hypnotherapy (25), regional sympathetic blockade (26), and cognitive behavioral therapy (27), [Table 4].

The study of cardiovascular fitness training [CFT] compared gradual incremental stationary biking to flexibility and stretching three times weekly. After 6 months, the patients in the CFT group had significant improvement in their aerobic fitness as well as a number of symptoms and tender point scores (23). Fifty percent of the patients in the CFT group but only 10% of the flexibility treatment group noted moderate or marked improvement. However, at 19 months follow-up, only 6 of the 20 patients in the cardiovascular treatment group continued to regularly exercise. This demonstrates that it is difficult to motivate patients to initiate and to continue in a regular exercise routine.

Unfortunately, the other non-medicinal therapeutic trials were rather small and had other methodological problems. Each of these approaches, including biofeedback, hypnotherapy, and cognitive behavioral therapy, is commonly utilized in the treatment of chronic pain disorders. The initial efficacy observed with these treatment modalities in fibromyalgia need to be confirmed by other groups.

OUTCOMES, FUTURE THERAPEUTIC APPROACHES

Unfortunately, most longitudinal studies have reported the persistence of significant pain and other symptoms in fibromyalgia, despite ongoing treatment. There has been little evidence of remission and any remissions have been of short duration (28). We found that moderate or marked pain was present in two-thirds of patients surveyed three years after treatment was started (29). Functional outcome and disability in fibromyalgia are comparable to that in rheumatoid arthritis (30).

New medications and different approaches to medicinal and nonmedic-

TABLE 4. Controlled theraputic trials of effective interventions in fibromyalgia

Author	Therapy
McCain	Cardiovascular fitness training
Ferraccioli	EMG-biofeedback
Haanen	Hypnotherapy
Bengtsson	Regional sympathetic blockade
Goldenberg	Cognitive behavioral therapy

inal treatment of fibromyalgia should be evaluated. Future pharmacological studies should concentrate on novel medications that are targeted at specific neurohormones or at peripheral nociceptors. "Combinations" of analgesics, anti-inflammatory and central nervous system medications should be studied. Individualized dosing schedules and evaluation of treatment responsiveness in various patient subsets should be evaluated. Nonmedicinal approaches that have not yet been adequately studied in fibromyalgia include specific forms of manual therapy and chiropractic, injection of soft tissue trigger or tender points, and psychologically based treatment.

However, it is likely that no single medication or therapeutic modality will be highly effective in the majority of fibromyalgia patients. Therefore, as in many chronic pain disorders, a multidisciplinary treatment program may be most effective in the treatment of fibromyalgia. These programs usually employ combinations of education, cognitive behavioral therapy [CBT], physical therapy and cardiovascular exercise. The foundation of successful therapy in such programs is education [Table 5]. This includes a frank discussion of what the syndrome "is" as well as what it "is not." An approach that makes the patient understand the interaction of the mind and body, not viewing chronic pain disorders as "physical" or "mental" and that emphasizes patient independence will be most effective. Cognitive restructuring is used to change the patients' perception that the pain and disability of fibromyalgia is beyond their control. Relaxation techniques such as deep breathing, meditation, and biofeedback may directly influ-

TABLE 5. Multidisciplinary treatment in fibromyalgia

Education
Validate the diagnosis
Explain mind-body association
Introduce therapeutic approaches
Discuss chronic pain, mood disturbances
Introduce the role of family and social support

Cognitive-behavior, stress-reduction training

Physical therapy and other myofascial pain reduction techniques

Cardiovascular fitness training, stretching

Medications to improve sleep, reduce pain, or treat associated mood disturbances

ence pain and sense of mastery over the disorder. These techniques are integrated into a program that uses physical therapy and trains patients in carefully controlled cardiovascular fitness exercises. Low-impact exercises such as fast-walking, biking, swimming or water aerobics with stretching techniques have been the most helpful. Mental health professionals, physiatrists, and physical therapists have been important members of the team. Preliminary results from our program (27) and that at the University of Oregon Health Sciences (31) has demonstrated the efficacy of a multidisciplinary approach to treatment in fibromyalgia.

In conclusion, the treatment of fibromyalgia, as with other common chronic idiopathic pain disorders, has been difficult to study and not highly effective. Controlled studies have demonstrated the efficacy of low doses of tricyclic medications, such as amitriptyline and cyclobenzaprine, but major improvement has been noted in only one-third of patients. Non-medicinal treatment, such as cardiovascular fitness training and relaxation techniques may be helpful adjuncts. A multidisciplinary team management program may prove to be the best approach to treatment, especially in patients referred to tertiary programs. However, a caring physician who validates the diagnosis and educates the patient and family about the disorder must be at the core of any successful treatment.

REFERENCES

1. Goldenberg DL: Fibromyalgia syndrome. An emerging but controversial condition. JAMA 257: 2782-2787, 1987.

2. Wolfe F, Smythe HA, Yunus MB, Bennett RM, Bombardier C, Goldenberg DL, Tugwell P, Abeles M, Campbell M, Clark P, Fam AG, Farber SJ, Fiechtner JJ, Franklin CM, Gatter RA, Hamaty D, Lessard J, Lichtbroun AS, Masi AT, McCain GA, Reynolds WJ, Romano TJ, Russell IJ, Sheon R: The American College of Rheumatology 1990 Criteria for the Classification of Fibromyalgia: Report of the Multicenter Criteria Committee. Arthritis Rheum 33: 160-172, 1990.

3. Burckhardt CS, Clark SR, Bennett RM: The Fibromyalgia Impact Questionnaire–development and validation. J Rheumatol 18: 728-733, 1991.

4. Simms RW, Felson DT, Goldenberg DL: Development of preliminary criteria for response to treatment in fibromyalgia syndrome. J Rheumatol 18: 1558-1563, 1991.

5. Carette S, McCain GA, Bell DA, Fam AG: Evaluation of amitriptyline in primary fibrositis. A double-blind, placebo-controlled study. Arthritis Rheum 29: 655-659, 1986.

6. Goldenberg DL, Felson DT, Dinerman H: A randomized, controlled trial of amitriptyline and naproxen in the treatment of patients with fibromyalgia. Arthritis Rheum 29: 1371-1377, 1986.

7. Scudds RA, McCain GA, Rollman GB, Harth M: Improvements in pain responsiveness in patients with fibrositis after successful treatment with amitriptyline. J Rheumatol (Suppl 19): 98-103, 1989.

8. Jaeschke R, Adachi J, Guyatt G, Keller J, Wong B: Clinical usefulness of amitriptyline in fibromyalgia: The results of 23 N-of-1 randomized controlled trials. J Rheumatol 18: 447-451, 1991.

9. Bennett RM, Gatter RA, Campbell SM, Andrews RP, Clark SR, Scarola JA: A comparison of cyclobenzaprine and placebo in the management of fibrositis. A double-blind controlled study. Arthritis Rheum 31: 1535-1542, 1988.

10. Quimby LG, Gratwick GM, Whitney CD, Block SR: A randomized trial of cyclobenzaprine for the treatment of fibromyalgia. J Rheumatol 19: 140-143, 1989.

11. Yunus MB, Masi AT, Aldag JC: Short term effects of ibuprofen in primary fibromyalgia syndrome: a double blind, placebo controlled trial. J Rheumatol 16: 527-532, 1989.

12. Russell IJ, Fletcher EM, Michalek JE, Mcbroom PC, Hester GG: Treatment of primary fibrositis/fibromyalgia syndrome with ibuprofen and alprazolam–A double-blind, placebo-controlled study. Arthritis Rheum 34: 552-560, 1991.

13. Caruso I, Sarzi Puttini PC, Boccassini L, Santandrea S, Locati M, Volpato R, Montrone F, Benvenuti C, Beretta A: Double-blind study of dothiepin versus placebo in the treatment of primary fibromyalgia syndrome. J Int Med Res 15: 154-159, 1987.

14. Goldenberg DL: Treatment of fibromyalgia syndrome. Rheum Dis Clin North Am 15: 61-71, 1989.

15. Carette S, Bell M, Reynolds J, Haraoui B, McCain G, Bykerk V, Edworthy S, Baron M, Koehler B, Fam A, Bellamy N, Gulmont C: A controlled trial of amitriptyline, cyclobenzaprine and placebo in fibromyalgia. Arthritis Rheum 35 (Suppl 9): 112, 1992

16. Reynolds WJ, Moldofsky H, Saskin P, Lue FA: The effects of cyclobenzaprine on sleep physiology and symptoms in patients with fibromyalgia. J Rheumatol 18: 452-454, 1991.

17. Vaeroy H, Abrahamsen A, Frre O, Kass E: Treatment of fibromyalgia (fibrositis syndrome): a parallel double blind trial with carisoprodol, paracetamol and caffeine (Somadril comp) versus placebo. Clin Rheumatol 8: 245-250, 1989.

18. Caruso I, Sarzi Puttini P, Cazzola M, Azzolini V: Double-blind study of 5-hydroxytrptophan versus placebo in the treatment of primary fibromyalgia syndrome. J Int Med Res 18: 201-209, 1990.

19. Jacobsen S, Danneskiold-Samsoe B, Andersen RB: Oral S-adenosylmethionine in primary fibromyalgia. Double blind clinical evaluation. Scand J Rheumatol 20: 294-302, 1991.

20. Drewes AM, Andreasen A, Jennum P, Nielsen KD: Zopiclone in the treatment of sleep abnormalities in fibromyalgia. Scand J Rheumatol 20: 288-293, 1991.

21. Max MB, Lynch SA, Muir J, Shoaf SE, Smoller B, Dubner R: Effects of desipramine, amitriptyline, and fluoxetine in diabetic neuropathy. N Engl J Med 326: 1250-1256, 1992.

22. Clark S, Tindall E, Bennett RM: A double blind crossover trial of prednisone versus placebo in the treatment of fibrositis. J Rheumatol 12: 980-983, 1985.

23. McCain GA, Bell DA, Mai FM, Halliday PD: A controlled study of the effects of a supervised cardiovascular fitness training program on the manifestations of fibromyalgia. Arthritis Rheum 31: 1135-1141, 1988.

24. Ferraccioli GF, Fontana S, Scita F, Chirelli L, Nolli M: EMG-biofeedback in fibromyalgia syndrome. J Rheumatol 16: 1013-1014, 1989.

25. Haanen HCM, Hoenderdos HTW, Van Romunde LKJ, Hop WCJ, Mallee C, Terwiel JP, Hekster GB: Controlled trial of hypnotherapy in the treatment of refractory fibromyalgia. J Rheumatol 18: 72-75, 1991.

26. Bengtsson A, Bengtsson M: Regional sympathetic blockade in primary fibromyalgia. Pain 33: 161-167, 1988.

27. Goldenberg DL, Kaplan KH, Nadeau MG: The impact of cognitive-behavioral therapy on fibromyalgia. Arthritis Rheum 34 (suppl 9): S 190, 1991.

28. Cathey MA, Wolfe F, Kleinheksel SM, Hawley DJ: Socioeconomic impact of fibrositis. A study of 81 patients with primary fibrositis. Amer J Med 81: 78-84, 1986.

29. Felson DT, Goldenberg DL: The natural history of fibromyalgia. Arthritis Rheum 29: 1522-1526, 1986.

30. Cathey MA, Wolfe F, Kleinheksel SM, Miller S, Pitetti KH: Functional ability and work status in patients with fibromyalgia. Arthritis Care Res 1: 85-98, 1988.

31. Bennett RM, Campbell S, Burckhardt C, Clark S, O'Reilly C, Wiens A: The contemporary management of fibromyalgia: a multidisciplinary approach. J Musculoskel Dis 8: 21-32, 1991.

The Management
of Myofascial Pain Syndromes

Robert D. Gerwin

SUMMARY. Objective: To present an approach to the management of the Myofascial Pain Syndrome [MPS] based on clinical experience, addressing the problems posed by the specific nature of primary myofascial trigger point pain, and the problem of chronic myofascial pain.

Results: Specific trigger point therapy is designed to inactivate the myofascial trigger point by means of manual techniques, intermittent cold and stretch, and invasive trigger point needling or injection with a local anesthetic. Management of recurrent MPS requires addressing the perpetuating factors of mechanical imbalances [structural, postural, compressive] and systemic abnormalities which interfere with the ability of muscle to recover or which continuously stress muscle reactivating the trigger point. The common systemic factors associated with MPS are hypothyroidism, folic acid insufficiency and iron insufficiency. The relationship of many of the perpetuating factors to MPS is clinically apparent, but has yet to be established firmly by statistically rigorous clinical studies. Corrective measures to prevent the reactivation of trigger points, physical reconditioning and psychological re-education help maintain improvement.

Conclusion: MPS is a condition which is treatable by eliminating the specific trigger points that are the immediate cause of pain, and correcting those factors that predispose to recurrence.

Robert D. Gerwin, MD, is Assistant Professor of Neurology, Johns Hopkins University, 7500 Hanover Parkway, Suite 201, Greenbelt, MD 20770.

[Haworth co-indexing entry note]: "The Management of Myofascial Pain Syndromes." Gerwin, Robert D. Co-published simultaneously in the *Journal of Musculoskeletal Pain* (The Haworth Press, Inc.) Vol. 1, No. 3/4, 1993, pp. 83-94; and: *Musculoskeletal Pain, Myofascial Pain Syndrome, and the Fibromyalgia Syndrome* (ed: Søren Jacobsen, Bente Danneskiold-Samsøe, and Birger Lund) The Haworth Press, Inc., 1993, pp. 83-94. Multiple copies of this article/chapter may be purchased from The Haworth Document Delivery Center [1-800-3-HAWORTH; 9:00 a.m. - 5:00 p.m. (EST)].

KEYWORDS. Myofascial pain, trigger points, muscle diseases

INTRODUCTION

Management of the *MYOFASCIAL PAIN SYNDROME* [MPS] requires both general measures for treatment of the structural and systemic perpetuating factors, and specific measures for treatment of the *Myofascial Trigger Point* [MTrP] itself. Treatment is based on the concept that the pain in MPS, as well as the taut band, local twitch response, referred pain, restricted motion, and weakness and autonomic phenomena, is caused by the trigger point within the muscle. The goal of treatment is to inactivate the MTrP, and to prevent its reoccurrence. The specific measures used to inactivate the MTrP are intermittent cold and stretch, and Trigger point [TrP] injections. The general measures are directed towards the perpetuating factors to correct the structural asymmetries and imbalances, and the systemic disorders which lead to muscle stress or overuse, and which perpetuate MTrPs and the MPS. Finally, corrective action must be taken to reduce the risk of reactivation of MTrPs and recurrence of MPS.

DIAGNOSIS

The first task is to make an accurate and complete diagnosis of MPS and of any pertinent associated condition such as cervical spondylosis, fibromyalgia, or specific nutritional or hormonal insufficiency state. The physical examination for MTrPs should determine if the MPS is localized to one regional functional group of muscles which work together as synergists or antagonists, or if it is widespread, affecting many functional muscle groups. The more chronic MPSs tend to spread through the development of *secondary* TrPs within the functional group, or through the development of *satellite* TrPs within zones of referred pain at distant sites (1, see Vol.1: 12-17).

PERPETUATING FACTORS

Factors that maintain chronic MTrPs can be divided into Mechanical factors and Systemic factors. These should be corrected insofar as possible prior to treating the MTrP specifically. If left uncorrected, reactivation of the MTrP is likely.

Mechanical Perpetuating Factors

The mechanical factors include structural inadequacies, (1, see Vol.1: 41-63), postural stresses and muscle compression. The most common structural inadequacies are the short leg syndrome or leg-length discrepancy, the small hemipelvis, which produces the same effect as the short leg syndrome, the long second metatarsal bone, and short upper arms.

The short leg syndrome [Figure 1]. The most common structural inadequacy is lower limb inequality. As with other mechanical stresses, this is usually well tolerated until an injury or illness destabilizes previous compensatory mechanisms. When one leg is shorter than the other, the pelvis tilts, causing the spine to tilt towards the short leg side. The spine then curves to right the head and level the eyes. If the inequality is slight, less than 1/2", a C-shaped scoliosis develops, causing the shoulder to rise on the side of the short leg. With a greater inequality, the scoliosis is often S-shaped, and the low shoulder may be on the side of the short leg. In the case of C-shaped scoliosis caused by leg-length discrepancy, a heel lift can level the pelvis and the shoulders, relieving the stress on the lower and upper back muscles, the trapezius, the levator scapulae, scaleni, and sternocleidomastoid muscles.

The small hemipelvis. This condition, caused by an asymmetry in the height of the two halves of the pelvis, causes a functional scoliosis when sitting that is similar to that described for the short leg syndrome. The stress on muscle is the same as in the short leg syndrome, as the head is maintained in the erect posture. An ischial or butt lift under the ischial tuberosity will level the pelvis and provide a similar correction as a heel lift.

The long second metatarsal bone (2). The first metatarsal bone is commonly longer than the second, allowing a stable tripod support of the foot by the heel and the heads of the first two metatarsal bones. When the second metatarsal bone is longer, the foot balances along a line from the heel to the second metatarsal head, creating an unstable knife-edge effect. As weight is transferred from the second to the first metatarsal head, the foot pronates, internally rotating the leg at the knee and hip. This causes MTrPs to develop and persist in the peroneus longus [ankle pain], the vastus medialis [knee pain], and the gluteus medius [low back pain]. Secondary TrPs in the gluteus minimis refer pain to the posterior thigh and calf. The condition can be corrected by an orthotic selectively supporting the first metatarsal head, thereby recreating the usual tripod support (1, see Vol.1: 110-112; Vol.2: 381-392).

Short upper arms. Persons with relatively short upper arms experience postural stresses on shoulder girdle muscles when sitting in chairs which

FIGURE 1. Lower limb inequality with a short right leg. A. Uncorrected, the right iliac crest is lower than the left, tilting the spine to the right. Compensatory contraction of the left quadratus lumborum muscle brings the left rib cage downward towards the left iliac crest, curving the thoracic spine back to the left and dropping the left shoulder. The right lateral cervical muscles right the head, leveling the eyes. B. Corrected with a lift under the right foot, leveling the pelvis and shoulder axes, relieving the stress on the quadratus lumborum, levator scalenus, trapezius, scaleni and sternocleidomastoid muscles. C. Incorrect placement of a lift under the longer left leg, accentuating the scoliosis. (From Travell JG, and Simons DG: Myofascial Pain and Dysfunction: The Trigger Point Manual, volume 2. Williams & Wilkins, Baltimore, 1992. Used with permission.)

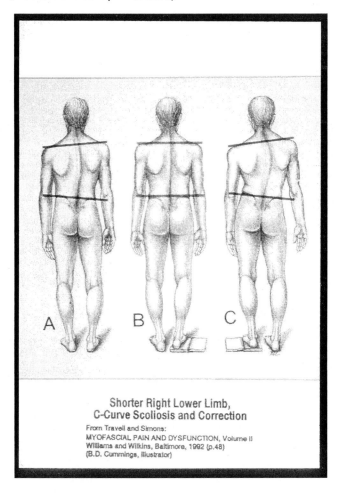

Shorter Right Lower Limb,
C-Curve Scoliosis and Correction

From Travell and Simons:
MYOFASCIAL PAIN AND DYSFUNCTION, Volume II
Williams and Wilkins, Baltimore, 1992 (p.48)
(B.D. Cummings, Illustrator)

do not give adequate arm support. Leaning to one side or slouching activates MTrPs in the quadratus lumborum causing low back pain. Inadequate shoulder support maintains MTrPs in the trapezius muscles. Adjustment of armrest height or desk height, or slanting the work surface, can alleviate this condition.

Other postural stresses that occur at work or at home can be discovered through a detailed history, or by examining photographs of the individual at different activities.

Chronic compression of muscle can cause MTrPs to persist. Tight brassiere straps, tight collars, and compression of the hamstring muscles by a seat edge are examples of readily correctable causes of muscle compression.

Systemic Perpetuating Factors

Metabolic, endocrine, toxic, inflammatory, and other systemic disorders can stress muscle, and impair its ability to heal. The most common systemic factors that we encounter among persons with MPS are hypothyroidism, folic acid inadequacy and iron insufficiency. The relationship of these factors to persistent MPS seems clinically evident, but has not been established by statistically rigorous studies. Among systemic illnesses, fibromyalgia deserves special mention because it causes widespread muscle discomfort, and may be confused with MPS.

Subclinical or marginal *hypothyroidism* (3) is often overlooked. Symptoms, which can be subtle, include widespread MTrPs, cold intolerance, fatigue, and constipation. Serum cholesterol can be elevated. Hyperactivity is a unexpected sign, caused by constant body movement in a attempt to generate heat. Muscle cramps, stiffness and pain occur as a result of muscle overactivity. The most useful test is the highly sensitive thyroid stimulating hormone assay. A level in the upper range of normal and a low or low normal T4 should lead to further investigation and consideration of a trial of thyroid hormone replacement therapy. Previously unresponsive MPS may improve when marginal hypothyroidism is corrected.

Nutritional inadequacy states must be considered in terms of optimum function of enzyme systems, rather than absolute deficiency states (4). Vitamins act as cofactors in different enzyme systems that may be functioning at different rates at any one time. The optimum level of a vitamin is that which permits maximum function for each enzyme for which it is an essential cofactor. The vitamin requirements therefore change with time and circumstances. The daily vitamin intake should thus support optimum function. The daily requirement is therefore affected by host factors such as smoking or by competitive inhibition from drugs.

The most common vitamin inadequacy in persons with MPS in my experience is that of *folic acid* (5). Persons with folic acid levels in the lower quartile of normal often feel cold, but tend to have a low cholesterol level in contrast to hypothyroidism. They have diarrhea, rather than constipation as seen in vitamin B12 inadequacy. The fast-twitch type 2 muscle fibers of the upper body are more likely to develop MTrPs. Headache, disturbed sleep and restless legs can be seen. Folate is present in food as reduced polyglutamates. The stable inactive, oxidized form pteroylglutamate used pharmacologically must be reduced to the active form tetrahydrofolate by dihydrofolate reductase. A vitamin B12 dependent enzyme transport system brings folate into bone marrow, where it can bind to a red cell surface membrane receptor. Measurement of serum folate, serum vitamin B12 and red blood cell folate gives the most complete assessment of folate status. Impairment of DNA synthesis by either vitamin B12 or folic acid deficiency leads to megaloblastic anemia. In persons with intrinsic factor deficiency parenteral B12 is administered. In persons with restricted intake of animal food products, vitamin B12 supplementation is essential, since it is available only from animal sources.

Iron inadequacy (6) is also frequently seen in persons with MPS, usually premenopausal women who have inadequate iron intake to replace menstrual blood loss. Persons chronically taking NSAIDs can also have microscopic gastrointestinal blood loss, leading to depletion of iron stores. Unusual fatigue, exercise-induced muscle cramps, and cold intolerance are characteristic symptoms. Tissue iron stores are best assayed by measuring serum ferritin levels. Iron is important in heme-enzyme functions such as the cytochrome-oxidase system essential for oxidative phosphorylation.

Many persons with MPS are cold or cold intolerant. Inadequate levels of thyroid hormone, folic acid or tissue iron (7) can be associated with this feeling. Iron is essential for the conversion of T4 to the active form of T3, which may be one link between these conditions.

Rheumatoid arthritis, gout, polymyalgia rheumatica, recurrent *Candida albicans* infections, other nutritional insufficiency states, and psychological stresses are among the many other medical conditions that may perpetuate MTrPs.

Fibromyalgia [FM] (8,9) causes generalized muscle pain, fatigue and an alpha-delta sleep disorder. Muscle involvement in FM is homogeneous, affecting muscles in all body areas uniformly. Muscle involvement in MPS is heterogeneous, affecting different muscle groups, and affecting muscle fibers differently within each muscle. MTrPs can occur in FM, creating an overlap condition. When this happens, the MTrPs are treated in the same manner as usual.

MTrP INACTIVATION

The specific treatment of MPS is the inactivation of the MTrP, most commonly by intermittent cold and stretch (10,11), and by TrP needling or injection.

Before initiating treatment, the patient must first be made comfortable and relaxed [Figure 2]. Functional scoliosis is corrected and arm and leg support is provided to prevent tension on the shoulder and hip muscles. The patient is often treated lying down to avoid postural hypotension which can accompany injection therapy.

Intermittent cold and stretch (1, Vol.1: 63-74) [Figure 3]. Vapocoolant spray or ice accompanied by stretch utilizes a tactile and thermal stimulus to inhibit spinal cord mediated reflex muscle contraction as muscle is

FIGURE 2. Positioning the patient in the lateral decubitus position in preparation for examination and treatment with either intermittent cold and spray or trigger point injections. Pillows are placed to support the head and the uppermost arm and leg. The room is kept warm and glare is avoided.

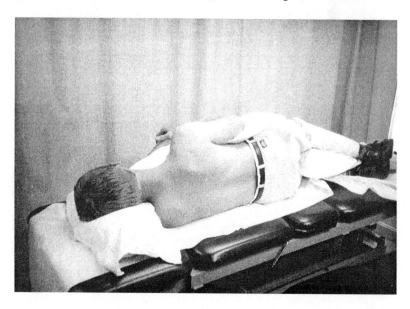

FIGURE 3. Intermittent cold and stretch. The vapocoolant used in this case is held about 40-50 cm from the muscle to be treated. The spray is applied at an acute angle to the skin, moving at 10 cm per second from the trigger point area over the muscle towards and over the zone of referred pain. Stretch is applied as the skin is sprayed. Moist heat is applied after the spray and stretch is completed, following which active and passive range of motion is performed to the part treated. X's mark common trigger point sites in the infraspinatus muscle. The arrows show the direction of spray over the muscle and into the zone of referred pain, including the arm and hand. The large short arrow shows the angle of application of the vapocoolant. The small short arrow indicates the stretch that is the essential action that inactivates the trigger point.

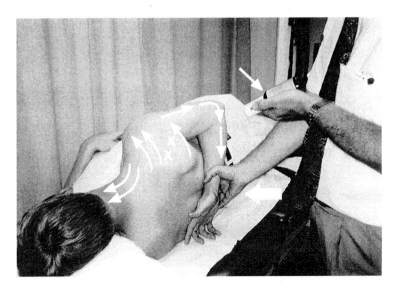

stretched. The combination of cold and the accompanying tactile stimulation produced by the fine jet spray or the touch of the ice produces a noxious stimulus which may excite the off-cells that suppress nociceptor transmission in the spinal cord. In this way, intermittent cold applied while stretching a muscle may inhibit a pain-initiated spasm or contraction. Stretching to the full length of the muscle is the essential action that inactivates the TrP. The cold stimulus is applied in parallel sweeps from the TrP over the functional muscle group to the zone of referred pain. There may be a diagnostic as well as therapeutic decrease in pain and increase in range of motion. Each muscle has a specific direction of action; the movement applied to stretch a muscle is opposite the muscle's direction of action. After stretching, the muscle is rewarmed with moist heat. This technique is particularly suitable for treating large areas of the body, when MTrPs involve many muscles.

Trigger point injection (1, Vol.1: 74-86) [Figure 4]. Dry needling a MTrP or injecting it with a local anesthetic is a highly effective way of inactivating a TrP. The procedure may act by disrupting the sarcolemmal membrane causing a change in intra- and extra-cellular calcium concentrations. Inactivation of the MTrP by injection is reversed by intravenous naloxone (12), suggesting that the procedure modifies the endogenous opioid system in the central nervous system. Dilute procaine is the preferred anesthetic (13), as it has low myotoxicity, a short half-life, and is metabolized peripherally by procaine esterase. An inadvertent nerve block is quite transient. Bacteriostatic saline can be used for those allergic to procaine.

The MTrP is located by palpation and fixed between the fingers. A 25 gauge needle is inserted at an oblique angle into the TrP. A local twitch response and transient pain may be elicited. Referred pain and transient

FIGURE 4. A and B. The needle is inserted obliquely through the skin after fixing the trigger point between the palpating fingers. Trigger points frequently occur in clusters, so that the muscle must be probed in a circular manner in order to identify and inactivate them all. The muscle is treated with intermittent spray and stretch after the injections are completed.

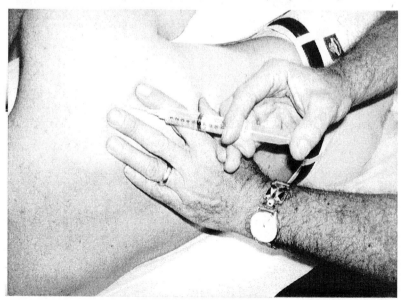

FIGURE 4 (continued)

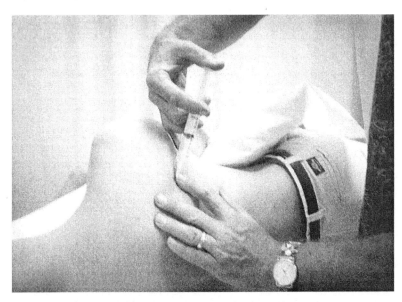

dysesthesia of short duration can be felt. MTrPs often occur in clusters and all must be treated. Satellite TrPs need to be treated either by injection or by stretch. Intermittent cold and stretch followed by moist heat is performed after the injections.

TrP injection is an invasive procedure with the risk of hemorrhage, pneumothorax, allergic reactions and vasodepressive syncope. Emergency care should be available in case of a complication. Failure of TrP injections to succeed can be due to injecting an inactive, not active, MTrP; to injecting the taut band, not the TrP; missing the TrPs in related muscles, to inadequate hemostasis, and to failure to actively stretch the muscle after injection.

Manual myofascial release techniques. In addition to ultrasound and electrical stimulation, other manual techniques have been effective in inactivating the TrP. Ischemic compression of a MTrP for 30-60 seconds can relax a TrP, presumably by depriving the muscle of oxygen and glucose through compression of capillary vessels. Rhythmic percussion of the TrP at about 2 second intervals will often inactivate a TrP, the percussion acting as a counterirritant in a manner similar to electrical stimulation or the application of heat or cold, possibly stimulating endorphin production or activating the off-cells that suppress nociceptive transmission centrally. Post-isometric relaxation (14), isometrically contracting a stretched muscle against resistance, relaxing it and then stretching it can be taught to the patient. Rhythmic stabilization utilizing reciprocal inhibition through alternating contraction of agonist and antagonist muscles against resistance will gradually lengthen muscle and increase range of motion. Other techniques such as friction massage can be effective in skilled hands.

Drug therapy. There is no specific drug therapy for MPS. Sleep disturbance can be corrected pharmacologically. Analgesia may be provided by aspirin, acetaminophen or by NSAIDs. Use of tricylic antidepressants are well established in management of chronic pain states, and can also help lessen insomnia.

Finally, the patient must be taught to recognize those activities that aggravate the pain, and to understand the distribution of pain from affected muscles. Corrective activities must be learned, and a home exercise program is prescribed to first stretch and then strengthen muscle. When muscle is injured, the body learns adaptive, protective behavior. Psychological reeducation and muscle conditioning is essential for long term recovery.

REFERENCES

1. Travell JG, Simons DG: Myofascial Pain and Dysfunction: The Trigger Point Manual. Williams & Wilkins, Baltimore, volume 1, 1983; volume 2, 1992.

2. Morton DJ: The Human Foot. Columbia University Press, New York, 1935.

3. Cooper DS: Subclinical hypothyroidism. JAMA 258: 246-247, 1987. (Editorial)

4. Levine M, Hartzell W: Ascorbic acid: the concept of optimum requirements. Third Conference on Vitamin C. Annals NY Acad Sci 498: 424-444, 1987.

5. Herbert VD, Colman N: Folic acid and vitamin B12. Modern Nutrition in Health and Disease, ed 7. Edited by ME Shils and BR Young. Lea and Febiger, Philadelphia, 1988, pp. 388-416.

6. Dallman PR: Biochemical basis for the manifestations of iron deficiency. Annu Rev Nutr 6: 13-40, 1986.

7. Beard J, Borel M: Iron deficiency and thermoregulation. Nutrition Today 23: 41-45, 1988.

8. Bennett R: Myofascial pain syndromes and the fibromyalgia syndrome: a comparative analysis. Myofascial Pain and Fibromyalgia. Edited by JR Fricton and EA Awad. Raven Press, New York, 1990, pp. 43-66.

9. Boissevain MD, McCain GA: Toward an integrated understanding of the fibromyalgia syndrome. I. medical and pathophysiological aspects. II. psychological and phenomenological aspects. Pain 45: 227-248.

10. Mennell JM: Spray and stretch for the relief of pain from muscle spasm and myofascial trigger points. J Am Podiatry Assoc 66: 873-876, 1976.

11. Nielson AJ: Spray and stretch for myofascial pain. Physical Therapy 58: 567-569, 1983.

12. Fine PG, Milano R, Hare BD: The effects of myofascial trigger point injections are naloxone reversible. Pain 32: 15-20, 1988.

13. Benoit PW, Belt WD: Some effects of local anesthetic agents on skeletal muscle. Exp Neurol 34: 264-278, 1972.

14. Lewit K, Simons DG: Myofascial pain: relief by post isometric relaxation. Arch Phys Med Rehabil 65: 452-456, 1984.

The Origin of Myopain:
An Integrated Hypothesis of Focal Muscle Changes and Sleep Disturbance in Patients with the Fibromyalgia Syndrome

Robert M. Bennett

SUMMARY. Objectives: Current ideas regarding the pathogenesis of the fibromyalgia syndrome espouse 2 major theories, the central and the peripheral. Herein a review of both theories is presented and an attempt made to integrate several apparently unrelated observations into a coherent hypothesis.

Results: The peripheral component of musculo-skeletal in fibromyalgia is generally considered to arise in muscle. However no *global* muscle defect has ever been demonstrated. On the other hand several studies have suggested *focal* muscle changes in terms of: reduced high energy phosphates, scattered red-ragged fibers, focal changes in oxygen tension and repetitive "contraction bands." These changes may result from muscle micro-trauma [MMT]–a universal experience after unaccustomed exercise. MMT causes a disruption of the sarcolemmal membrane leading to an influx of Ca^{++}

Robert M. Bennett, MD, FRCP, FACP, is Professor of Medicine and Chairman, Division of Arthritis and Rheumatic Diseases, Oregon Health Sciences University, Portland, OR, USA.

Address correspondence to: Prof. Robert M. Bennett, Dept. Medicine [L329A], Oregon Health Sciences University, 3181 SW Sam Jackson Park Road, Portland, OR 97201 USA.

[Haworth co-indexing entry note]: "The Origin of Myopain: An Integrated Hypothesis of Focal Muscle Changes and Sleep Disturbance in Patients with the Fibromyalgia Syndrome." Bennett, Robert M. Co-published simultaneously in the *Journal of Musculoskeletal Pain* (The Haworth Press, Inc.) Vol. 1, No. 3/4, 1993, pp. 95-112; and: *Musculoskeletal Pain, Myofascial Pain Syndrome, and the Fibromyalgia Syndrome* (ed: Søren Jacobsen, Bente Danneskiold-Samsøe, and Birger Lund) The Haworth Press, Inc., 1993, pp. 95-112. Multiple copies of this article/chapter may be purchased from The Haworth Document Delivery Center [1-800-3-HAWORTH; 9:00 a.m. - 5:00 p.m. (EST)].

ions and contraction of the involved units–the cause of the palpable band? ATP dependent Ca^{++} pumps attempt to correct the influx and in the process deplete sarcolemmal stores of high energy phosphates. Involvement of muscle spindles in the vicinity of sarcomeric contraction would reset muscle tension, giving rise to a sensation of stiffness. It is envisaged that there is a genetic polymorphism in susceptibility to MMT, and that fibromyalgia patients are at one extreme end of the curve. Most susceptible individuals will not develop fibromyalgia unless they also develop the alpha-delta sleep anomaly. This is an acquired central defect which may provide a "double-hit" in the form of impaired growth hormone [GH] secretion–seen clinically as low levels of somatomedin-C. GH is essential for normal muscle homeostasis and repair of MMT. As GH is produced during stage 4 sleep, its impaired secretion may be the link between sleep and myopain.

Conclusions: An analysis of contemporary research suggests that myopain in fibromyalgia may result from a convergence of both a peripheral factor–an increased susceptibility to muscle micro-trauma, and a central factor–the suboptimal secretion of growth hormone secondary to the alpha-delta sleep anomaly.

KEYWORDS. Fibromyalgia, muscle micro-trauma, growth hormone, sleep disturbance

The American College of Rheumatology guidelines for diagnosing fibromyalgia emphasizes a widespread musculoskeletal pain and the presence of widespread tender points (1). However it is quite evident that fibromyalgia is a much more complex problem than trying to understand muscle pain (2-4). Indeed, the very presence of multiple poorly defined symptoms often lacking a well defined pathophysiology has invited the diagnosis of a somatoform disorder (5). According to the Diagnostic and Statistical Manual for Mental Disorders [DSM IIIR], this diagnosis is based upon symptoms suggesting a physical disorder [hence, somatoform] for which there are no demonstrable organic findings or physiological mechanisms (6). Further there should be a strong presumption, that the symptoms are linked to psychological factors or conflicts. Unlike factitious disorder or malingering, the symptom production in somatoform disorders is not intentional, i.e., the patient does not experience a sense of controlling the production of the symptoms. In other words, although the symptoms are "physical," in the absence of a generally agreed upon pathophysiological arrangements, the symptoms are most readily conceptualized by means of psychological constructs. On the other hand, if well defined pathophysiological aberrations can be demonstrated to account for symptomatology, the notion of a somatoform disorder becomes invalid. With these thoughts in mind, a review of contemporary fibromyalgia studies is provided, and an attempt made to integrate the peripheral and central mechanisms into a plausible hypothesis.

CENTRAL MECHANISMS

There has been a profusion of studies which have explored psychological factors, neurotransmitters, neuroendocrine axis aberrations and sleep disturbance.

Contemporary Psychological Studies

The concept that stress is all pervasive in the workplace and in the home is a popular topic of everyday conversation and numerous magazine articles. It is well accepted in the lay mind that stress may be associated with problems such as headache, fatigue, peptic ulceration, lack of concentration, altered bowel function and heart attacks. The majority of fibromyalgia patients readily acknowledge that their symptomatology is often worsened by stress. Robbins et al. compared fibromyalgia patients with rheumatoid arthritis patients and noted that symptomatology and disability was largely determined by the patients worry about having a serious disease (5). The notion that worrying about illness was found to be strongly correlated with physical disability in fibromyalgia patients was used to support the hypothesis of a significant cognitive component to disability in this condition. The alternative concept, that fibromyalgia may exacerbate an inability to deal with stress, due to fatigue and pain has not been studied. Birnie et al. examined psychological aspects of 36 patients with fibromyalgia and compared them to 99 patients with chronic pain [39% low back, 48% lower extremities, 35% neck and shoulder] and 34 people with no pain (7). Interestingly, there was no significant difference between fibromyalgia patients and chronic pain patients with the exception of somatization on the Symptom Checklist 90R questionnaire. It was concluded that many of the psychological aspects of fibromyalgia are the psychological sequelae of chronic pain. Such an interpretation may be the result of studying patients from a tertiary referral setting–with a resultant bias towards more severely involved and long standing disease. A study comparing 35 fibromyalgia patients with 33 rheumatoid patients and 31 patients without pain, using a Diagnostic Interview Schedule, found no differences in the lifetime history of any psychiatric disorder (8). However, fibromyalgia patients had an elevation on the somatization scale which correlated with a history of psychiatric disorder. The reporting of multiple symptoms by fibromyalgia patients which would fit the current DSM III diagnosis of undifferentiated somatoform disorder has been difficult to explain without evoking a psychological mechanism. Hudson and Tate have recently proposed that fibromyalgia belongs to a family disorders with a common pathophysiology, which they call the "affective spectrum disorder" (9). The other conditions encompassed by this diagnosis include panic disorder, depression, obsessive/compulsive disorder, attention deficit disorder, bulimia nervosa, migraine and irritable bowel syndrome. The justification for placing these conditions into one diagnostic category is based on the common denominators of: 1. an association with depression, 2. a high comorbidity with one another 3. a tendency to familial aggregation and 4. a beneficial response to antidepressants. These ideas are not universally accepted and must be interpreted in the light of widely differing reports on the extent of depression in fibromyalgia and equivocal results with the dexamethasone suppression test (10-12).

Sleep and the Neuroendocrine Axis

The seminal observations of Moldofsky et al. that fibromyalgia patients have an abnormality of stage 4 sleep in the form of an alpha-delta rhythm has been a major stimulus for the scientific study of this syndrome (13). The intriguing follow up study in which a transient fibromyalgia-like state was induced by disturbing stage 4 sleep in healthy volunteers has never been repeated or refuted (14). Thus nearly two decades later, it is still not known whether the sleep disturbance is primary [as suggested by Moldofsky's second study] or secondary–i.e., the pain and other distractions of having fibromyalgia compromise restorative sleep. Irrespective of these considerations, virtually all fibromyalgia patients complain of non-restorative sleep and it has been assumed that this is due to the alpha-delta sleep anomaly. More recently there has been some interest in the idea that the disturbed sleep may affect the neuroendocrine axis. McCain reported that fibromyalgia patients had less variations between peak and trough values of plasma cortisol levels compared to rheumatoid arthritis patients (10). Ferraccioli et al. noted a hyperprolactinemic response [10 times basal value] after stimulation with thyrotropin releasing hormone in 33% of 24 fibromyalgia patients (15). In another recent study Neeck et al. reported a suboptimal response of TSH/thyroid hormones and a hyperprolactinemic response to thyrotropin releasing hormone (16)–as also noted by Ferraccioli. Bennett et al. have recently reported significantly lower levels of somatomedin-C in the serum of fibromyalgia patients compared to healthy controls (17). Somatomedin-C is produced by the liver in response to the pulsatile secretion of growth hormone and is the major mediator of growth hormone's anabolic actions. In particular, it has important effects on muscle homeostasis and its stimulation by the provision of exogenous growth hormone has been shown to have remarkable effects on muscle mass and function in middle aged and elderly men (18-20). Approximately 80% of growth hormone is produced during stage 4 sleep (21) and thus one might expect its secretion to be abnormal in patients with the alpha-delta sleep anomaly.

Neurotransmitters

A central tenant of the somatization concept is that patients overreact to normal bodily sensations. Although most studies have stressed that fibro-myalgia patients are more tender over the so-called tender points compared to control points, there is some evidence that when compared to healthy normals they are somewhat more tender over control points albeit to a lesser degree than the tender points (1,22,23). Moldofsky was the first to suggest that abnormalities of serotonin metabolism may be relevant to understanding of fibromyalgia syndrome. In a preliminary study he reported that there was a weak but definite association of symptomatology with low levels of plasma tryptophan (24). Tryptophan is the precursor of serotonin which is now known to be an important neurotransmitter involved in an inhibitory pathways modulating pain, as well as pathways involved in stage 4 sleep. In a recent study, Yunus et al. noted normal levels of plasma tryptophan in fibromyalgia compared to healthy controls but found a significantly reduced transport ratio of tryptophan in fibromy-algia (25)–[the transport ratio is the molar concentration of tryptophan divided by the sum of molar concentrations of other plasma aminoacids]. On the other hand, Russell et al. reported lower concentrations of serum tryptophan, as well as 9 other aminoacids, in 20 fibromyalgia patients compared to 20 matched controls (26). Interestingly, Russell has also noted an up regulation of 3H-imipramine binding to platelets in fibromyal-gia patients (27). As imipramine binds specifically to platelet serotonin receptors an increased density of receptors would be expected as a normal physiological response to low tryptophan levels. A metabolic product of brain tryptophan metabolism 5-hydroxy-indoleacetic acid [5-HIAA] has been shown to be lower in the CSF of fibromyalgia patients compared to controls (28,29); supporting the notion that there may be a central deficit of serotonin. Vaeroy et al. have found high levels of substance P in the CSF of fibromyalgia patients compared to healthy controls and other chronic pain patients (30). Although it wasn't clear from the paper whether the measurements in the healthy controls and chronic pain patients were taken from the literature or the result of parallel assays.

PERIPHERAL MECHANISMS

If fibromyalgia is not a somatization disorder, one would expect unequivocal evidence that there is a peripheral component to the pain experienced by patients. The general perception of most patients with fibromyalgia is that their pain is arising from muscles. However, some patients describe pain and even swelling of their joints [however the swelling is never verified by competent rheumatologists and technetium joint scans have been negative (31)]. Some fibromyalgia patients seem to have unduly sensitive skin; this may be another tissue that provides a nociceptive component to fibromyalgia pain.

Tender Points

Probably the most compelling evidence for a peripheral nociceptive component to fibromyalgia pain comes from the observation of increased tenderness over specific locations (1,32-35). In general, these locations correspond to the insertion of muscles into ligaments or bone and are hence at a location where muscular force is transmitted through a small cross sectional area; this is a common site for both minor and major muscle tears. Tender areas often have an increased consistency, compared to surrounding muscle–the so-called palpable band or fibrositic nodule. Sometimes pressure over one of these areas causes referred pain in a distal distribution; in which case, it is often referred to as a trigger point. It should also be noted that asymptomatic but tender areas in the muscle may be found in apparently healthy individuals as evidenced by the study of Sola who found tender areas in 54% of women and 45% of male Air Force recruits (36). Such asymptomatic tender points have been referred to as "latent trigger points" (37). A complete understanding of the peripheral component of pain in fibromyalgia will have to encompass all of these observations.

Nociceptive Pain

There is a rich innervation of skeletal muscle; pain sensitive end organs have been shown to relay their impulses through unmyelinated type C fibers. Blockage of this impulse either in the periphery or at the level of the spinal cord should lead to a significant reduction of pain. The injection of tender points and trigger points with a local anesthetic has enjoyed wide success as a palliative treatment in the patients with myofascial pain syndrome (37-39). The very fact that one can inject a tender area with a local anesthetic causes significant reduction in pain is compelling evidence that there is a peripheral component to the musculoskeletal pain in these patients. It seems unlikely that this is a placebo response or "an attempt to please reaction" as these injections are painful; one cannot imagine many patients returning for repeat injections in the absence of a worthwhile effect. An attempt to block the pain impulse in fibromyalgia patients at the level of the spinal cord was reported by Bengtsson et al. using an epidural block (40). An almost complete disappearance of pain was noted with a local anesthetic and a significant reduction with opiods. The ability to modulate fibromyalgia pain both at the level of pain nociceptors and the level of the spinal cord provides powerful evidence there is a critical peripheral nociceptive component to fibromyalgia pain.

Muscle Histology, Biochemistry and Metabolism

The notion that fibromyalgia patients have a *generalized* abnormality of muscle, such as a metabolic myopathy, has not been supported by several studies (41-44). Exercise studies of fibromyalgia patients have shown that they reach an anaerobic threshold and achieve a reasonable workload (45): these findings are not consistent with a metabolic defect in the glycolytic, Krebs' or electron transport chain pathways (46). More recently, NMR studies at both resting and exercise muscle has failed to show any global defect in muscle metabolism. The changes that are seen in global muscle diseases such as polymyositis and muscular dystrophy–chronically increased levels of muscle enzymes and distinctive EMG findings–are not present in fibromyalgia patients (47,48). On the other hand, there is evidence that there may be a *focal* muscle defect in fibromyalgia patients. A seminal study in this regard was that of Bengtsson et al. who sampled the tender areas in the trapezius muscles of fibromyalgia patients (49). There was a 17% reduction in ATP and a 21% reduction of phosphoro-creatine compared to normals. Interestingly, an increase in ragged red fibers has also been noted by the same group in fibromyalgia tender points (42). Ragged red fibers are due to a proliferation of mitochondria and indicate metabolic distress. Similar findings have been noted in patients with a myofascial pain syndrome involving the shoulder girdle muscles (50); this suggests that tender points and trigger points share a similar pathophysiology. Jacobsen et al. have recently described repetitive transverse bands in individual muscle fibers taken from the quadriceps muscle of fibromyalgia patients (25). A blinded evaluation of the morphological feature gave a specificity of 71% and a sensitivity of 63% when applied to fibromyalgia patients in comparison to controls. Bartels et al. have described a similar rubber band morphology in an earlier study (51). It is possible that these bands could disrupt the capillary network to muscle, and Lund et al. have reported an asymmetric distribution of oxygen tension over the trapezius tender points (52). In another study of exercising muscle blood flow, fibromyalgia patients had reduced values compared to age, sex and fitness matched controls (45).

Connective Tissue Changes

There is some preliminary evidence that fibromyalgia patients have an increased prevalence of both hypermobility syndrome (53) and mitral valve prolapse (54). This may be an important clue to a possible genetic predisposition to the fibromyalgia syndrome as described by Pellegrino et al. (55). Jacobsen et al. have described low levels of procollagen type III amino terminal peptide in a subgroup of fibromyalgia patients with relentless disease characterized by a particularly severe sleep disturbance, numerous tender points and reduced muscle strength (55A). Interestingly the synthesis of this protein is closely linked to growth hormone production (56), hence Jacobsen's observations may be the end result of a severe alpha-delta sleep anomaly disrupting growth hormone secretion.

AN INTEGRATED HYPOTHESIS TO EXPLAIN MYOPAIN IN FIBROMYALGIA

A consideration of the studies described herein, makes it difficult to explain fibromyalgia symptomatology solely on the basis of somatization. One interpretation of the findings presented in the last two sections is that muscle pain in fibromyalgia results from *focal* areas of muscle micro-trauma (17,57-59)–referred to here as MMT. Muscle micro-trauma is a universal experience and its extent is related to the intensity and duration of exercise (60-63). It is more likely to occur at high loads during impact type exercises, particularly when eccentric muscle contractions are involved (64-67); although any part of a muscle may be involved, there is a predominance at muscle-tendon and muscle-bone junctions. It is hypothesized that muscle micro-trauma occurs in fibromyalgia patients at unusually low levels of exertion and that they are not repaired in an efficient manner. As fibromyalgia usually starts in child-bearing years, it is unlikely that there is a single genetic locus responsible for its initiation. More likely, a convergence of both *genetic* and *acquired* components will be required to generate the complete syndrome. It is common experience, that from a very early age some people have a greater athletic potential than others, and that some individuals hurt more than others after strenuous exercise. Based on this simple everyday observation, it is envisaged that there is a genetic susceptibility to muscle micro-trauma with the typical Gaussian distribution seen in polygenic inheritance [Figure 1]. If this notion is correct, one would expect to find quantitative and possibly qualitative differences in one or more proteins of the sarcolemmal membrane of fibromyalgia patients compared to athletic controls. One logical "candidate protein" would be the ATP dependent calcium transporters which are essential for maintaining the low levels of ionized calcium [10-7 M] that are found in resting muscle cells.

FIGURE 1. It is envisaged that there is a polygenic inheritance pattern for susceptibility to muscle microlesions [MMT]. People destined to develop fibromyalgia would be at one extreme end of the normal distribution curve—the "critical range." However, by itself, this genetic predisposition to MMT does not usually lead to the development of widespread muscle pain unless some acquired factors emerge. This "double-hit" theory is thought to be the basis of many diseases which have a non-dominant genetic background.

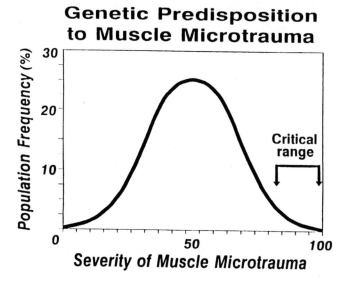

Physiological muscle contraction proceeds via excitation–contraction–coupling; every sarcomere of a muscle fiber contracts synchronously as a result of neurally induced calcium release from the sarcoplasmic reticulum–Figure 2. Sarcolemmal injury leads to an influx of calcium ions from extra-cellular fluid [concentration 10-3 M] which in turn causes *non-physiological* contraction of the involved sarcomeres (68,69). It is hypothesized that the focal contraction of several contiguous sarcomeres will lead to the band like appearance described by Bartels and Jacobsen (25,51); see Figure 3. The focal contraction could account for the indurated areas of muscle commonly found in association with tender points and trigger points. Such focal contractions of muscle would cause a functional shortening of the muscle fiber which could account for the reduced range of motion which is often seen in fibromyalgia patients. If the involved area encompassed muscle spindles, the dynamic tension of the muscle would be reset, thus accounting for the common symptom of muscle stiffness. The intriguing finding of increased EMG activity during the short pauses necessary for efficient dynamic exercise (70) may also result from focal sarcomeric contractions involving muscle spindles. Furthermore, the influx of calcium ions activates a calcium sensitive protease and phospholi-

FIGURE 2. Physiological muscle contraction proceeds via excitation–contraction–coupling; *every* sarcomere of a muscle fiber contracts synchronously as a result of neurally induced calcium release from the sarcoplasmic reticulum. This cause a 2 fold increase of Ca^{++} from 10^{-7} M to 10^{-5} M and the interaction of Ca^{++} with troponin C initiates the ATP dependent interdigitation of the actin and myosin filaments.

Excitation-Coupling Contraction

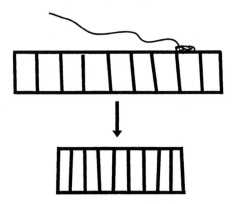

pase. This results in activation of the cyclo-oxygenase/lipoxygenase pathways and the production of free oxygen radicals from the peroxidation of free fatty acids (71). The resulting enzymatic attack on the sarcolemmal membrane perpetuates and amplifies the effects of the original injury–see Figure 4. The influx of ionized calcium into a sarcomere will lead to an overactivity of the ATP dependent calcium transporters in an effort to restore the milieu intérieur; this will result in a focal reduction in ATP, as found by Bengtsson et al. (49), as well as ragged red fibers (42)–as a reaction to metabolic distress.

The recent finding of low levels of somatomedin-C in fibromyalgia patients may represent an *acquired central* defect, as the growth hormone somatomedin-C axis is important in normal muscle homeostasis (17-20,72). Growth hormone is produced predominantly during stage 4 sleep (21,73,74), and thus this central defect may be the missing link between disturbed sleep and muscle pain. The other major stimulus for growth hormone secretion is exercise (75,76). Most fibromyalgia patients

FIGURE 3. This depicts the injury of 4 contiguous sarcomeres. The resultant influx of calcium from the extra-cellular fluid [Ca^{++} 10^{-3}] causes a non-physiological contraction of the involved sarcomeres. A microscopic appearance similar to this "contraction band" has been described by Jacobsen et al. in muscle biopsies from fibromyalgia patients [see reference #25].

Injury induced Contraction

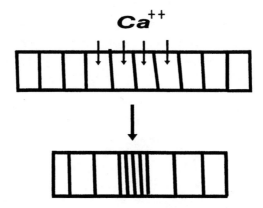

FIGURE 4. Not only does an influx of Ca^{++} ions cause non-physiological contraction, it also results in a calcium dependent activation of a protease and phospholipase. The protease will directly result in further damage to the sarcolemmal membrane and intra-cellular structures. Phospholipase liberates free fatty acids [FFA] from the sarcolemmal membrane which in turn leads to the production of free oxygen radicals–these are extremely toxic and further catalyze the peroxidation of FFA. In this schema sarcolemmal injury becomes a self amplifying process. The mechanisms responsible for minimizing this damage and effecting eventual repair are not well characterized.

Calcium activated muscle damage

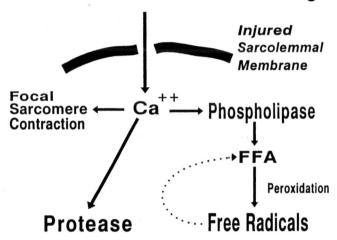

have a reduced exercise capacity (45), and this may further exacerbate suboptimal GH production. Muscle deconditioning is known to increase the susceptibility to muscle micro-trauma; and this may represent another *acquired* component to the syndrome. Some of these ideas are depicted in Figure 5.

Regarding other central mechanisms, contemporary evidence suggests that abnormalities of tryptophan metabolism may be relevant to the sleep disturbance as well as enhancing the experience of peripheral nociceptive pain (77). In this respect, it is important to note that serotoninergic pathways have been implicated in both the descending pathways inhibiting peripheral pain appreciation and in the complex pathways involved in the generation of the sleep. One of the intriguing aspects of the fibromyalgia syndrome is the apparent diverse nature of its initiating stimuli. Whether it

FIGURE 5. It is hypothesized that myopain in fibromyalgia patients results from the effects of muscle micro-trauma [MMT] as depicted in other figures. A "double-hit" may be required to initiate the syndrome—both a genetic predisposition to MMT and defective repair mechanisms, such as defective growth hormone [GH] production. Another acquired factor in some patients may be chronic deconditioning which further enhances proneness to MMT, as well as removing a stimulus for GH secretion. The alph-delta sleep anomaly is thought to have many potential triggers—not shown here. Central mechanisms are thought to enhance the perception of pain and drive the sleep anomaly.

An integrated hypothesis

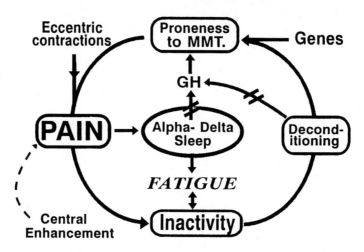

be set off by physical lesions (78) or an infectious agent (79,80), once the switch is activated it remains in the "on" position—long after the initial stimulus is past. To discover the biochemical correlates of this "switch" will be the holy grail of fibromyalgia researchers in the next decade.

REFERENCES

1. Wolfe F, Smythe HA, Yunus MB, Bennett RM, Bombardier C, Goldenberg DL, Tugwell P, Campbell SM, Abeles M, Clark P, Fam AG, Farber SJ, Fiechtner JJ, Franklin CM, Gatter RA, Hamaty D, Lessard J, Lichtbroun AS, Masi AT, McCain GA, Reynolds WJ, Romano TJ, Russell IJ, Sheon RP: The American College of Rheumatology 1990 criteria for the classification of fibromyalgia: Report of the Multicenter Criteria Committee. Arthritis Rheum 33:160-172, 1990.

2. Goldenberg DL: Fibromyalgia syndrome. An emerging but controversial condition. JAMA 257:2782-2787, 1987.

3. Yunus MB, Masi AT, Aldag JC: A controlled study of primary fibromyalgia syndrome: clinical features and association with other functional syndromes. J Rheumatol Suppl 19:62-71, 1989.

4. Bennett RM: Confounding features of the fibromyalgia syndrome: A current perspective of differential diagnosis. J Rheumatol 16 Suppl. 19:58-61, 1989.

5. Robbins JM, Kirmayer LJ, Kapusta MA: Illness worry and disability in fibromyalgia syndrome. Int J Psychiatry Med 20:49-63, 1990.

6. Diagnostic and statistical manual of mental disorders. 3rd edition. Washington, D.C., American Psychiatric Association, 1987.

7. Birnie DJ, Knipping AA, van Rijswijk MH, de Blécourt AC, de Voogd N: Psychological aspects of fibromyalgia compared with chronic and nonchronic pain. J Rheumatol 18:1845-1848, 1991.

8. Ahles TA, Khan SA, Yunus MB, Spiegel DA, Masi AT: Psychiatric status of patients with primary fibromyalgia, patients with rheumatoid arthritis, and subjects without pain: a blind comparison of DSM-III diagnoses. Am J Psychiatry 148:1721-1726, 1991.

9. Hudson JI, Pope HG,Jr.: Fibromyalgia and psychopathology: Is fibromyalgia a form of "affective spectrum disorder?" J Rheumatol 16 Suppl. 19:15-22, 1989.

10. McCain GA, Tilbe KS: Diurnal hormone variation in fibromyalgia syndrome: a comparison with rheumatoid arthritis. J Rheumatol Suppl 19:154-157, 1989.

11. Hudson JI, Pliner LF, Hudson MS, Goldenberg DL, Melby JC: The dexamethasone suppression test in fibrositis. Biol Psychiatry 19:1489-1493, 1984.

12. Goldenberg DL: Psychiatric and psychologic aspects of fibromyalgia syndrome. Rheum Dis Clin North Am 15:105-114, 1989.

13. Moldofsky H: Sleep and fibrositis syndrome. Rheum Dis Clin North Am 15:91-103, 1989.

14. Moldofsky H, Scarisbrick P: Induction of neurasthenic musculoskeletal pain syndrome by selective sleep stage deprivation. Psychosom Med 38:35-44, 1976.

15. Ferraccioli G, Cavalieri F, Salaffi F, Fontana S, Scita F, Nolli M, Maestri D: Neuroendocrinologic findings in primary fibromyalgia (soft tissue chronic pain syndrome) and in other chronic rheumatic conditions (rheumatoid arthritis, low back pain). J Rheumatol 17:869-873, 1990.

16. Neeck G, Riedel W: Thyroid function in patients with fibromyalgia syndrome. J Rheumatol 19:1120-2, 1992.

17. Bennett RM, Clark SR, Campbell SM, Burckhardt CS: Low levels of somatomedin-C in patients with the fibromyalgia syndrome: A possible link between sleep and muscle pain. Arth Rheum 35:1113-1116, 1992.

18. Crist DM, Peake GT, Loftfield RB, Kraner JC, Egan PA: Supplemental growth hormone alters body composition, muscle protein metabolism and serum

lipids in fit adults: characterization of dose-dependent and response-recovery effects. Mechanisms of Ageing and Development 58:191-205, 1991.

19. Fryburg DA, Louard RJ, Gerow KE, Gelfand RA, Barrett EJ: Growth hormone stimulates skeletal muscle protein synthesis and antagonizes insulin's antiproteolytic action in humans. Diabetes 41:424-429, 1992.

20. Yarasheski KE, Campbell JA, Smith K, Rennie MJ, Holloszy JO, Bier DM: Effect of growth hormone and resistance exercise on muscle growth in young men. Am J Physiol Endocrinol Metab 262:E261-E267, 1992.

21. Holl RW, Hartman ML, Veldhuis JD, Taylor WM, Thorner MO: Thirty-second sampling of plasma growth hormone in man: correlation with sleep stages. J Clin Endocrinol Metab 72:854-861, 1991.

22. Scudds RA, Rollman GB, Harth M, McCain GA: Pain perception and personality measures as discriminators in the classification of fibrositis. J Rheumatol 14:563-569, 1987.

23. Quimby LG, Block SR, Gratwick GM: Fibromyalgia: generalized pain intolerance and manifold symptom reporting. J Rheumatol 15:1264-1270, 1988.

24. Moldofsky H, Warsh JJ: Plasma tryptophan and musculoskeletal pain in non-articular rheumatism ("fibrositis syndrome"). Pain 5:65-71, 1978.

25. Jacobsen S, Bartels EM, Danneskiold-Samsøe B: Single cell morphology of muscle in patients with chronic muscle pain. Scand J Rheumatol 20:336-343, 1991.

26. Russell IJ, Michalek JE, Vipraio GA, Fletcher EM, Wall K: Serum amino acids in fibrositis/fibromyalgia syndrome. J Rheumatol 16 Suppl. 19:158-163, 1989.

27. Yunus MB, Dailey JW, Aldag JC, Masi AT, Jobe PC: Plasma tryptophan and other amino acids in primary fibromyalgia: a controlled study. J Rheumatol 19:90-94, 1992.

28. Houvenagel E, Forzy G, Cortet B, Vincent G: 5-Hydroxy indol acetic acid in cerebro spinal fluid in fibromyalgia. Arth Rheum 33:S55, 1990.

29. Russell IJ, Vaeroy H, Javors M, Nyberg F: Cerebrospinal fluid biogenic amine metabolites in fibromyalgia/fibrositis syndrome and rheumatoid arthritis. Arthritis Rheum 35:550-556, 1992.

30. Vaeroy H, Helle R, Forre O, Kass E, Terenius L: Elevated CSF levels of substance P and high incidence of Raynaud phenomenon in patients with fibromyalgia: new features for diagnosis. Pain 32:21-26, 1988.

31. Yunus MB, Berg BC, Masi AT: Multiphase skeletal scintigraphy in primary fibromyalgia syndrome: A blinded study. J Rheumatol 16:1466-1468, 1989.

32. Smythe HA, Moldofsky H: Two contributions to understanding of the "fibrositis" syndrome. Bull Rheum Dis 28:928-931, 1977.

33. Yunus M, Masi AT, Calabro JJ, Miller KA, Feigenbaum SL: Primary fibromyalgia (fibrositis): clinical study of 50 patients with matched normal controls. Semin Arthritis Rheum 11:151-171, 1981.

34. Wolfe F, Cathey MA: Prevalence of primary and secondary fibrositis. J Rheumatol 10:965-968, 1983.

35. Campbell SM, Clark S, Tindall EA, Forehand ME, Bennett RM: Clinical characteristics of fibrositis. 1. A "blinded," controlled study of symptoms and tender points. Arthritis Rheum 26:817-824, 1983.

36. Sola AE, Rodenberger ML, Gettys BB: Incidence of hypersensitive areas in posterior shoulder muscles. Am J Phys Med 34:585, 1955.

37. Travell JG, Simons DG: Myofascial pain and dysfunction: the trigger point manual. Baltimore, Williams & Wilkins, 1983.

38. Sheon RP, Moskowitz RW, Goldberg VM: Intralesional soft tissue injection technique, Soft Tissue Rheumatic Pain: Recognition, Management, Prevention. Philadelphia, Lea & Febiger, 1987 p. 293.

39. Bennett RM: Nonarticular rheumatism and spondyloarthropathies. Similarities and differences. Postgrad Med 87:97-9, 102-4, 1990.

40. Bengtsson M, Bengtsson A, Jorfeldt L: Diagnostic epidural opioid blockade in primary fibromyalgia at rest and during exercise. Pain 39:171-180, 1989.

41. Yunus MB, Kalyan-Raman UP: Muscle biopsy findings in primary fibromyalgia and other forms of nonarticular rheumatism. Rheum Dis Clin North Am 15:115-134, 1989.

42. Bengtsson A, Henriksson KG, Larsson J: Muscle biopsy in primary fibromyalgia. Light-microscopical and histochemical findings. Scand J Rheumatol 15:1-6, 1986.

43. Yunus MD, Kalyan-Raman UP, Masi AT, Aldag JC: Electromicroscopic studies of muscle biopsy in primary fibromyalgia syndrome: a controlled and blinded study. J Rheumatol 16:97-101, 1989.

44. Jacobsen S, Wildschiodtz G, Danneskiold-Samsøe B: Isokinetic and isometric muscle strength combined with transcutaneous electrical muscle stimulation in primary fibromyalgia syndrome. Journal of Rheumatology 18:1390-1393, 1991.

45. Bennett RM, Clark SR, Goldberg L, Nelson D, Bonafede RP, Porter J, Specht D: Aerobic fitness in patients with fibrositis. A controlled study of respiratory gas exchange and 133xenon clearance from exercising muscle. Arthritis Rheum 32:454-460, 1989.

46. Bennett RM: Physical fitness and muscle metabolism in the fibromyalgia syndrome: an overview. J Rheumatol Suppl 19:28-29, 1989.

47. Kraft GH, Johnson EW, LaBan MM: The fibrositis syndrome. Arch Phys Med Rehabil 49:155-162, 1968.

48. Zidar J, Bäckman E, Bengtsson A, Henriksson KG: Quantitative EMG and muscle tension in painful muscles in fibromyalgia. Pain 40:249-254, 1990.

49. Bengtsson A, Henriksson KG, Larsson J: Reduced high-energy phosphate levels in the painful muscles of patients with primary fibromyalgia. Arthritis Rheum 29:817-821, 1986.

50. Larsson SE, Bengtsson A, Bodegard L, Henriksson KG, Larsson J: Muscle changes in work-related chronic myalgia. Acta Orthop Scand 59:74-78, 1988.

51. Bartels EM, Danneskiold Samsøe B: Histological abnormalities in muscle from patients with certain types of fibrositis. Lancet 1:755-757, 1986.

52. Lund N, Bengtsson A, Thorborg P: Muscle tissue oxygen pressure in primary fibromyalgia. Scand J Rheumatol 15:165-173, 1986.

53. Goldman JA: Hypermobility and deconditioning: important links to fibromyalgia/fibrositis. South Med J 84:1192-1196, 1991.

54. Pellegrino MJ, Van Fossen D, Gordon C, Ryan JM, Waylonis GW: Prevalence of mitral valve prolapse in primary fibromyalgia: a pilot investigation. Arch Phys Med Rehabil 70:541-543, 1989.

55. Pellegrino MJ, Waylonis GW, Sommer A: Familial occurrence of primary fibromyalgia. Arch Phys Med Rehabil 70:61-63, 1989.

55A. Jacobsen S, Jensen LT, Foldager M, Danneskiold-Samsøe B: Primary fibromyalgia: clinical parameters in relation to serum procollagen type III aminoterminal peptide: Br J Rheumatol 29:174-177, 1990.

56. Jensen LT, Jorgensen OL, Risteli J, Christiansen JS, Lorenzen I: Type I and III procollagen in growth hormone-deficient patients: effects of increasing doses of GH. Acta Endocrinol 124:278-282, 1991.

57. Bennett RM: Etiology of the fibromyalgia syndrome: a contemporary hypothesis. Internal Medicine for the Specialist 11:48-61, 1990.

58. Bennett RM: Muscle physiology and cold reactivity in the fibromyalgia syndrome. Rheum Dis Clin North Am 15:135-147, 1989.

59. Bennett RM: Beyond fibromyalgia: ideas on etiology and treatment. J Rheumatol Suppl 19:185-191, 1989.

60. Edwards RHT: Hypotheses of peripheral and central mechanisms underlying occupational muscle pain and injury. Eur J Appl Physiol 57:275-281, 1988.

61. Newham DJ, McPhail G, Mills KR, Edwards RH: Ultrastructural changes after concentric and eccentric contractions of human muscle. J Neurol Sci 61:109-122, 1983.

62. Friden J, Kjorell U, Thornell LE: Delayed muscle soreness and cytoskeletal alterations: an immunocytological study in man. Int J Sports Med 5:15-18, 1984.

63. Friden J: Muscle soreness after exercise: implications of morphological changes. Int J Sports Med 5:57-66, 1984.

64. Friden J, Sfakianos PN, Hargens AR: Muscle soreness and intramuscular fluid pressure: comparison between eccentric and concentric load. J Appl Physiol 61:2175-2179, 1986.

65. Friden J, Sfakianos PN, Hargens AR, Akeson WH: Residual muscular swelling after repetitive eccentric contractions. J Orthop Res 6:493-498, 1988.

66. Newham DJ: The consequences of eccentric contractions and their relationship to delayed onset muscle pain. Eur J Appl Physiol 57:353-359, 1988.

67. Newham DJ, Mills KR, Quigley BM, Edwards RH: Pain and fatigue after concentric and eccentric muscle contractions. Clin Sci 64:55-62, 1983.

68. Edwards RH, Newham DJ, Jones DA, Chapman SJ: Role of mechanical damage in pathogenesis of proximal myopathy in man. Lancet 1:548-552, 1984.

69. Duncan CJ: Role of intracellular calcium in promoting muscle damage: a strategy for controlling the dystrophic condition. Experientia 34:1531-1535, 1978.

70. Elert JE, Rantapää-Dahlqvist SB, Henriksson-Larsën K, Lorentzon R, Gerdlë BU: Muscle performance, electromyography and fibre type composition in fibromyalgia and work-related myalgia. Scand J Rheumatol 21:28-34, 1992.

71. Jackson MJ, Jones DA, Edwards RHT: Experimental skeletal muscle damage: the nature of the calcium-activated degenerative process. Eur J Clin Invest 14:369-374, 1984.

72. Cuneo RC, Salomon F, Wiles CM, Hesp R, Sonksen PH: Growth hormone treatment in growth hormone-deficient adults. II. Effects on exercise performance. J Appl Physiol 70:695-700, 1991.

73. McCain GA: Non-medicinal treatments in primary fibromyalgia. Rheum Dis Clin N Amer 15:73-90, 1989.

74. Holl RW, Hartman ML, Veldhuis JD, Taylor WM, Thorner MO: Thirty-second sampling of plasma growth hormone in man: Correlation with sleep stages. J Clin Endocrinol Metab 72:854-861, 1991.

75. Weltman A, Weltman JY, Schurrer R, Evans WS, Veldhuis JD, Rogol AD: Endurance training amplifies the pulsatile release of growth hormone: Effects of training intensity. J Appl Physiol 72:2188-2196, 1992.

76. De Vries JH, Noorda RJP, Voetberg GA, Van der Veen EA: Growth hormone release after the sequential use of growth hormone releasing factor and exercise. Horm Metab Res 23:397-398, 1991.

77. Russell IJ: Neurohormonal aspects of fibromyalgia syndrome. Rheum Dis Clin North Am 15:149-168, 1989.

78. Greenfield S, Fitzcharles MA, Esdaile JM: Reactive fibromyalgia syndrome. Arthritis Rheum 35:678-681, 1992.

79. Simms RW, Zerbini CA, Ferrante N, Anthony J, Felson DT, Craven DE: Fibromyalgia syndrome in patients infected with human immunodeficiency virus. The Boston City Hospital Clinical AIDS Team. Am J Med 92:368-374, 1992.

80. Leventhal LJ, Naides SJ, Freundlich B: Fibromyalgia and parvovirus infection. Arthritis Rheum 34:1319-1324, 1991.

EPIDEMIOLOGY AND NATURAL HISTORY–MYOFASCIAL PAIN AND FIBROMYALGIA

Review of the Epidemiology and Criteria of Fibromyalgia and Myofascial Pain Syndromes: Concepts of Illness in Populations as Applied to Dysfunctional Syndromes

Alfonse T. Masi

SUMMARY. Objectives: To review epidemiologic methodology and concepts in the study of fibromyalgia and myofascial pain syndromes. To identify studies of the prevalence and relative frequency of fibromyalgia and myofascial pain in community and clinic popu-

Alfonse T. Masi, MD, DR, PH, FACP, is Professor of Medicine, University of Illinois College of Medicine at Peoria [UICOM-P], One Illini Drive, Peoria, IL 61656.

[Haworth co-indexing entry note]: "Review of the Epidemiology and Criteria of Fibromyalgia and Myofascial Pain Syndromes: Concepts of Illness in Populations as Applied to Dysfunctional Syndromes." Masi, Alfonse T. Co-published simultaneously in the *Journal of Musculoskeletal Pain* (The Haworth Press, Inc.) Vol. 1, No. 3/4, 1993, pp. 113-136; and: *Musculoskeletal Pain, Myofascial Pain Syndrome, and the Fibromyalgia Syndrome* (ed: Søren Jacobsen, Bente Danneskiold-Samsøe, and Birger Lund) The Haworth Press, Inc., 1993, pp. 113-136. Multiple copies of this article/chapter may be purchased from The Haworth Document Delivery Center [1-800-3-HAWORTH; 9:00 a.m. - 5:00 p.m. (EST)].

lations. To compare etiologic mechanisms and concepts of classical diseases versus dysfunctional syndromes. To draw analogies between irritable bowel syndrome [IBS] and fibromyalgia syndrome [FMS] with respect to the rationale for patient subgrouping in order to achieve improved classification schema.

Findings: Prevalences of fibromyalgia in community populations differ widely, i.e., from about 1% to 10%. Differences may be due to variations in age, sex, occupation, socioeconomic status and other personal factors, but are more likely due to differences in criteria or other methodology used. The classical epidemiologic concept of agent, host and environmental causes of disease does not apply well to dysfunctional syndromes, e.g., FMS or myofascial pain syndrome [MPS]. These syndromes are more complex etiologically than the classical diseases, have multifactorial illness dynamics and considerable individualized variability.

Conclusions: Population surveys with standardized definitions [e.g., the 1990 American College of Rheumatology criteria for fibromyalgia] promise to identify important overall demographic and socio-environmental risk factors in FMS and MPS. However, more specific analytical studies of risk factors are also needed. These will require further patient subgroupings which can better reflect personalized illness dynamics. Improved conceptual models of dysfunctional disorders need to be developed. Integrated systems research approaches [e.g., force field analysis] can accommodate the complex host dynamics, i.e., somatic, emotional and behavioral mechanisms, and potential risk factors in the environment.

KEYWORDS. Fibromyalgia syndrome, myofascial pain syndrome, epidemiology, etiology, dysfunction

INTRODUCTION

Since the initial presentation in 1985, of concepts of illness in populations as applied to fibromyalgia syndromes, at the first North American symposium on the fibrositis/fibromyalgia syndrome (1), significant research has been accomplished. This review summarizes various aspects relevant to the epidemiology and criteria of fibromyalgia and myofascial pain syndromes. Emphasis is given to clinical-epidemiological issues which are central to the family of dysfunctional syndromes as opposed to the classical, "organic" diseases with defined tissue pathogenesis.

Literature was searched to identify studies of the prevalence in community populations and relative frequency in clinic patients of fibromyalgia and myofascial pain syndromes. Etiological and epidemiological characteristics of classical diseases and dysfunctional syndromes are compared. Analogies are drawn between irritable bowel syndrome [IBS] and fibromyalgia syndrome [FMS] with respect to the rationale for patient subgrouping in order to better define risk factors.

EPIDEMIOLOGIC PRINCIPLES

Epidemiologic methodology may be broadly categorized into descriptive, analytical and interventional or other types of research, including classification and course of illness [Table 1]. The accurate definition of an illness and correct formulation of its criteria are the first logical steps in a series of interrelated investigations. In reality, however, criteria usually develop operationally, in a step-wise, evolving pro-

TABLE 1

CATEGORIZATION OF EPIDEMIOLOGICAL METHODS IN RESEARCH ON FMS AND MPS

METHODOLOGICAL APPROACHES	CHARACTERISTIC STUDIES
I. Descriptive:	
Population frequencies and concordance in other disorders	Prevalence in populations Incidence in populations Relative prevalence in clinics Concordance, e.g., "overlaps" with IBS, CFS
II. Analytical:	
Etiologic or risk factors	Psychosocial-behavioral factors Neuroendocrine factors Physical-functional capacity Family and twin studies Other (e.g., immunogenetic)
III. Interventional and Others	
Clinical trials, classification and course of illness	Controlled therapy trials Criteria (general & subsets) Course and prognosis Costs analysis

IBS is irritable bowel syndrome, CFS is chronic fatigue syndrome.

cess, as improved knowledge of the disorder is acquired. Differing perspectives and interpretations of complex illnesses often delay establishment of optimal criteria. Therefore, accuracy of criteria improves as better understanding of the condition is achieved and valid concepts of the illness are derived.

The concept of severity gradients of illness (1) is a fundamental, widely-accepted principle in both epidemiological research and clinical therapeutics. Some prominent exceptions of mainly fatal diseases are untreated rabies and AIDS. Both result from infection of susceptible, unprotected hosts with virulent agents. Most other illnesses, e.g., hypertension, have a broad gradient of severity, which merges into the normal range, in the mild cases, to a severe extreme, in the "malignant" phase.

A corollary issue is the spectrum of illnesses within a broader category of overlapping disorders, e.g., the various soft tissue rheumatism [STR] syndromes [Table 2]. A critical question, both clinically and epidemiologically, is to what extent do the more limited syndromes, e.g., myofascial pain syndrome [MPS], represent a milder form of physiological abnormalities than are found in the more generalized fibromyalgia syndrome [FMS]? Alternatively, do the more localized syndromes result from different combinations of contributory factors, e.g., physical, psychological-behavioral and sleep mechanisms, than does fibromyalgia? Should these syndromes be considered unified, with appropriate subgroupings, or should they be separate? Issues and dilemmas of this kind result from incomplete understanding of the dynamics of these dysfunctional disorders. In turn, the conceptual limitations directly im-

TABLE 2

SUSPECTED FACTORS IN SOFT TISSUE RHEUMATISM [STR]

STR Syndromes	Suspected Contributory Factors[+]		
	Physical	Psychologic-Behavioral	Sleep
Sports-related injury	* * *	?	?
Localized syndromes:			
shoulder pain	* *	*	*
low back pain	* *	* *	* *
myofascial pain	* *	* *	*
Fibromyalgia syndrome	*	* *	* * *

[+] Presumed degrees of intensity

pact upon efficacy of classification criteria, frequency studies and other research.

REVIEW OF FIBROMYALGIA SYNDROME [FMS]

Prevalence of Fibromyalgia in Community Population Studies

Published Reports [Table 3]: Since 1989, three reports were published on the prevalence of fibromyalgia in Scandinavian community populations (2-4), with widely differing results among women. The earlier two reports (2,3) were based upon data collected from men and women in multistage surveys not designed or executed specifically to determine the prevalence of fibromyalgia. Criteria of Yunus MB et al. (5,6) were retrospectively applied to the already collected data (2,3). In contradistinction, the most recent report (4) gathered data longitudinally with incorporation of the necessary elements of the 1990 American College of Rheumatology [ACR] fibromyalgia criteria (7), as well as the criteria of Yunus MB et al. (5,6) [latter data not reported]. The objective was to specifically determine

TABLE 3

PERCENTILE PREVALANCES OF FIBROMYALGIA IN PUBLISHED COMMUNITY POPULATION STUDIES

Populations Studied, First Author, Year, Refs.	Study Design and Criteria Used, Refs.	Number of Respondents and Percentile Prevalances [ ]		
		Female	Male	Total
Sweden, Malmö 50-70 years [Jacobsson L, 1989], (2)	1984 & 1985 interviews plus examination surveys: Yunus MB et al 1981 criteria (5)	442 [1.8]	434 [0.2]	876 [1.0]
Finland, national sample 30+ years [Mäkelä M, 1991], (3)	1977-80 executed multistage survey: Yunus MB et al 1989 criteria (6)	3,895 [1.0]	3,322 [0.5]	7,217 [0.75]
	30-44 years sample			2,716 [0.07]
Norway, Arendal 20-49 years women [Forseth KO, 1992], (4)	1989-90 executed multistage survey: 1990 ACR criteria (7)	2,498 [10.5]	--	--

fibromyalgia prevalence in women 20 to 49 years of age. As expected, the prevalence in women was far higher in the most recent study (4), estimated at 10.5 percent. Essentially all detected cases were "primary" (5,6), i.e., not "secondary" to or "concomitant" with other disorders. The frequency differences could not be attributed to use of different criteria (5-7). Similarly high prevalences were found in the most recent study (4) when the criteria of Yunus MB et al. (5,6) were used [data not shown in publication].

A minuscule frequency [0.07%] of fibromyalgia was found among persons 30-44 years of age in the earliest survey conducted between 1977-80 (3). Importantly, no person within any age group in this survey (3) was found to have "primary" fibromyalgia (5,6)! Furthermore, no case was found among 1,596 white collar workers. The conclusion from that retrospective study (3) was, "Descriptive epidemiological data offer little support for the concept of fibromyalgia." This interpretation of the retrospective data seems to be erroneous and due to the insensitive detection of only non-primary cases.

The female to male [F:M] sex ratio of prevalences in the two retrospective surveys were 2:1 (3) and 9:1 (2). The lower ratio in the earlier survey (3) most likely reflects a greater influence of non-primary fibromyalgia found among males. No studies of incidence have yet been reported, but are important to determine risk factors (8).

MYOPAIN '92 Presented Studies [Table 4]: Studies presented at the MYOPAIN '92 symposium mainly support the view of a relatively high prevalence of FMS or widespread pain among women in community populations (9-12). In a South African small town (9), 5.5% of women 35 years of age or older had 11 or more tender points specified in the 1990 ACR criteria (7). Interestingly, only 7 of these 35 women with generalized tender points admitted to having widespread pain as defined in those criteria (7). Thus, the full ACR criteria were satisfied in only about 1% of these women. Remarkably, no tender points or widespread pain case was found in men!

In a German town (10), the overall prevalence of FMS among adult men and women was 2.3%. Eight of the ten cases found were in females. The F:M sex ratio of detected FMS cases was about 4:1, i.e., 8 cases found in women and 2 in men.

In Denmark, however, the detected FMS prevalence was considerably lower (11). Out of 1,219 subjects interviewed from eastern Denmark, 118 persons responded positively to questions screening for generalized muscular pain and were invited to participate in the FMS survey. Among the

118 persons, 65 agreed to examination and 8 were positive for 1990 ACR criteria. None of the eight detected FMS cases occurred in men (11). Thus, a minimum prevalence of 8 [0.65%] of 1,219 persons originally surveyed was found. However, the prevalence in women would have been several fold higher among a completely examined sample.

Interestingly, the prevalence of generalized myalgias (11) or widespread pain (12), as defined by ACR criteria (7), was relatively high, both in Denmark, i.e., 118 [9.7%] of 1,219, and in suburban Cheshire, England, i.e., 13.2% (12). A lower prevalence in Denmark may have reflected spontaneous reporting of generalized myalgias (11). The higher prevalence in Cheshire may have resulted from more active assessment of widespread pain using shadings in mannequins (12). Widespread pain in

TABLE 4

PERCENTILE PREVALENCES OF FIBROMYALGIA [FMS] OR WIDESPREAD PAIN:

COMMUNITY POPULATION STUDIES PRESENTED AT MYOPAIN '92*

Populations Studied, Investigators, Refs.	Study Design and Criteria Used	Number of Respondents and Percentile Prevalances [ ]		
		Female	Male	Total
South Africa, small town 35+ years [Lyddell C. et al], (9)	Subjects interviewed and examined for 1990 ACR criteria	639 [5.5]**	463 [0.0]	1,102 [3.2]**
Germany, Bad Säckinger 25-74 years [Raspe H et al], (10)	Multistage survey: Regional pain plus 17+ TPs of 34, but < 3 control points [Among 80 persons examined]	8 FMS	2 FMS	438 [2.3] FMS 10 FMS
Denmark, random sample 16+ years [Prescott E. et al] (11)	Multistage survey: Generalized myalgias plus ACR TP criteria [Among 65 persons examined]	8 FMS	0 FMS	1,219 118 8 FMS [0.66] FMS
England, suburban Cheshire 20-85 years [Croft PR et al] (12)	Widepsread pain survey, according to 1990 ACR fibromyalgia criteria [No tender point examination]			1,340 [13.2]+

* See text for explanations
**35 women satisfied tender point criteria, but only 7 of whom admitted to diffuse pain.
+ Widespread pain was twice as common in women as in men.

the latter study was twice as common in women as in men. No examination was performed for tender points in this survey (12).

Relative Prevalences of Fibromyalgia in Clinic Patient Populations

Primary Care Clinics [Table 5]: Only two reports were published of fibromyalgia prevalences relative to patients attending primary care or specialty medicine clinics, excluding rheumatology (13,14). The term "relative prevalence" is intended to indicate that the sampling base is selective and not considered to be representative of the community population at large. In both studies, data were collected longitudinally to specifically determine these frequencies. Prevalences of FMS among adult men and women were 3.7% (13), according to criteria of Campbell SM et al. (13), and 1.9% (14), according to criteria of Yunus MB et al. (5). Chronic, diffuse unexplained muscular aching was found in 4.8% of one clinic population (14) and was four times as frequent in women [6.7%] as in men [1.5%]. These non-rheumatology clinic frequencies of FMS are consistent with population surveys presented at MYOPAIN '92 (9-12) and as shown in Table 4.

Rheumatology Clinics [Table 6]: One may expect a higher relative frequency of FMS in rheumatology clinics than in other medical settings or in the general population. Patients with both "primary" and "non-primary" fibromyalgia are selectively referred to such clinics. Total fibromyalgia, i.e., "primary," "secondary," and more importantly, "concomitant" (5-7), was usually at least 10% or more among rheumatology clientele [Table 6]. The only exception was a report of 1981 (15), which antedated the first quantitatively-derived criteria for fibromyalgia (5). No case of fibromyalgia was reported as such (15). However, one may suspect that FMS patients were included among those diagnosed as uncertain or undetermined [11.3%], myofascial pain syndrome [4.7%] or psychogenic rheumatism [3.3%].

The issue of "primary" vs. "secondary" or "concomitant" fibromyalgia is unsettled and requires further analysis. The two reports which differentiated these categories (18,20) showed close concordance. Both used the same criteria (18) and found about 3-4% "primary" and about 8-10% "secondary." However, another report of only "primary" fibromyalgia (19) found a relative prevalence of 17.4% using criteria of Yunus MB et al. of 1981 (5). Although not reported, it was estimated that "secondary" or "concomitant" fibromyalgia occurred in about another 10% of this clinic population (19). The age and sex distributions of "primary" and "second-

TABLE 5

RELATIVE PERCENTILE PREVALENCES OF FIBROMYALGIA IN PRIMARY CARE CLINICS

Clinic Patients Studied, First Author, Year, Refs.	Study Design and Criteria Used, Refs.	Patients Surveyed and Prevalences [ ]		
		Female	Male	Total
USA, Portland, OR, Medical [excluding rheumatology] clinics Adult patients [Campbell SM, 1983], (13)	Multitistage survey: positive question- naire response and 12+ of 17 TPs (13)			596 [3.7] FMS
USA, Hershey, PA, Family practice clinic 21-70 years [Hartz A, 1987], (14)	1986 executed multistage survey: Published and lib- eralized criteria used to define "chronic diffuse un- explained muscular aching" as well as	418 [6.7]	274 [1.5]	692 [4.8]
	Yunus MB et al 1981 FMS criteria (5)			[1.9] FMS

ary" or "concomitant" fibromyalgia are expected to be significantly different (2,3,5,18). This finding necessitates patient subclassification when comparing different populations.

Since 1982, the relative prevalence of fibromyalgia reported among adults in all clinic populations, i.e., both primary care (13,14) and rheumatology (16-20), has been less variable than data derived from community surveys (2-4, 9-12). One may presume a greater inter-observer consistency in application of criteria among physicians experienced in FMS, than was true in retrospective community surveys. No data were provided on relative frequencies by sex from rheumatology clinic studies. However, ample clinical series (5-7) indicate an F:M sex ratio of about 9:1 or greater among fibromyalgia patients seen in rheumatology settings.

Age, Sex and Race Frequencies of Juvenile Fibromyalgia

Few reliable data are available on detailed demographic features of juvenile fibromyalgia. The primary clinical report of juvenile FMS (21)

TABLE 6

RELATIVE PERCENTILE PREVALENCES OF FIBROMYALGIA IN RHEUMATOLOGY CLINICS

Rheumatology Patients Studied, First Author, Year, Refs.	Study Design and Criteria Used	Patients Reviewed [Percent "FMS"]
USA, Newport Beach, CA [Bohan A, 1981], (15)	First 2 years of practice: Uncertain or undetermined diagnosis; Myofascial pain syndrome, Psychogenic rheumatism. No criteria were specified	1,000 [11.3] [4.7] [3.3]
USA, Cleveland, OH [Mazanec DJ, 1982], (16)	First year of practice: Fibrositis, NOS	150 [16]
Mexico, Mexico City [Alarcon-Segovia D, 1983], (17)	Consecutive patients: Muscular rheumatism/fibrositis, NOS	1,000 [17.5]
USA, Wichita, KS [Wolfe F, 1983], (18)	Database review of 1980-82 new patients: Diffuse musculoskeletal aching plus 7+ of 14 TPs (18)	1,473 [3.7]* [10.9]** [14.6]
USA, Peoria, IL [Yunus MB, 1986], (19)	Chart review of 1979 & 1982-83 new patients: Yunus MB et al 1981 criteria (5)	816 [17.4]*
Spain, Barcelona [Colabozo RM, 1990], (20)	Database review of 1988 new patients to a hospital clinic: Diffuse musculoskeletal aching plus 7+ of 14 TPs (18)	673 [2.9]* [7.8]** [10.7]

*   "Primary" fibromyalgia
**   "Secondary" or "concomitant" fibromyalgia
NOS, Not otherwise specified

indicated a F:M ratio of 15:1. Interestingly, all 33 cases presented between ages 10-17 years. However, 9 cases were believed to have had onset between 5 and 9 years of age. Two patients were black, but control expectation was not specified.

Other methodologic issues in the epidemiology of FMS are reviewed elsewhere (1,22-24).

REVIEW OF MYOFASCIAL PAIN SYNDROME [MPS]

Epidemiologic Problems in Myofascial Pain Syndromes [MPS]

Characteristics and epidemiology of MPS have been reviewed recently (25). Summation of data is more difficult than in FMS. Standardized criteria (26) have not usually been employed. Another factor is the difficulty in examination techniques of these varied regional pain disorders. A major issue is whether or not the myofascial "trigger" points (25-27) are different or related manifestations to the fibromyalgia "tender" points (28-30)? A listing of reported characteristics of "trigger" and "tender" points (25-30) shows similarities and differences [Table 7]. The one main differentiating feature is that the active "trigger" point is a source of reproducible referred pain, whether or not it is firmly palpated.

A recent study (30) showed considerable similarity in the frequency of pain related to active "trigger" points among MPS and FMS patients [i.e., about 18%]. Also, local tenderness [i.e., "tender" points] was common in both groups [65-82%]. However, in this study (30) and another recent one (31), different examiners were unable to reliably determine when a "trigger" point was present, which is essential to diagnosing MPS.

Population studies of MPS require objective, reliable and standardized criteria, in order to generate valid data for reasonable comparability across surveys. It appears that if accurate research is to be conducted in the field of MPS, investigators will need to acquire general expertise with this challenging syndrome and special training in the reliable detection of "trigger" points (30,31).

The prevalence of myofascial pain in general internal medicine practice (32) may be higher than the reported frequency of FMS (13,14) [Table 5]. Among a series of 172 patients who presented to a university practice, 16 [9.3%] satisfied criteria for a clinical diagnosis of myofascial pain (32). These 16 MPS patients were similar in age, sex and intensity of pain as assessed by a visual analog scale to the other 38 [22.1%] patients who also presented with a primary complaint of pain. However, those with MPS were more likely to have upper body pain. Regional MPS seems to be an important cause of pain complaints in general internal medicine practice. In this study (32), physicians rarely recognized the syndrome prior to diagnosis in the referral clinic.

TABLE 7

MYOFASCIAL "TRIGGER" POINTS VS FIBROMYALGIA "TENDER" POINTS

Characteristic Features	Myofascial "Trigger" Points	Fibromyalgia "Tender" Points
Focal deep tenderness on palpation	Yes	Yes
Source of reproducible referred pain	Active	No*
Result of a distant pain source	No	Yes
Pain site predominance	Upper body	None
Tissue origin	Muscle	Multiple
Restricts muscle range of motion	Yes	No
History of muscle strain	Frequent	Variable
Local twitch response	"Yes"	"No"
Responsiveness to physical measures	Often	Variable
Occurrence in asymptomatic persons	Rare	50% have 1+
Gender predominance	No	Females
Associated symptoms	25-75%	70-100%
Systemic perpetuating factors [e.g., sleep]	Variable	Often
Number needed for diagnosis	1+	Many

*Hypothetical construct - a tender point may refer pain on firm palpation

Craniomandibular Disorders [CMD], Including Temporomandibular Dysfunction [TMD]

Epidemiologic Considerations: As an example of epidemiologic research in MPS, one may review some aspects of recent studies on one of the more common entities, i.e., craniomandibular disorders [CMD], including temporomandibular dysfunction [TMD]. Although regional, these cranial syndromes are both common and complex (25). They illustrate many of the methodologic problems also found in FMS (1,22-24). This article does not allow review of the other MPS entities (25-27,32), most of which have been less extensively surveyed than CMD and TMD.

Considerable gradients of severity are manifested in CMD. Also, the variability in primary and associated symptoms and signs (25,33) contribute to selection bias (24) and diagnostic problems (33) in community (34)

and clinic surveys (35). Variations in subject sampling and complexities of classification make comparisons among studies difficult. For example, in a telephone survey of a metropolitan community population (34), any one of the five primary symptoms of TMD [i.e., nocturnal bruxing, joint noise with use, soreness on waking, soreness with use, and diurnal clenching] ranged from 8% to 12% and about 30% of respondents reported one or more features. Associated pain was infrequent, but more commonly reported by respondents with four or five of the primary symptoms. However, in a hospital clinic population (35), pain manifestations are considerably more frequent and bothersome among patients seeking relief, e.g., TMJ pain [55%], painful chewing [47%], painful opening [37%] and jaw muscle pain [23%].

Sex Distribution: Symptoms were equally prevalent among women and men in the community telephone survey (34). However, females outnumbered males by 2:1 in the hospital clinic patients (35). A suspected factor which might predispose women to CMD is general joint hypermobility (36). However, neither this association nor the relative sex frequency of CMD or TMD are established.

Age-Specific Patterns: The age distributions of CMD and TMD have not been determined accurately over a broad age range of many decades. Population surveys of TMD usually focus on narrow age ranges in childhood (37,38), adolescence (37-40) or young adults (41). Usually, one or more TMD symptoms or signs are found at any one time in about one-third to one-half of these young subjects. However, manifestations are not stable on longitudinal follow-up of community populations (38-40). For example, in a 3-year longitudinal survey of Japanese adolescents (39), only 9% of the junior and 13% of the senior high school students had one or more signs of TMD [e.g., TMJ sounds] at each of the 3 annual examinations. Most of these manifestations were mild and did not require medical intervention.

The frequency of symptoms and signs of TMD seem to increase with age in minors from childhood to adolescence (37,39,40), reaching a peak in senior high school (39) or junior college students (41). Then, the frequency seems to decrease somewhat in the older university students, to the level of teenagers (41). Such patterns of usually mild manifestations are believed to reflect growth factors in the different ages (42). Among adults, TMD symptoms were more prevalent among younger respondents (34).

Occlusal Factors and CMD: Despite the large number of studies of CMD and occlusal interferences, no firm documentation of this relationship has been provided (38,41,43,44). One may suspect a dilemma wherein the actual determinant[s] of CMD and TMD may also be contributing to masticatory dysfunctions, e.g., certain malalignments. Thus, various associations found between mechanical factors and CMD may not have causal implications, but both may be "outcome" manifestations, i.e., co-morbidity events.

Longitudinal observational studies (42-45) are more likely to rationalize these associational relationships than cross-sectional surveys (37,41). However, they are still susceptible to methodologic pitfalls (23,24). Selection biases may occur, leading to nonrepresentative samples being studied. Also, interval corrective treatments of occlusal interferences can obscure associations.

One longitudinal, double-blind, placebo-controlled study was performed over a 3-year interval (44). Results in the third year suggest a significant association between the number of occlusal interferences and signs of CMD. These conclusions are also supported by a statistical model of the etiology of temporomandibular pain dysfunction syndrome (45). Those results (45) suggest that the most important factors in TMD are malocclusions, occlusal interferences and impaired general state of health. Constitutional joint factors and anxiety also seem to play a lesser role.

Emotional Factors and CMD: The relationship of anxiety, stress and tension to CMD and TMD is important, but difficult to ascertain. Various selection factors may influence subject sampling and reporting of symptoms. Among white children selected for CMD and malocclusion, comparison of symptoms and signs was made between 26 boys and 20 girls classified by their parents as "calm" versus the same number of subjects considered "not calm" [total of 92 children] (46). Muscle and TMJ tenderness were significantly higher among the "not calm" group. Such findings may suggest that temporomandibular muscle tensing may be a contributory factor to these manifestations [and possibly also to masticatory dysfunctions].

Among Taiwanese university students, those with evidence of TMD showed a higher score on emotional factors, such as Type A personality, anger and stress, compared to their cohorts (41). However, scores were not significantly higher on competition, anxiety and tension among students with evidence of TMD. Authors concluded that psychoemotional factors are as important as dental factors in relation to the TMD symptomatology, if not more important (41). As indicated above, another study (45) inferred that anxiety was playing a role in TMD, but was less important than occlusal factors.

Future Research in MPS: This limited review of recent epidemiological studies of CMD and TMD, as examples of MPS, indicate the considerable methodological challenges facing investigators of these regional pain syndromes. Similar or greater problems exist with other less extensively surveyed MPS entities. Nevertheless, one may hope for progress to be made in future MPS research. The various epidemiological approaches outlined in Table 1 will need to be rigorously employed.

CONCEPTS OF ILLNESS IN POPULATIONS AS APPLIED TO DYSFUNCTIONAL SYNDROMES

Classical Disease Biology vs. Dysfunctional Syndrome Dynamics [Table 8]

Since the last presentation in 1985 (1), it has become increasingly evident that a new conceptual paradigm for etiology is needed for FMS (47) and other dysfunctional syndromes, e.g., irritable bowel syndrome [IBS] (48,49), or problems seen in primary care practice settings (50). The classical, pathophysiologic model of agent, host and environmental risk factors [i.e., the classical triad or "triangle" schema] is not sufficiently inclusive or structured to critically investigate personalized factors (1,50). The pathobiology of classical diseases is focused upon specific etiologic agents and their tissue effects which differ from the dynamics of dysfunctional syndromes. Many critical features differentiate the "organic" diseases from the "dysfunctional" syndromes, which are relevant both for research and patient management [Table 8]. In dysfunctional syndromes, the focus is upon the individual person and his or her constellation of constitutional, psycho-behavioral and socio-environmental circumstances.

Dysfunctional syndromes are associated more with presumed determinants, e.g., a person's perceptions, reactivities and coping skills in dealing with stressful living circumstances (51), than exposure to specific pathogenic agents or toxic environments. About 4 in 10 American workers said that they were highly stressed (51) and many of them suffer from fatigue or exhaustion [65%], tight neck or shoulder muscles [63%] or insomnia [45%]. Work place stress affects women more than men (51).

Conceptually, dysfunctional syndromes are far more complex than the classical diseases. They require more sophisticated analytic methodology (52,53). Formulation of valid concepts or models of dysfunctional syndromes are essential to productive research. New and valid paradigms will offer better understanding of the complex mechanisms of illness, allow for improved criteria to be developed as well as more targeted research and enhanced patient management, hopefully leading to prevention and control of the illnesses [Table 9].

TABLE 8

PATHOBIOLOGY OF CLASSICAL DISEASES VS DYNAMICS OF DYSFUNCTIONAL SYNDROMES

Differentiating Characteristics	Pathobiology of Classical Diseases	Dynamics of Dysfunctional Syndromes
Diagnostic features	Specific pathophysiology	Subjective dysfunctions
Etiologic factors	Specific agent, host, or environmental pathogens	Multifactorial risk determinants
Factor relationships to illness	Necessary or sufficient pathogenic linkages	Predominating factors within subgroups
Major determinants to onset	Sufficient "dose" of the etiologic factor	Personal reactivity to circumstances
Course of illness	Outcome reflects host ability to control pathogen	Function reflects person's ability to deal with risks
Research designs and analyses	Traditional factor-oriented approaches	New personalized systems orientation

A Personalized Model of Dysfunctional Disorders [Figure 1]

A classical model of agent, host and environmental factors in disease was proposed previously for conceptualizing FMS [Figure 3, Ref. 1], although it was specifically qualified [and revised from a "triangle" to a "circle"]. However, this model is not sufficiently broad or structured to properly assess personalized determinants in dysfunctional syndromes and needs to be further modified.

New models should explicitly indicate that multiple, simultaneous risk factors exist. Furthermore, they operate via indirect and complex mechanisms, i.e., through currently undefined pathways [i.e., a "box"] and not necessarily as primary pathways. They operate via reactions of the person as a "whole," i.e., the "persona," rather than via specific tissue damage [Figure 1].

The sum of potential risk factors affecting a particular person is highly personalized and variable. Under ideal conditions, most of these factors are not harmful and may promote full dynamic functioning. However, under other "similarly appearing" circumstances, among other persons, the factors may result in suffering and behavioral dysfunction. The net effects of the multitudinous factors operating upon different persons cannot be calculated by simple accounting techniques of adding "positives"

TABLE 9

BENEFITS OF A VALID CONCEPT OR MODEL OF ILLNESS*

- Better understanding of illness dynamics
- Improved criteria development [minimizes "circularity"]
- More productive research directions
- Greater effectiveness in patient management
- Insights in prevention and illness control

---

* New paradigms are needed for dysfunctional syndromes

and "negatives." Neither, can other linear function analytic techniques be used simply to determine a persons risk status of developing FMS.

In specific diseases, etiologic factors tend to "over-ride" personalized, functional reactivities, i.e., the "persona." The process of identifying individual risk factors is more complex in dysfunctional syndromes. Matrix and simultaneously interacting systems concepts, with different hierarchical control levels, are needed to interpret such complex mechanisms (47,52,53). Due to such complexities, appropriate stratification and subgrouping of persons and factors becomes vital. Such process helps to identify more homogeneous groups of persons experiencing dysfunctional syndromes and to identify determinants of risk and mechanisms of illness.

Importance of Stratifying and Subgrouping Patients [Figure 2]

In IBS, various interacting dysfunctions have been identified which contribute to manifestations, e.g., abnormal motility, increased visceral perceptions [sensory awareness] and psychologic distress (48). Patient subgrouping, based upon the particular type of dysfunction that may predominate in a particular individual, has allowed improved targeting for both investigation and therapy (48,49). Similarly, in FMS and MPS, major dysfunctional mechanisms need to be identified in order to formulate patient subgroupings which will allow greater homogeneity for purposes of more focused studies or managements.

Presently, the classification of FMS is empirical. It is useful to differentiate major categories of "primary," "concomitant" and the rare "secondary" forms which markedly affect its epidemiologic characteristics. Further differentiation of the "primary" patients is presently intuitive.

FIGURE 1. Numerous constitutional, psychological-behavioral and socio-environmental factors operate continuously on the whole person ["persona"] through complex, integrated mechanisms. The constellations may promote well-being and good function in certain persons or suffering and dysfunction in others. The major determinants may disturb the integrated person or a particularly susceptible pathway ["box"] and may vary in number and magnitude of the personalized influences. Traditional, single-factor research approaches and analytic methodology are not suited to such complexities and are not likely to reveal the true dynamics of dysfunctional disorders. Personalized, integrated systems approaches [e.g., force field analysis] offer greater promise in addressing such complex problems.

Factors Contributing to Health vs. Dysfunctional Disorders: A Personalized Model

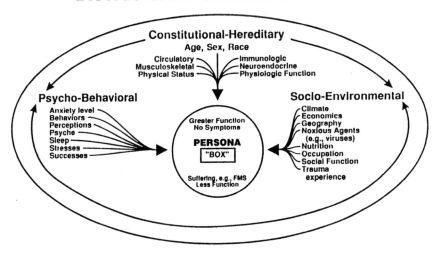

Criteria need to be established scientifically for valid subsetting. Once accomplished, more homogeneous groups of FMS patients may be identified for more targeted research and therapy.

CONCLUSIONS AND FUTURE RESEARCH DIRECTIONS

The objectives of this review were mainly to address central concepts and issues of dysfunctional syndromes, e.g., FMS and MPS, as well as to summarize available frequency data. Other methodological and statistical

FIGURE 2. The enormous variability in FMS may be empirically structured into its major classification subcategories [i.e., "primary," "concomitant" and the rare "secondary" forms]. Intuitive subsetting of the "primary" patients may allow improved detection of suspected determinants which may influence the onset, course and severity of this disorder. Valid patient classification and subsetting systems will need to be derived scientifically in order to establish true determinants of this disorder.

Classification And Subsetting Of FMS:
A Personalized Perspective To Target Determinants

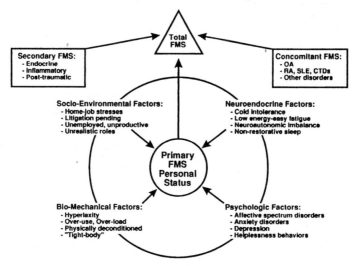

problems in the epidemiology of FMS and MPS have been addressed previously (1,22-25).

Available published data suggest that FMS is probably more prevalent in the community than was previously appreciated, especially in women, where it seems to be a common condition (4). More studies are needed with proper design to determine the true range of prevalence of FMS in populations. Data must be collected longitudinally in a fashion which allows proper application of standardized classification criteria (7), in order for results to be comparable.

Results of the most recent population studies presented at MYOPAIN '92 (9-12) again suggest that methodologic factors probably account for a considerable variation in the prevalence of FMS or widespread pain as determined in community surveys.

Overall, fibromyalgia prevalences reported from primary care clinics

(13,14) are consistent with those community population studies in which fibromyalgia criteria data were also collected longitudinally (4,9), rather than analyzed retrospectively (2,3).

Age-specific prevalences of fibromyalgia among adults, particularly stratified by "primary" or "concomitant" rheumatic disease status, have not been well-studied. Data are scant in terms of detailed ages of onset or ages of first diagnosis and further study is needed. Clinical impression suggests that fibromyalgia most frequently has its clinical onset in women during the decade of the 30's, with most frequent presentation to a specialist in the 40's. Further research on the actual age-specific frequency of FMS onset and presentation may provide clues to risk factors influencing the development or course of this condition.

Gender has not been critically studied in FMS, aside from the few data on prevalence studies in community or clinic populations mentioned above. Opportunity exists for critical analytic studies [Table 1], comparing male and female patients and their respective determinants of risk.

Race and ethnic factors similarly have been little studied. The prevalence report from South Africa (9) is most welcomed and suggests that FMS may not be rare in black females or among populations living in less-developed cultures. The relationship of widespread pain to generalized tender points seems to differ by populations (9,11) and needs further definition.

Regarding MPS, a high priority should be given to developing reliable classification criteria, such as those which have evolved in FMS (5-7). Controlled studies using such criteria need to be performed in various clinic populations, as have been accomplished in FMS (5,7,22-24). Armed with results of such controlled and criteria studies, more meaningful, descriptive population research may be accomplished. Population frequencies may be determined by age, sex, race, ethnic and geographic factors. More specific analytic research can then be designed to determine risk factors in the various MPS entities.

Research in MPS should remain integrated with FMS, to the extent that is feasibly possible. These regional and generalized disorders may share important overlapping determinants and be segments within a common spectrum of dysfunctional disorders, whatever may be their etiologies.

Improved conceptual models of dysfunctional disorders need to be developed. Integrated systems research approaches can accommodate the complex host dynamics, i.e., somatic, emotional and behavioral mechanisms, and potential risk factors in the environment. Personalized experiences and characteristics must be analyzed in order to optimally apply such concepts to a particular individual [Figures 1,2]. Investigators in FMS and MPS have an opportunity to provide leadership in formulating new paradigms for the study and management of dysfunctional syndromes.

AUTHOR NOTE

Author wishes to express sincere appreciation to Debbie Harper for her excellent typing of this manuscript, to Walter Wilkins for his generous help with literature searches and documentation, to Mitchell Anheir and Jon Spacht for their expert photography and art work, and to secretary, Margaret Walsh, for her generous ongoing assistance. Also, appreciation is expressed to Dr. Muhammad B. Yunus for his review of this manuscript and helpful suggestions.

REFERENCES

1. Masi AT, Yunus MB: Concepts of illness in populations as applied to fibromyalgia syndromes. Am J Med 81 [3A]: 19-25, 1986.

2. Jacobsson L, Lindgärde F, Manthorpe R: The commonest rheumatic complaints of over six weeks' duration in a twelve-month period in a defined Swedish population: prevalences and relationships. Scand J Rheumatol 18: 353-360, 1989.

3. Mäkelä M, Heliövaara M: Prevalence of primary fibromyalgia in the Finnish population. Brit Med J 303: 216-219, 1991.

4. Forseth KØ, Gran JT: The prevalence of fibromyalgia among women aged 20-49 years in Arendal, Norway. Scand J Rheumatol 21: 74-78, 1992.

5. Yunus M, Masi AT, Calabro JJ, Miller HA, Feigenbaum SL: Primary fibromyalgia [fibrositis]: clinical study of 50 patients with matched normal controls. Semin Arthritis Rheumatol 11: 151-171, 1981.

6. Yunus MB, Masi AT, Aldag JC: Preliminary criteria for primary fibromyalgia syndrome [PFS]. Multivariate analysis of a consecutive series of PFS, other pain patients, and normal controls. Clin Exp Rheumatol 7: 63-69, 1989.

7. Wolfe F, Smythe HA, Yunus MB, et al: The American College of Rheumatology 1990 criteria for the classification of fibromyalgia: Report of the Multicenter Criteria Committee. Arthritis Rheum 33: 160-172, 1990.

8. Masi AT and Medsger TA, Jr.: Epidemiology of the rheumatic diseases, Arthritis and Allied Conditions. Edited by DJ McCarty. Lea & Febiger, Philadelphia, 1989, 11th edition, pp 16-54.

9. Lyddell C, Meyers OL: The prevalence of fibromyalgia in a South African community. MYOPAIN '92: Abstracts from the 2nd World Congress on Myofascial Pain and Fibromyalgia, Copenhagen, Denmark, August 17-20, 1992, Abstract 143. Scand J Rheum Suppl 94, 1992.

10. Raspe H, Baumgartner Ch: The epidemiology of the fibromyalgia syndrome [FMS] in a German town. ibid, Abstract 38.

11. Prescott E, Jacobsen S, Danneskiold-Samsøe B, Bülow P: Prevalence of fibromyalgia in the adult Danish population. ibid, Abstract 155.

12. Croft PR, Schollum J, Rigby AS, Boswell RF, Silman AJ: Chronic widespread pain in the general population. ibid, Abstract 84.

13. Campbell SM, Clark S, Tindall EA, Forehand ME, Bennett RM: Clinical characteristics of fibrositis. 1. A 'blinded,' controlled study of symptoms and tender points. Arthritis Rheum 26: 817-825, 1983.

14. Hartz A, Kirchdoerfer E: Undetected fibrositis in primary care practice. J Fam Pract 25: 365-369, 1987.

15. Bohan A: The private practice of rheumatology: the first 1,000 patients. Arthritis Rheum 24: 1304-1307, 1981.

16. Mazanec DJ: First year of a rheumatologist in private practice [letter]. Arthritis Rheum 25: 718-719, 1982.

17. Alarcón-Segovia D, Ramos-Niembro F, González-Amaro RF: One thousand private rheumatology patients in Mexico City [letter). Arthritis Rheum 26: 688-689, 1983.

18. Wolfe F, Cathey MA: Prevalence of primary and secondary fibrositis. J Rheumatol 10: 965-968, 1983.

19. Yunus MB, Kudmani NA, Masi AT: A rheumatology practice in a community-based medical school. Illinois Med J 170: 317-320, 1986.

20. Calabozo Raluy M, Llamazares González AI, Munoz Gallo MT, Alonso-Ruiz A: Síndrome de fibromialgia [fibrositis]: tan frecuente como desconocido. Med Clin [Barc] 94: 173-175, 1990.

21. Yunus MB, Masi AT: Juvenile primary fibromyalgia syndrome: a clinical study of thirty-three patients and matched normal controls. Arthritis Rheum 28: 138-145, 1985.

22. Felson DT: Epidemiologic research in fibromyalgia. J Rheumatol 16 (Suppl 19): 7-11, 1989.

23. Wolfe F: Methodological and statistical problems in the epidemiology of fibromyalgia. Pain Res Ther 27: 147-163, 1990.

24. Wolfe F: Fibromyalgia. Rheum Dis Clin North Am 16: 681-698, 1990.

25. Fricton JR: Myofascial pain syndrome: characteristics and epidemiology. Pain Res Ther 17: 107-127, 1990.

26. Travell JG, Simons DG: Myofascial Pain and Dysfunction: The Trigger Point Manual. Williams & Wilkins, Baltimore, 1983, pp. 431-439.

27. Simons DG: Fibrositis/fibromyalgia: a form of myofascial trigger points? Am J Med 81[3A]: 93-98, 1986.

28. Smythe H: Tender points: evolution of concepts of the fibrositis/fibromyalgia syndrome. ibid 2-6.

29. Campbell SM: Is the tender point concept valid? ibid 33-37.

30. Wolfe F, Simons DG, Fricton J, Bennett RM, Goldenberg DL et al: The fibromyalgia and myofascial pain syndromes: a preliminary study of tender points and trigger points in persons with fibromyalgia, myofascial pain syndrome and no disease. J Rheumatol 19: 944-951, 1992.

31. Nice DA, Riddle DL, Lamb RL, Mayhew TP, Rucker K: Intertester reliability of judgements of the presence of trigger points in patients with low back pain. Arch Phys Med Rehabil 73: 893-898, 1992.

32. Skootsky SA, Jaeger B, Oye RK: Prevalence of myofascial pain in general internal medicine practice. West J Med 151: 157-160, 1989.

33. Ficarra BJ, Nassif NJ: Temporomandibular joint syndrome: diagnostician's dilemma: a review. J Med 22: 97-121, 1991.

34. Duckro PN, Tait RC, Margolis RB, Deshields TL: Prevalence of temporomandibular symptoms in a large United States metropolitan area. Cranio 8: 131-138, 1990.

35. Chua EK, Tay DK, Tan BY, Yuen KW: A profile of patients with temporomandibular disorders in Singapore: a descriptive study. Ann Acad Med Singapore 18: 675-680, 1989.

36. Westling L, Mattiasson A: Background factors in craniomandibular disorders: reported symptoms in adolescents with special reference to joint hypermobility and oral parafunctions. Scand J Dent Res 99: 48-54, 1991.

37. Pakhala R, Laine T: Variation in function of the masticatory system in 1,008 rural children. J Clin Pediatr Dent 16: 25-30, 1991.

38. Egermark-Eriksson I, Carlsson GE, Magnusson T, Thilander B: A longitudinal study on malocclusion in relation to signs and symptoms of cranio-mandibular disorders in children and adolescents. Eur J Orthod 12: 399-407, 1990.

39. Morinushi T, Ohno H, Ohno K, Oku T, Ogura T: Two year longitudinal study of the fluctuation of clinical signs of TMJ dysfunction in Japanese adolescents. J Clin Pediatr Dent 15: 232-240, 1991.

40. Ohno H, Morinushi T, Ohno K, Oku T, Ogura T: A longitudinal study on individual fluctuation of signs in accordance with TMJ dysfunction syndrome in adolescents. Shoni Shikagaku Zasshi 27: 64-73, 1989.

41. Shiau YY, Kwan HW, Chang C: Prevalence of temporomandibular disorder syndrome (TMD) in university students: a third year report of the epidemiological study in Taiwan. Chung-hua Ya I Hsueh Hui Tsa Chih 8: 106-116, 1989.

42. Dibbets JM, van der Weele LT: Prevalence of TMJ symptoms and x-ray findings. Eur J Orthod 11: 31-36, 1989.

43. Helm S, Petersen PE: Mandibular dysfunction in adulthood in relation to morphologic malocclusion at adolescence. Acta Odontol Scand 47: 307-314, 1989.

44. Kirveskari P, Alanen P, Jämsä T: Association between craniomandibular disorders and occlusal interferences. J Prosthet Dent 62: 66-69, 1989.

45. Vägö P: Linear model of the etiology of temporomandibular pain dysfunction syndrome. Dtsch Stomatol 40: 366-368, 1990.

46. Vanderas AP: Prevalence of craniomandibular dysfunction in white children with different emotional states: Part III. A comparative study. ASCD J Dent Child 59: 23-27, 1992.

47. Masi AT, Yunus MB: Fibromyalgia—which is the best treatment? A personalized, comprehensive, ambulatory, patient-involved management program. Baillière's Clinical Rheumatology: Controversies in the Management of Rheumatic

Diseases. Edited by N Bellamy. Harcourt Brace Jovanovich, Inc., London 1990, Volume 4: 333-370.

48. Camilleri M, Prather CM: The irritable bowel syndrome: mechanisms and a practical approach to management. Ann Intern Med 116: 1001-1008, 1992.

49. Drossman DA, Thompson WG: The irritable bowel syndrome: review and a graduated multicomponent treatment approach. Ann Intern Med 116: 1009-1016, 1992.

50. Odegaard CE, Inui TS: A 1992 manifesto for primary physicians. Pharos 55: 2-6, 1992.

51. Northwestern National Life: Employee burnout: causes and cures, Part 1/employee stress levels, a research report 1992. Copyright 1992 Northwestern National Life Insurance Company, pp 1-13.

52. Von Bertalanffy L: General Systems Theory. Braziller. New York, 1968.

53. Pinter GG, Pinter V: A search for the certitude of scientific facts with Vico, Giambattista and Popper, Karl–The importance of integrative physiology. Perspect Biol Med 35: 436-442, 1992.

The Epidemiology of Fibromyalgia

Frederick Wolfe

SUMMARY. Objectives: To review current estimates of fibromyalgia prevalence in the clinic and community from studies recently published or in progress.

Results: Data from 9 studies are available, two of which have been previously published. Studies which use reliable ascertainment methods and criteria [emphasizing tender points and pain] tend to show community prevalence to be about 2-4%. Prevalence in children is 6.2%. Greater than 90% of cases in adults occur in women, 67% in girls. Psychological and socio-demographic characteristics are associated with fibromyalgia symptoms and diagnosis. Cases in the community resemble cases seen in the clinic.

Conclusion: Fibromyalgia is common in the community [2-4%] both in adults and children. Cases are similar to those seen in the clinic.

KEYWORDS. Fibromyalgia, prevalence, epidemiology

Frederick Wolfe, MD, is affiliated with the Arthritis Research Center [St. Francis Research Institute], and is Clinical Professor of Internal Medicine and Family and Community Medicine, University of Kansas School of Medicine, Wichita, KS.

Address correspondence and reprint requests to: Frederick Wolfe, MD, Arthritis Research Center, 1035 N. Emporia, STE 230, Wichita, KS 67214.

Supported in part from a grant from the Los Angeles Chapter, Arthritis Foundation.

[Haworth co-indexing entry note]: "The Epidemiology of Fibromyalgia." Wolfe, Frederick. Co-published simultaneously in the *Journal of Musculoskeletal Pain* (The Haworth Press, Inc.) Vol. 1, No. 3/4, 1993, pp. 137-148; and: *Musculoskeletal Pain, Myofascial Pain Syndrome, and the Fibromyalgia Syndrome* (ed: Søren Jacobsen, Bente Danneskiold-Samsøe, and Birger Lund) The Haworth Press, Inc., 1993, pp. 137-148. Multiple copies of this article/chapter may be purchased from The Haworth Document Delivery Center [1-800-3-HAWORTH; 9:00 a.m. - 5:00 p.m. (EST)].

The coming of age of clinic fibromyalgia during the last decade has spawned several critical questions [Table 1].

1. Is fibromyalgia a clinic phenomenon only or does it exist in the community?
2. What is the prevalence of fibromyalgia in the community?
3. What are the characteristics of persons with fibromyalgia in the community?

A number of investigators have performed studies to answer these questions. In all instances investigators have shared with me their data and manuscripts [when requested] so that I might review the topic here. Their individual presentations provide detail.

For background [Table 2], fibromyalgia appears to be present [by various definitions] in about 8% of unselected medical patients (1,2), and between 12 and 20% of rheumatic disease clinic patients (3,4).

To enumerate fibromyalgia one requires a definition of the syndrome and, of course, criteria; requirements that should be met before the study is begun. While this seems obvious, it has not always been. Surveys among rheumatologists (5) and at least one community survey (6) have neither had definition nor criteria, or as in the case of the community study, definition or reasonable criteria.

By the time of the publication of the 1990 American College of Rheumatology criteria for the classification of fibromyalgia (7) a generally uniform definition of fibromyalgia had emerged [Widespread pain, multiple tender points, and characteristic symptoms] [Figure 1 and Table 3].

Equally important was the sense that the major criteria sets in use [including the criteria from Professor Müller's group (8)] identified generally similar patients and had adequate sensitivity and specificity *in the clinic* (4,7). As I have noted elsewhere (9), the two trends in criteria sets were to emphasize either pain and tenderness *or* pain and symptoms [the Yunus et al. criteria [Table 4] (4)].

TABLE 1. Critical issue concerning fibromyalgia in the community

1. Is fibromyalgia a clinic phenomenon only or does it exist in the community?

2. What is the prevalence of fibromyalgia in the community?

3. What are the characteristics of persons with fibromyalgia in the community?

TABLE 2. Prevalence of fibromyalgia in the clinic

Setting	Author	Fibromyalgia Classification	Prevalence
Hospital	Müller(18)	Primary	7.5
Family Practice Clinic	Hartz(19)	Primary	2.1
General Medical Clinic	Campbell(2)	Primary	5.7
Rheumatology Clinic	Yunus(4)	Primary	20.0
Rheumatology Clinic	Wolfe(3)	Primary	2.7
Rheumatology Clinic	Wolfe(3)	Primary & concomitant	10.9

Modified from Wolfe, F: Fibromyalgia. Rheum Dis Clin North AM:16:681-698, 1990.

It might be expected that the pain-tenderness criteria would function equally well in the clinic and the community in identifying subjects with fibromyalgia. But the pain-symptom criteria might operate differently in the two settings since the relative relationship of symptoms, pain, and tenderness are allowed to vary in these criteria, and the relative proportion of subjects with the pain, tenderness, and symptoms, respectively, might differ between the clinic and the community.

This appears to be the case. Walewski (10) reports that the Yunus et al. criteria yielded the highest "morbidity." Raspe indicates that those criteria identified 3.3 times as many cases as the ACR criteria (11) and 5 times as many cases as Professor Raspe's own criteria [which exclude subjects with significant "control site" response]. These observations tend to suggest that criteria that place reliance on symptoms do not work well in the community, though they do in the clinic.

When criteria are applied to community subjects do they identify subjects who have similar characteristics to those seen in the clinic? This is an important question since it is possible to identify subjects with criteria, but find they do not resemble clinic patients. Such criteria, of course, would not be valid. Preliminary data from our own study is available at this time to partially answer this question. Additional studies from Raspe's survey in Bad Sächingen, Germany (11), Croft et al. in the U.K. (12), from Lyddell et al. in South Africa (13), Walewski et al. (10), and Prescott et al. (14) are completed or nearing completion, but their data are not yet available concerning this point. Our in-progress report concerns our communi-

TABLE 3. The 1990 criteria for the classification of fibromyalgia (7)

---

1. History of widespread pain.

Definition: Pain is considered widespread when all of the following are present: pain in the left side of the body, pain in the right side of the body, pain above the waist and pain below the waist. In addition, axial skeletal pain [cervical spine or anterior chest or thoracic spine or low back] must be present. In this definition shoulder and buttock pain is considered as pain for each involved side. "Low back" pain is considered lower segment pain.

2. Pain in 11 of 18 tender point sites on digital palpation.

Definition: Pain, on digital palpation, must be present in at least 11 of the following 18 tender point sites:

Occiput: bilateral, at the suboccipital muscle insertions.

Low cervical: bilateral, at the anterior aspects of the inter-transverse spaces at C5-C7.

Trapezius: bilateral, at the midpoint of the upper border.

Supraspinatus: bilateral, at origins, above the scapula spine near the medial border.

2nd rib: bilateral, at the second costochondral junctions, just lateral to the junctions on upper surfaces.

Lateral epicondyle: bilateral, 2 cm distal to the epicondyles.

Gluteal: bilateral, in upper outer quadrants of buttocks in anterior fold of muscle.

Greater trochanter: bilateral, posterior to the trochanteric prominence.

Knees: bilateral, at the medial fat pad proximal to the joint line

Digital palpation should be performed with an approximate force of 4 kg.

For a tender point to be considered "positive" the subject must state that the palpation was painful. "Tender" is not to be considered painful.

---

* For classification purposes patients will be said to have fibromyalgia if both criteria are satisfied. Widespread pain must have been present for at least 3 months. The presence of a second clinical disorder does not exclude the diagnosis of fibromyalgia.

FIGURE 1. Tender point sites of the 1990 American College of Rheumatology criteria for the classification of fibromyalgia (7)

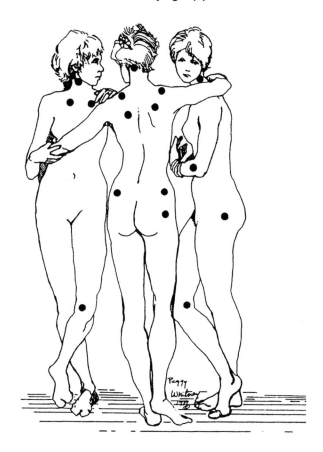

ty study which has now surveyed > 1,676 subjects. Table 5 compares our data to those published in the ACR criteria study (7).

Although the patients are older in the community survey, there is a remarkable concordance of symptom frequencies between the two studies. In fact, all of the major symptom characteristics of fibromyalgia seem to be identified at the expected proportion by the application of the ACR criteria to the community. Data such as these offer support for the validity of pain-tenderness criteria applied to community research. Our data are, however, preliminary, and are based only on 14 subjects, so final conclusions are premature.

TABLE 4. Symptoms emphasized in the Yunus et al. criteria (4)

Sleep Disturbance
Fatigue
Anxiety
Headache
Irritable Bowel Syndrome
Subjective Swelling
Numbness
Modulation of symptoms by physical activity
Modulation of symptoms by Weather factors
Aggravation of symptoms by anxiety or stress

TABLE 5. Selected characteristics of fibromyalgia patients in the American College of Rheumathology 1990 classification study and in a community survey using the ACR criteria

Characteristic	ACR N=293	Wichita Community N=14 [54]*
Sex [% Female]	88.7	93.0
Age [Years]	49.1	57.0
Fatigue [%]	81.4	78.6
Sleep Disturbance [%]	74.6	85.7
Morning Stiffness [%]	77.0	71.4
Paresthesias [%]	62.8	64.3
Irritable Bowel Syndrome [%]	29.6	21.4
Past Depression [%]	31.5	42.9

*Based on a sample of 14 of 54 subjects with fibromyalgia.

The prevalence of fibromyalgia [Table 6]. Jacobsson's 1989 study was the earliest population based survey of fibromyalgia (15). Studying 455 available subjects [ages 50-70] from a sample of 900 subjects studied previously almost 10 years earlier, they found a prevalence of only 1.1%. There are several reasons to suspect that the prevalence should have been much higher. First, fibromyalgia prevalence is increased in the age group studied. Second, the Yunus criteria have high rates of identification in community surveys. Although not stated in the text, if the Yunus criteria were rigorously adapted so that only those with "primary" fibromyalgia [no other concomitant disease] were identified, then the prevalence might

TABLE 6. Population surveys of fibromyalgia prevalence

Investigator	Year	Criteria	Age	N	Male	Fem	Both	
Jacobsson(15)	1989	Yunus	50-70	445	0.43	1.86	1.1	'Primary', incomplete sample
Makela(6)	1991	Invalid					0.75	Retrospective population survey, invalid criteria and examination
Forseth(20)	1992	ACR	20-49	2038		10.5		Non-widespread pain included, equal prevalence assumed for non-responders
Buskila(17)	1992	ACR	9-15	338	3.9	8.8	6.2	8.3% met ACR tender point criterion
Croft(12)	1992-3?	ACR	18-85	2034				Widespread pain = 11.2%
Walewski(10)	1992-3	Many	Elderly	1105		13.0	4.4	Own criteria reported here. Sampling incomplete
Prescott(14)	1992-93	ACR +-	> 15	6000			0.66	Widespread Pain = generalized muscular pain = 1.1%
Raspe(11)	1992-3?	Many	25-74	541			2.8	1.9% when those with [+] control points are excluded
Wolfe	1993	ACR	>18	1676		6-7	3.2	Widespread pain = 11.7%
Lyddell(13)	1992-3?	ACR+-	≥ 35	1278			3.2	Only 7/35 with 11/18 tender points had widespread pain
Aerflot	1993	ACR+-	40-42	7391				Widespread pain = 15.1%

be artificially low. To a large extent this depends on how "primary" was defined, something we were unable to determine from the text.

In 1992 Forseth and Gran published a study of 2,498 women aged 20-49 who had been surveyed during 1989/90. At the time of that survey they were asked if they had had pain for at least 3 months during the past year in at least 1 of 4 sites: a. the joints, b. the muscle, c. the back, and d. all over. If they answered positive to one of these questions they were considered a positive responder. Positive responders who during an examination of 37 "active" tender point sites satisfied the ACR tender point examination criterion were considered to have fibromyalgia. It is not stated in the text, but I am assuming that the 11 tender point criterion was satisfied from the 18 tender points of the ACR criteria rather than from the 37 sites examined. The authors estimated the prevalence of fibromyalgia to be 10.5%, considerably higher than they had expected. In fact the rate seems even higher than 10.5% when one considers that the average age of patients with fibromyalgia in a number of clinic studies and populations studies is greater than 49 years!

There are some explanations for this high rate. First the authors made a number of assumptions about non-responders that were not likely to be true, leading to conclusions that fibromyalgia in non-responders was likely to occur at the same rate as among responders. Non-responders in population studies are known to be younger and healthier (16), and therefore less likely to have fibromyalgia. We, in fact, observed this phenomenon in performing our own population survey: the more the study identifies previous non-responders, the lower becomes the prevalence of widespread pain and fibromyalgia. Even so, if we do some worse case calculations [assuming all non-responders are disease free], the rate falls only to 8.5%. Another contributing factor might lie in their definition of "responder." As it seems from reading the Forseth and Gran report, subjects did not necessarily satisfy the ACR "widespread pain" criterion. We noted that non-widespread but chronic pain occurred in 24.1% of subjects. In contrast our group found widespread pain in 11.7%, and Croft found it in 11.2% (12). We noted that about 3% of those with non-widespread chronic pain met the tender point criterion. Therefore, it is possible that a small number of subjects with non-widespread pain were identified by the Forseth and Gran study. Finally, most fibromyalgia patients are women. Thus the overall high rate is not a surprise. My estimate of the overall prevalence of fibromyalgia, considering the factors above suggest that if a more conservative estimate of the prevalence among non-responders is used ["corrected" prevalence = 9.5%], then reduced 25% for non-widespread pain ["corrected" prevalence = 7.125], then adjusted for sex assuming

90% of cases occur among women, the final "corrected" prevalence for both sexes is about 4%. By these figures I don't mean to suggest that the authors are wrong in their estimate, but only to suggest how some differing assumptions could lead to different estimates.

In 1991 Makela and colleagues made use of a previously performed Finnish population pain survey. Some of the Yunus symptom data were available, but, in general, joint rather than tender point data were available. The authors used all available data, and using the well known method of Procrustes came up with a prevalence estimate of 0.75%. No attempt to validate their criteria was made, and the criteria they used bore little resemblance to the original Yunus criteria. This study was not valid and the results are uninterpretable.

Buskila (17) and colleagues examined 338 Israeli children, using dolorimetry. Widespread pain was not assessed. Using ACR 11 of 18 tender points as the criterion for fibromyalgia, 7.3% of boys and 9.4% of girls had fibromyalgia. Assessments were also made with dolorimetry, and were strongly correlated with digital examination results. This important study objectifies tenderness while at the same time removing it from the stress and turmoil of adult life.

A number of studies are ongoing for which the results are not yet complete. Croft et al. (12) are assessing fibromyalgia prevalence in a survey of 2,034 subjects in the U.K. Data in press are available regarding pain and other symptoms. The prevalence of widespread pain standardized to the population of northern England and Wales was 11.2%. It is of interest, as noted above, that we found a prevalence of widespread pain of 11.7% and Aarflot found 15.2%. Both Croft's group and our own study found widespread pain [as well as the tender point count] to be more common in women, to increase with age, and to be associated with psychological distress.

Walewski and Szczepanski from the University Medical School in Lublin, Poland present the results of a study of 1,105 rural and urban "elderly" subjects (10). The overall prevalence of fibromyalgia, using their own criteria was 4.5%, but was 13.0% in women. Between the ages of 45 and 74, the highest prevalence [10.0%] was noted. Not all persons with pain were examined, and prevalence rates may be upwardly biased by study methodology.

Prescott et al. used the 1990/91 screening questionnaire of 6,000 Danish subjects to screen for fibromyalgia (14). A sample of 1,740 was identified of whom 1,318 agreed to be interviewed. One hundred twenty-nine subjects had "generalized musculoskeletal pain [9.35%]" and 78 were selected for examination. Eight, all women, met the ACR tender point criterion yielding a prevalence of 0.66%.

Raspe et al. surveyed 541 persons from Bad Säckingen (11). Using their definition of widespread pain [pain in one or more joints and back and/or neck pain and/or chest wall pain] they identified 24% who were questionnaire positive. Various criteria yielded varying results. Raspe et al.'s own criteria which excluded those with 3 or more control points positive yielded a prevalence of 1.9 percent. ACR criteria equaled 2.8%, Müller's criteria 4.6%, and Yunus's criteria 9.2%.

We report preliminary data from our own survey in Wichita, KS, U.S. As part of an ongoing community surveyed we have to date surveyed 1,676 persons. Widespread pain was noted in 11.7% and chronic non-widespread pain in 24.1%. Using ACR criteria, fibromyalgia prevalence of 3.2% was noted. Approximately 3% of those with chronic non-widespread pain satisfied the tender point criterion as opposed to 30% of those with widespread pain.

Perhaps the most interesting report comes from an extremely careful population survey performed by Lyddell et al. in a small rural South African community (13). Subjects were "very unsophisticated, with virtually no formal education." One thousand one hundred two of 1,278 persons were examined. Widespread pain was rare in this group. Thus the investigators determined the prevalence of fibromyalgia by the ACR tender point criterion. A prevalence of 3.2% was noted, and only females were identified. Only 7 of 35 persons with the requisite tenderness had widespread pain. If the widespread pain criterion were to be applied to this group, the prevalence figure would be 0.64%. The absence of pain in this population is striking, suggesting the importance of physical, cultural, and psychological factors to the syndrome of fibromyalgia.

One additional study, by Aarflot et al., is now in progress [Trygve Aarflot: personal communication]. Using the Nordic Form Body Map which can be configured to be similar to the ACR definition of widespread pain, 7,391 adults between the ages of 40-42 were surveyed in Østfold county. Fifteen point one [15.1] percent [19.5 female, 10.3 male] had widespread chronic pain. Various Yunus et al. 1981 symptom criteria were also available. When 3 pain regions and 3 of 10 minor criteria and modulating factors were applied, 13.4% were identified. Tender point examinations have not yet been carried out, and the data presented here are preliminary.

This review represents preliminary results of many authors who shared with me their data. I have purposely not gone into detail about the individual studies since the authors themselves should and will do so. I have also not included confidence intervals and other measures of precision in this review, deferring such data and their interpretation to the authors and readers. But what, then, can we conclude about prevalence. Based on the many results, it is likely that the true prevalence of fibromyalgia [using a definition of the syndrome approximate to the ACR criteria and definition] is between 2 and 4%. As in the clinic, more than 90% of persons with fibromyalgia are women.

All studies show striking female predominance, usually in excess of 90%. Interestingly, there was a tendency for this to be true in children as well. The study of tenderness in childhood by Buskila and colleagues (17) demonstrated that 67% of fibromyalgia cases occurred among girls. Similarly, pain threshold was lower in girls than boys, regardless of age. While fibromyalgia has often been linked to life stresses in women, particularly during the child bearing years, these data suggest that other factors play a central role. Whether there are important behavioral factors present in children, however, as there are in adults has not been determined.

Similarly interesting is the finding by Lyddell et al. (13) in their rural, essentially uneducated African community of tenderness but little pain. Their findings suggest the importance of physical activity, cultural factors, and pain behavior in the development of fibromyalgia.

Studies from the U.K., Germany, Poland, and the U.S. suggest an importance in psychological factors. There is an increasing level of psychological distress with each level of increase in pain, going from no pain, to regional pain, to widespread pain, and to fibromyalgia. Our data, for example, indicate that 57% of persons with fibromyalgia in the community consider themselves depressed compared with 18% without pain. The *mean* AIMS depression score is high, and the SCL-90 depression T-Score is greater than 60. Although the number of patients involved is small and the psychological results might represent a sampling error, the level of psychological abnormality appears to be greater than what is seen in the clinic.

Studies from the many centers suggest that both tenderness and pain location may represent a continuum, and that rigorous cut off points may form artificial boundaries. Even so, patients identified in epidemiological surveys strikingly resemble those seen in the clinic and offer evidence that fibromyalgia exists in the community as it does in the clinic.

REFERENCES

1. Wolfe F: The epidemiology of fibromyalgia. *Rheum Dis Clin North Am* 16:681-698, 1990.

2. Campbell SM, Clark S, Tindall EA, Forehand ME, Bennett RM: Clinical characteristics of fibrositis. I. A "blinded," controlled study of symptoms and tender points. *Arthritis Rheum* 26:817-824, 1983.

3. Wolfe F, Cathey MA: Prevalence of primary and secondary fibrositis. *J Rheumatol* 10:965-968, 1983.

4. Yunus MB, Masi AT, Calabro JJ, Miller KA, Feigenbaum SL: Primary fibromyalgia [fibrositis]: clinical study of 50 patients with matched normal controls. *Semin Arthritis Rheum* 11:151-171, 1981.

5. Epstein WV, Henke CJ: The nature of U.S. rheumatology practice, 1977. *Arthritis Rheum* 24:1177-1187, 1981.

6. Makela M, Heliovaara M: Prevalence of primary fibromyalgia in the Finish population. *BMJ* 303:216-219, 1991.

7. Wolfe F, Smythe HA, Yunus MB, et al: The American College of Rheumatology 1990 Criteria for the Classification of Fibromyalgia: Report of the Multicenter Criteria Committee. *Arthritis Rheum* 33:160-172, 1990.

8. Lautenschlager J, Bruckle W, Seglias J, Muller W: Lokalisierte druckschmerzen in der diagnose der generalisierten tendomyopathie [fibromyalgie]. *Z Rheumatol* 48:132-138, 1989.

9. Wolfe F: Fibromyalgia: On diagnosis and certainty. *J Musculoske Pain* [In Press], 1993.

10. Walewski W, Szczepanski L: Epidemiological Studies of Fibromyalgia Syndrome Morbidity. *Scand J Rheumatol Suppl* 94:S138 [Abstract], 1992.

11. Raspe H, Baumgartner Ch: The Epidemiology of the fibromyalgia syndrome in a German town. *Scand J Rheumatol* 94:S38 [Abstract], 1992.

12. Croft P, Rigby AS, Boswell R, Schollum J, Silman AJ: The prevalence of widespread pain in the general population. *J Rheumatol* [In Press], 1993.

13. Lyddell C: The prevalence of fibromyalgia in a South African community. *Scand J Rheumatol [Suppl]* 94:S143 [Abstract], 1992.

14. Prescott E, Jacobsen S, Danneskiold-Samsøe B, Bulow P: Prevalence of fibromyalgia in the adult danish population. *Scand J Rheumatol [Suppl]* 94:S115 [Abstract], 1992.

15. Jacobsson L, Lindgärde F, Manthorpe R: The commonest rheumatic complaints of over six weeks' duration in a twelve-month period in a defined Swedish population. Prevalences and relationships. *Scand J Rheumatol* 18:353-360, 1989.

16. Eaton WW, Anthony JC, Tepper S, Dryman A: Psychopathology and Attrition in the Epidemiologic Catchment Area Surveys. *Am J Epidemiol* 135:1051-1059, 1992.

17. Buskila D, Press J, Gedalia A, et al.: Assessment of nonarticular tenderness and prevalence of fibromyalgia in children. *J Rheumatol* 20: 368-370, 1993.

18. Muller W: The fibrositis syndrome: diagnosis, differential diagnosis and pathogenesis. *Scand J Rheumatol [Suppl]* 65:40-53, 1987.

19. Hartz A, Kirchdoerfer E: Undetected fibrositis in primary care practice. *J Fam Pract* 25:365-369, 1987.

20. Forseth KO, Gran JT: The Prevalence of Fibromyalgia Among Women Aged 20-49 Years in Arendal, Norway. *Scand J Rheumatol* 21:74-78, 1992.

The Epidemiology
of the Fibromyalgia Syndrome [FMS]:
Different Criteria–
Different Results

Heiner Raspe
Christoph Baumgartner

SUMMARY. Objectives: To estimate the prevalence of FMS and to examine the clinically derived concept of FMS in a population sample.

Methods: Five hundred forty-one German residents of Bad Säckingen, aged 25-74, were randomly selected for study from a target population of 6,100. Four hundred thirty-eight [81%] responded to a postal screening questionnaire. One hundred five of these reported chronic pain in at least one joint region *and* in the axial region [i.e., neck, back and/or thoracic pain]. All were invited to a medical examination: 80 attended. Cases of FMS were identified by counting active tender points [TP, n = 34] and non tender control points [CP, n = 10]. A proband was classified as FMS if she/he showed 17 or more active TPs and 2 or fewer tender CPs.

Heiner Raspe, MD, PhD, is Professor and Director of the Institute for Social Medicine, Medical University Lübeck, St.-Jürgen-Ring 66, D 2400 Lübeck.

Christoph Baumgartner, MD, is affiliated with the Hochrhein-Institut, Bergseestraße, D 7880 Bad Säckingen.

Address correspondence to: Dr. Heiner Raspe, Institute for Social Medicine, Medical University Lübeck, St.-Jürgen-Ring 66, D 2400 Lübeck.

The study was supported by a grant of the Hochrhein-Institut, Bad Säckingen.

[Haworth co-indexing entry note]: "The Epidemiology of the Fibromyalgia Syndrome [FMS]: Different Criteria–Different Results." Raspe, Heiner, and Christoph Baumgartner. Co-published simultaneously in the *Journal of Musculoskeletal Pain* (The Haworth Press, Inc.) Vol. 1, No. 3/4, 1993, pp. 149-152; and: *Musculoskeletal Pain, Myofascial Pain Syndrome, and the Fibromyalgia Syndrome* (ed: Søren Jacobsen, Bente Danneskiold-Samsøe, and Birger Lund) The Haworth Press, Inc., 1993, pp. 149-152. Multiple copies of this article/chapter may be purchased from The Haworth Document Delivery Center [1-800-3-HAWORTH; 9:00 a.m. - 5:00 p.m. (EST)].

Results: Eighteen subjects had 17 or more TPs. Eight of these had 3 or more tender CPs resulting in 10 FMS-cases and a minimal prevalence of 1.8%. The median age was 62; 8/10 were females. Assuming that the prevalence in the nonresponders and nonparticipants was similar to those who responded and participated, and that none of those with regional or no musculoskeletal pain fulfilled the TP/CP-criteria, the estimated prevalence would be 3.1% [95% CI 1.6-4.4]. Using the ACR-criteria (Wolfe et al. 1990) results in a rate of 2.0. The second assumption however may not be valid: in a small control group of 20 probands with only monolocular pain but a high amount of non-specific bodily complaints, 3 were found to fulfill our TP/CP-criteria for FMS.

Conclusions: Our study, though giving a prevalence estimate close to that of other FMS-surveys, raises questions about the rheumatologically defined nosologic and nosographic concept of the disorder.

KEYWORDS. Fibromyalgia, criteria, epidemiology

INTRODUCTION

Recent prevalence estimates of FMS are in the range of 0.75-10.5% (1,2,3) with more evidence for figures around 1%. Most of the variation seems to depend on differences in concepts and operational definitions. By referring to different criteria and examining a small control group we were able to give further evidence for a prevalence well below 10% and–more important–to specify some of the nosologic and nosographic problems of the clinically derived concept of FMS.

METHODS

Bad Säckingen is a spa-town in South-West Germany with about 6,100 residents between the ages of 25 to 74 years in the core city from which in autumn 1990 543 inhabitants were randomly selected for study. Five hundred forty-one contactable subjects [100%] received a postal questionnaire asking about a variety of rheumatic and bodily complaints. Four hundred thirty-eight [81%] responded after two reminders. Overall, 105 [24%] reported chronic pain in at least one joint region as well as neck, back and/or thoracic pain [our definition of "widespread pain"]. All were invited to a medical examination including a pain drawing and a tender point count [TP] as well as a control point count [CP] with 10 CPs. Tenderness was assessed by digital palpation with about 4 kp/cm^2 over 34 TPs. The TP-count includes all non-redundant

TPs described by Wolfe et al. 1990 (4), Yunus et al. 1989 (5) and Lautensch-laeger et al. 1989 (6). Eighty subjects with a pain history of at least 8 months participated. To distinguish FMS from regional as well as undifferentiated pain syndromes probands were classified as FMS if they fulfilled each of 3 criteria, i.e., giving a history of multiregional pain *and* showing at least 17 active TPs *and* not more than 2 active CPs.

RESULTS

The tender point and the control point count each followed a non-for-mal distribution with no indication of bimodality in either variable [TP: range 0 - 5, mean 1.1, sd 1.4, 0 = 53%]. The two counts correlated with r = 0.62. Eighteen of 80 subjects with a history of widespread pain showed 17+ active TPs. However, 8 of the 18 had 3 or more tender control points. Thus, only 10 fulfilled our FMS-criteria. This results in a minimal preva-lence of 10/541 or 1.8%. Eight of the 10 cases were female with a median age and a median disease duration of 62 and 19 years respectively. The widespread pain and TP definition of the ACR-criteria (4) lead to 7 FMS-cases and a minimal prevalence of 1.3%.

Assuming 1. that we would find an equal frequency of widespread pain among the non-responders and 2. an equal frequency of FMS-cases among the non participants with widespread pain and 3. no FMS-cases among those with only regional or even no pain one would expect a total of 17 cases among all 541 probands, resulting in an estimated true prevalence of 3.1% [11 cases or 2.0% according to the ACR-classification, estimating a prevalence of 12% for ACR-widespread pain and among them a preva-lence of 17% for 11+/18 TP].

The question is: are these three assumptions valid? We have no reason to question the first and second; it is however clear that the third is wrong. We invited 30 subjects who–on the postal questionnaire–showed a high amount of bodily complaints [i.e., were above the 90% percentile of a German symptom check-list (7)] without fulfilling our widespread pain criterion. Twenty followed the invitation. Three showed 17 or more TPs *and* 2 or less CPs. Should they be classified as FMS-cases according to the TP/CP-criterion in the presence of exclusively regional pain?

CONCLUSIONS

The potential value of population based epidemiologic studies is not limited to the enumeration of disease frequencies; they also allow us to clarify nosologic and nosographic concepts among subjects different from the patients who are usually involved in clinically based investigations to establish criteria sets.

Adhering to our criteria for FMS or those of the ACR this study gives prevalence estimates that are comparable to those that have been reported from other groups [3.1 and 2.0% resp. (1,2)]. In fact, FMS seems to be more frequent than rheumatoid arthritis. Our figures, however, are clearly lower than what has been reported by Forseth and Gran from Norway (3).

One may, however, question the concept and/or the operational definitions of FMS. We identified 3 main problems: 1. In the open population there seems to exist a continuum of soft tissue "disturbance" that makes all delimitations more or less arbitrary. So far we have no prognostic information that could help in defining cut-off points, for instance for TPs or CPs, as is the case in the measurement of blood pressure or bone mineral content. 2. The existence of TP-positive and CP-negative cases among persons with only regional pain questions the relevance and specificity of a history of widespread pain. 3. It questions also the concept of FMS as an exclusively rheumatic disorder. Could it be that FMS is part of a wider spectrum of functional disorders? Further epidemiologic studies of carefully selected samples from the open population will help to clarify these nosographic and nosologic questions.

REFERENCES

1. Mäkelä M, Heliövaara: Prevalence of primary fibromyalgia in the Finnish population. BMJ 303: 216-219, 1991.

2. Jacobsson LTH: Common rheumatic complaints. Medical Thesis. University of Lund. Malmö 1991.

3. Forseth KO, Gran JT: The prevalence of fibromyalgia among women aged 20-49 years in Arendal, Norway. Scand J Rheumatol 21: 74-78, 1992.

4. Wolfe F, Smythe HA, Yunus MB et al.: The American College of Rheumatology 1990 Criteria for the Classification of Fibromyalgia. Arthritis Rheum 33: 160-172, 1990.

5. Yunus MB, Masi AT, Aldag JC: Preliminary criteria for primary fibromyalgia syndrome (PFS): multivariate analysis of a consecutive series of PFS, other pain patients, and normal subjects. Clin Exp Rheumatol 7: 63-69, 1989.

6. Lautenschläger J, Brückle W, Seglias J, Müller W: Lokalisierte Druckschmerzen in der Diagnose der generalisierten Tendomyopathie (Fibromyalgie). Z Rheumatol 48: 132-138, 1989.

7. Zerssen v D and Koeller DM: Die Beschwerden-Liste. Beltz Test Weinheim 1976.

Preliminary Communication on the Prevalence of Fibromyalgia in the Adult Danish Population

Eva Prescott
Søren Jacobsen
Mette Kjøller
Per Martin Bülow
Bente Danneskiold-Samsøe
Finn Kamper-Jørgensen

SUMMARY. Objective: The purpose of this paper is to present preliminary results on the prevalence of fibromyalgia in the adult Danish population.

Methods: The reported study is based on a national health interview survey on musculoskeletal diseases carried out by the Danish

---

Eva Prescott, MD, Mette Kjøller, MD, Per Martin Bülow, MD, Bente Danneskiold-Samsøe, MD, PhD, and Finn Kamper-Jørgensen, MD, PhD, are affiliated with the Departments of Rheumatology, Frederiksberg and Hvidovre Hospital and Danish Institute for Clinical Epidemiology [DICE], Copenhagen, Denmark.

Søren Jacobsen, MD, is affiliated with the Department of Medicine TTA, Copenhagen University Hospital, Tagensvej 20, 2200 Copenhagen N, Denmark.

Address correspondence to: Eva Prescott, MD, Hasselvej 58, 2720 Vanløse, Denmark.

The authors wish to thank nurse Karen Lisbeth Jensen and laboratory technicians Jette Nielsen and Anna Kligert for valuable help. The study was supported economically by The Helse Foundation, The Valborg and Edith Larsen Award, The Bodil Pedersen Foundation, The Erna Hamilton Science and Art Award and The Oak Foundation.

[Haworth co-indexing entry note]: "Preliminary Communication on the Prevalence of Fibromyalgia in the Adult Danish Population." Prescott, Eva et al. Co-published simultaneously in the *Journal of Musculoskeletal Pain* (The Haworth Press, Inc.) Vol. 1, No. 3/4, 1993, pp. 153-157; and: *Musculoskeletal Pain, Myofascial Pain Syndrome, and the Fibromyalgia Syndrome* (ed: Søren Jacobsen, Bente Danneskiold-Samsøe, and Birger Lund) The Haworth Press, Inc., 1993, pp. 153-157. Multiple copies of this article/chapter may be purchased from The Haworth Document Delivery Center [1-800-3-HAWORTH; 9:00 a.m. - 5:00 p.m. (EST)].

153

Institute for Clinical Epidemiology in 1990/91 on approximately 6,000 randomly selected Danish citizens more than 15 years of age. For this study 1,219 subjects from the eastern part of Denmark aged 18 to 79 years were asked about widespread muscle pain and/or fibromyalgia. One hundred and twenty-three persons fulfilling our screening criteria were asked to participate in a clinical examination. Clinical examination for fibromyalgia could be performed on 65 persons.

Results: Eight female subjects out of 1,219 persons met the 1990 American College of Rheumatism criteria for fibromyalgia.

Conclusion: The minimum prevalence of fibromyalgia in the Danish population between 18-79 years of age was found to be 0.66% [95% confidence limits 0.28%-1.29%].

KEYWORDS. Epidemiologic survey, muscle pain, musculoskeletal disease

INTRODUCTION

The epidemiology of fibromyalgia has been studied using different settings, criteria and populations which makes it difficult to estimate the prevalence of fibromyalgia in the general population. Classification criteria for fibromyalgia have been suggested by the American College of Rheumatology in 1990 [ACR-90] (1). The subject of this paper is to present preliminary results on the prevalence of fibromyalgia according to the ACR-90 criteria in the adult Danish population.

SUBJECTS AND METHODS

Survey population. In 1990/91 a national health interview survey was carried out by the Danish Institute for Clinical Epidemiology on approximately 6,000 randomly selected Danish citizens more than 15 years of age. Data collection was done in three sessions through personal interviews performed in the homes of the subjects by professional interviewers. To clarify the inclusion procedure a flow chart is shown in Figure 1.

For practical and economical reasons the study population was limited to individuals aged 18 to 79 in the eastern part of Denmark which includes the capital, Copenhagen. This screening population [n = 1595] constituted approximately 44 percent of the whole survey population and was repre-

FIGURE 1. Flow chart for the inclusion procedure of a Danish epidemiologic survey on fibromyalgia performed in 1990/91.

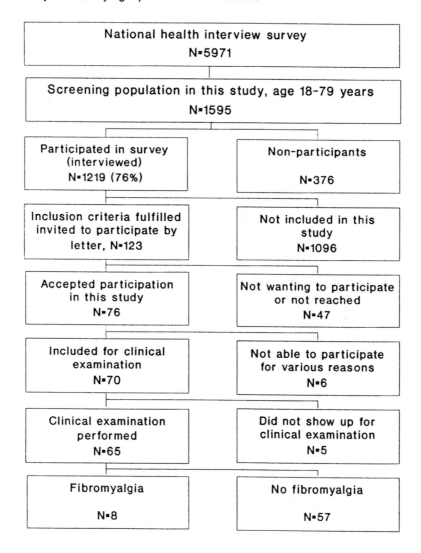

sentative of the overall Danish adult population with regard to gender, age and marital status. The number of subjects who agreed to participate and to be interviewed was 1,219 [76%]. The remaining 376 subjects either did not want to participate [14%], were not reached at home [6%] or could not participate due to other causes [4%].

Study inclusion. During the interview a survey questionnaire regarding musculoskeletal problems was filled in by the interviewer. Participants were screened for widespread pain by asking if they had had daily or longstanding [more than 30 days during the last 12 months but not daily] pain or discomfort in at least three regions that were represented both below and above the waist. Regions defined above the waist were neck, shoulders, upper back, elbows and hands/wrists. Regions defined below the waist were lower back, hips, knees and feet/ankles. Subjects classified by the interviewer as meeting inclusion criteria [n = 123] were invited to participate in the clinical continuation of the study. Oral and written information was presented, accompanied by an answer sheet and a stamped envelope, which they were asked to fill in and return.

Clinical examination. Of the 123 included subjects, 76 agreed to participate. Eleven subjects either did not show up for the clinical examination [n = 5], were excluded since they could not get to the place of examination on their own [n = 3] or for other reasons could not participate [n = 3], leaving 65 [86%] cases in which clinical examination was performed. The clinical examination followed a standard protocol which consisted of blood sampling, muscle strength measurement, blinded tender point palpation, physical examination and completion of a self-administered questionnaire, in the order mentioned. More detailed data on the selection procedures and the outcome of the clinical examination will be published elsewhere.

RESULTS

One hundred twenty-three subjects [10.1%] fulfilled the screening criteria for widespread pain. Out of the 65 study subjects who were clinically examined, 8 females fulfilled both the subjective criteria of widespread pain and the tender point count criteria according to the ACR-90 criteria for fibromyalgia. The observed rate of fibromyalgia in this sample of the Danish population between the ages of 18 and 79 was thus 8/1219 equalling 0.66% [95% confidence limits 0.28%-1.29%].

The eight fibromyalgia subjects that were identified had a median age of 54 years, ranging from 35 to 73 years. Median duration of their muscle pain was 10 years, ranging from 2 to 18 years.

DISCUSSION

Only few epidemiologic surveys have been performed to establish the prevalence of fibromyalgia in the general population. An overview of the presently available epidemiologic data on fibromyalgia concludes that the community prevalence of fibromyalgia is 2-4% (2). In the present study the prevalence of subjects meeting the ACR-90 criteria for fibromyalgia in the Danish population between 18 and 79 years of age was found to be 0.66%. The prevalence found in this study is a minimum estimate since non-participants may hide some fibromyalgia cases.

This paper is a preliminary communication of the results of the described study. However, further data are to be published which will further characterize the identified fibromyalgia subjects, yielding important information about the syndrome in non-patient community subjects.

REFERENCES

1. Wolfe F, Smythe HA, Yunus MB, Bennett RM, Bombardier C, Goldenberg DL, Tugwell P, Campbell SM, Abeles M, Clark P, Fam AG, Farber SJ, Fiechtner JJ, Franklin CM, Gatter RA, Hamaty D, Lessard J, Lichtbroun AS, Masi AT, McCain GA, Reynolds WJ, Romano TJ, Russell IJ, Sheon RP: The American College of Rheumatology 1990 criteria for the classification of fibromyalgia. Report of the multicenter criteria committee. Arthritis Rheum 33: 160-172, 1990.

2. Wolfe F. The epidemiology of fibromyalgia. J Musculoskel Pain 1(3/4):137-148, 1993.

Preliminary Results
of a 4-Year Follow-Up Study
in Fibromyalgia

Jesper Nørregaard
Per Martin Bülow
Eva Prescott
Søren Jacobsen
Bente Danneskiold-Samsøe

SUMMARY. Objectives: The objectives of this study were to examine the extent to which fibromyalgia patients later on developed somatic diseases which might account for the pain and to examine symptoms some years after the diagnosis of fibromyalgia was established.

Methods: A follow-up study of 91 patients registered under a diagnosis of primary fibromyalgia.

Results: Only in three of 91 did other somatic diseases, which might account for the pain, develop during the median 4 year follow-

Jesper Nørregaard, MD, Per Martin Bülow, MD, Eva Prescott, MD, and Bente Danneskiold-Samsøe, MD, PhD, are all affiliated with the Department of Rheumatology, Frederiksberg Hospital, Copenhagen, Denmark.

Søren Jacobsen, MD, is affiliated with the Department of Medicine TTA, Copenhagen University Hospital, Tagensvej 20, 2200 Copenhagen N, Denmark.

Address correspondence to: Jesper Nørregaard, Bomlærkevej 14, 2970 Hørsholm, Denmark.

The study was supported by grants from The Oak Foundation, and The Bodil Pedersen Foundation.

[Haworth co-indexing entry note]: "Preliminary Results of a 4-Year Follow-Up Study in Fibromyalgia." Nørregaard, Jesper et al. Co-published simultaneously in the *Journal of Musculoskeletal Pain* (The Haworth Press, Inc.) Vol. 1, No. 3/4, 1993, pp. 159-163; and: *Musculoskeletal Pain, Myofascial Pain Syndrome, and the Fibromyalgia Syndrome* (ed: Søren Jacobsen, Bente Danneskiold-Samsøe, and Birger Lund) The Haworth Press, Inc., 1993, pp. 159-163. Multiple copies of this article/chapter may be purchased from The Haworth Document Delivery Center [1-800-3-HAWORTH; 9:00 a.m. - 5:00 p.m. (EST)].

159

up period. Sixty out of 83 attending subjects reported worsened pain, 8 reported improvement of pain, 13 no change in pain. Only 20% of the patients were gainfully employed at the time of follow-up.

Conclusions: Other somatic diseases associated with pain rarely developed in our fibromyalgia patients during the follow-up period.

KEYWORDS. Fibromyalgia, follow-up, somatic diagnosis

INTRODUCTION

The existence of fibromyalgia as a separate diagnostic entity has recently been questioned in a Swedish retrospective study. During a 5 year period all 25 patients developed other, mainly psychiatric or thyroid diseases (1). Thus the patients did no longer have primary fibromyalgia. The distinction between primary and secondary fibromyalgia has recently been abandoned due to similarities in the clinical picture (2). However, from a therapeutic and a prognostic point of view the distinction still seems relevant.

Little is known about the natural history and long term prognosis of fibromyalgia. In a follow-up study from Norway 53% of patients with long lasting muscle pain received disability pension after 7 years (3). In an American study the majority of patients diagnosed as having fibromyalgia showed severe continuing symptoms during a 3 year follow-up (4).

The purpose of the study was to investigate the common existence or later appearance of other diseases in our patients, who earlier had a diagnosis of primary fibromyalgia, and to examine whether the patients reported the symptoms to improve or worsen during time.

SUBJECTS AND METHODS

First attendance. In our hospital all patients are registered by diagnostic codes. From the register all patients living in the area of Copenhagen with an earlier diagnosis of primary fibromyalgia at least one year previously were elected for the study. All were diagnosed by S.J. or B.D.S. as having primary fibromyalgia. A uniform set of diagnostic criteria was not used, but in general the criteria of Smythe and Yunus and a modification of these (5) were used. At their first attendance to our department all patients had the following blood tests performed to exclude other diseases: Erythrocyte sedimentation rate, blood cell count, thyroid parameters, creatine kinase, myoglobin, calcium, rheumatoid factor, anti-nuclear antibodies and hepatic enzymes.

Follow-up visit. By interview and palpation of tender points it was determined whether the patients fulfilled the 1990 ACR classification criteria for fibromyalgia (2). All patients were examined by the first mentioned author, 92% of the patients were also examined by another observer. The palpation examinations were performed without knowledge to patients' symptom severity and the subjects were not given any instruction before palpation.

Subjects answered a self-administered questionnaire which included questions regarding medication, changes in muscle symptoms, concomitant diseases or diagnoses and employment status during the last year.

The patients were asked whether they had had other diseases or diagnoses since their last visit. Specifically they were asked if they had ever suffered from thyroid diseases, a rheumatic disease or a psychiatric disorder or a depression. To further establish other diagnoses the initial blood analysis was repeated. If any of these assessments were abnormal further examinations were conducted to establish other concomitant diagnosis.

RESULTS

Attendance at follow-up. From our register, 91 patients with an earlier diagnosis of primary fibromyalgia were included in the follow-up. Two subjects had another diagnosis [rheumatoid arthritis, hypothyroidism] 2-3 months after the diagnosis of fibromyalgia, one female had committed suicide: All the remaining 88 called for a follow-up visit had contact with the department. There were 83 [71 females, 12 males] who attended the follow-up visit. Their median age was 53 years [range 29-77 years] and the median follow-up period was 47 months [range 12-72 months]. Five females did not return for the follow-up evaluation, but were interviewed by telephone. These 5 all had been diagnosed between 2 and 5 years previously and had almost unchanged muscle pain; one reported to have been treated for an endogenous depression.

Criteria of fibromyalgia. Only one subject reported no muscle pain. Seventy-eight [94%] fulfilled the clinical criteria of generalized muscle pain for more than 3 months. Fifty-four [69%] of the subjects with generalized muscle pain had 11 or more tender points by at least one observer. Forty-eight [62%] had a mean tender points count by the two observers of 11 or more. The mean tender point count is used in the following results.

Other diagnoses. Seven subjects reported to have suffered from thyroid diseases years before the first diagnostic examination, but they all had TSH and thyroid hormone levels in the normal range both at time of diagnosis and at the follow-up. Four received thyroid medication. In none of the subjects could the symptoms be explained by some other reported somatic disease. This evaluation was based upon information on the disease history and response on medication. Two suffered from severe diseases [renal insufficiency, benign intracranial hypertension] which might cause muscle symptoms. These diagnoses were all established before the diagnosis of fibromyalgia. One subject had a 10 fold elevation of creatine kinase and was further examined on suspicion of specific myopathy. All of the others had either normal blood tests or unspecific abnormalities without apparent clinical relevance. Twenty-five [30%] reported to have suffered from depression or psychiatric diseases. There was no attempt to relate the severities of the fibromyalgia and psychiatric symptoms nor to evaluate the time relationships between psychiatry and the pain symptoms.

Employment status. At the follow-up visit 16 of 82 [20%] patients were gainfully employed. Thirty-three [40%] received disability pension, 11 received old age pension, 6 were housewives, 16 were unemployed or received social insurance. [The employment status was not registered at the time of diagnosis.]

Severity of symptoms and treatment. Thirty-nine reported much worsening of pain during the last year, 21 slight worsening, 13 no change, and 8 reported improvement or no pain. In five [6%] the improvement was evaluated to be marked. The number of subjects reporting worsening was higher in the group with more than 11 tender points [41 of 48, P < 0.01]. The self-reported change in severity was not related to the employment status.

DISCUSSION

The main finding of our study was that the development of concomitant somatic disorders which might account for the pain in fibromyalgia was very uncommon and that pain was generally reported to be worsening.

Our study thus does not support the previous finding of common development of other diseases in patients with primary fibromyalgia during a follow-up (1). The high proportion of thyroid diseases in that study might indicate that our patients might be more carefully examined before a diagnosis of primary fibromyalgia was established. The high proportion of psychiatric diagnoses in the Swedish study (1) might to some degree reflect a presumption of the pain to be of psychic origin. Slight depression is a common reaction to chronic pain and the psychiatric studies of fibromyalgia patients have not been conclusive (6,7).

To determine the natural history of fibromyalgia prospective studies are needed. These should include repeated registrations of symptoms and measures of functional capacity. A newly designed questionnaire 'The fibromyalgia impact questionnaire' might be helpful for such purposes (8).

REFERENCES

1. Forslind K, Frederiksson KE, Nived O. Does primary fibromyalgia exist? Br J Rheumatol 29: 368-70, 1989.

2. Wolfe F, Smythe HA, Yunus MB et al. The american college of rheumatology 1990 criteria for the classification of fibromyalgia. Arthritis Rheum 33: 160-72, 1990.

3. Gunvaldsen UA, Melbye IM. Langvarige muskelsmerter. Tidskr Nor Laegeforen 111: 1096-9, 1991.

4. Felson DT, Goldenberg DL. The natural history of fibromyalgia. Arthritis Rheum 29: 1522-6, 1986.

5. Jacobsen S, Danneskiold-Samsøe B. Inter-relations between clinical parameters and muscle function in patients with primary fibromyalgia. Clin Exp Rheumatol 7: 493-8, 1989.

6. Merskey H. Psychiatry and chronic pain. Can J Psychiatry 34: 329-36, 1989.

7. Boissevain MD, McCain GA. Toward an integrated understanding of fibromyalgia syndrome. II Psychological and phenemenological aspects. Pain 45: 239-48, 1991.

8. Burckhardt CS, Clark SR, Bennett RM. The fibromyalgia impact questionnaire: Development and validation. J Rheumatol 18: 728-33, 1991.

PERIPHERAL AND CENTRAL MECHANISMS IN MUSCLE PAIN

Muscle Biopsy in Fibromyalgia

Henrik Daa Schrøder
Asbjørn Mohr Drewes
Arne Andreasen

SUMMARY. Objective: The study was initiated in order to see if muscle biopsy is helpful as a diagnostic test in fibromyalgia.

Methods: Needle biopsies from the quadriceps muscle of the right thigh were obtained from 25 patients with fibromyalgia symptoms for a median of 11.5 years and from 10 healthy age matched controls. Biopsies from patients and controls were processed for conventional staining, immunohistochemical staining and enzyme histochemistry.

Henrik Daa Schrøder, MD dr. med. S.C., is affiliated with the Department of Pathology, Odense University Hospital, DK-5000, Denmark.

Asbjørn Mohr Drewes, MD, is affiliated with the Department of Rheumatology, Aalborg Hospital, DK-9000, Denmark.

Arne Andreasen, MD, is affiliated with the Department of Rheumatology, Århus University Hospital, DK-8000, Denmark.

[Haworth co-indexing entry note]: "Muscle Biopsy in Fibromyalgia." Schrøder, Henrik Daa, Asbjørn Mohr Drewes, and Arne Andreasen. Co-published simultaneously in the *Journal of Musculoskeletal Pain* (The Haworth Press, Inc.) Vol. 1, No. 3/4, 1993, pp. 165-169; and: *Musculoskeletal Pain, Myofascial Pain Syndrome, and the Fibromyalgia Syndrome* (ed: Søren Jacobsen, Bente Danneskiold-Samsøe, and Birger Lund) The Haworth Press, Inc., 1993, pp. 165-169. Multiple copies of this article/chapter may be purchased from The Haworth Document Delivery Center [1-800-3-HAWORTH; 9:00 a.m. - 5:00 p.m. (EST)].

Results: The light microscopy studies demonstrated type 2 atrophy in 23/25 patients and 0/10 controls (P < 0,01).

Conclusion: Type 2 atrophy is a frequent, but nonspecific change in striated muscle, often seen in response to inactivity. Muscle biopsy therefore can not be used as a diagnostic test in fibromyalgia, but is still recommended in unclear cases where primary myopathy is a differential diagnosis.

KEYWORDS. Striated muscle, fibromyalgia, histopathology

INTRODUCTION

One of the central questions, considering the biology behind fibromyalgia, is if muscle pain can be referred to morphological changes in the striated muscle. Subsequently such changes could be regarded a primary change or a phenomenon secondary to an abnormal CNS influence.

For this reason, there has been an interest in studying muscle morphology in fibromyalgic patients (1,2,3). Moreover, a demonstration of specific muscle changes could establish an objective finding to support the fibromyalgia diagnosis.

We have studied 2 series of muscle biopsies from fibromyalgia patients. The first (3) focused on inflammatory and reactive changes by light microscopically and on the ultrastructure. The main finding was scattered atrophic fibres with redundant basement lamina sleeves. Prompted by this observation, we designed the second study to characterize further the atrophic muscle fibres.

MATERIAL AND METHODS

Muscle biopsies from quadriceps muscle of the right thigh were obtained from 25 fibromyalgia patients fulfilling the ACR 90 criteria. All patients were females, median age 49.5 [range 35-48] years with symptoms for median 11.5 [range 2.5-32] years. Controls were 10 women, median age 40.5 [range 37-56] years. They were recruited from the patients' circle of acquaintances and their physical activity was within normal range. The biopsies were taken with the Biopty needle biopsy system. One biopsy from each patient was frozen and cut for enzyme and immunocytochemical staining. Sections were stained with H&E and mod-ified Trichrome stain.

The enzyme stainings performed were ATP-ase at pH 4.2, 4.6 and 9.3 and NADH-tetrazolium reductase according to Dubowitz (4). The immunocytochemical technique used was a 2-layered peroxidase method with thiocarbazol as chromogen. The primary antibody was an anti-neuronal cell adhesive molecule [N-CAM] antibody [clone 13, DAKO-Patts]. This antigen is present in muscle fibre membranes if the fibres are denervated.

The biopsies were read by two of the authors [HDS, AMD], who were blinded to diagnosis.

RESULTS

The biopsies in this series presented a slight to moderate fibre atrophy in 23 of 25 patients compared to no atrophy in the controls [P < 0.01].

Enzyme histochemistry demonstrated a selective type 2 fibre atrophy [Figure 1]. There was no fibre grouping and no changes in the staining pattern in the NADH-staining that could indicate myofibrillar disorganization.

The immunohistochemical stainings for N-CAM were invariably negative.

FIGURE 1. Type 2 atrophy recognized as small rounded or angular light fibres in striated muscle from a fibromyalgia patient, NADH-tetrazolium reductase.

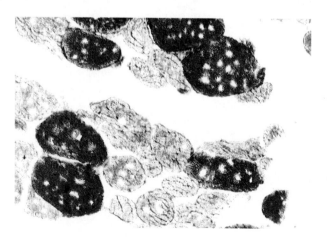

DISCUSSION

Several publications have dealt with morphological changes in muscle biopsies in patients with fibromyalgia (1,2,3,5,6,7). The changes described have been fibrillary disorganization presenting as motheaten fibres and indications of mitochondrial disorders, e.g., ragged red fibres (2,6) and structural mitochondrial changes (1). These observations could indicate a disturbed energy supply.

However, the observations were made in the heavily loaded trapezius muscle where similar changes were seen in the control groups.

Inflammatory changes have been sought for (1,3) but neither in routine stainings nor with immunohistochemical staining for inflammatory reactions (3) has evidence for inflammation been found.

The atrophy and basal lamina excess reported by Drewes et al. (3) are seen, e.g., in neurogenic atrophy. However, the present study could not confirm a neurogenic element in the fibromyalgia muscle changes.

The "rubberband" changes described in teased muscle fibre preparations (5) was initially thought to be coupled to fibromyalgia, but the basis for these changes has not been clarified and later studies have not found them (8).

The only established changes in fibromyalgia muscle appear to be the type 2 atrophy demonstrated in the present study in 23 of 25 patients and in the study of Kalyan-Raman et al. (1) in 7 of 12.

Type 2 atrophy is a nonspecific finding, but rather is frequently attributed to disuse of striated muscle. It must be concluded that muscle biopsy does not contribute to the diagnosis of fibromyalgia. However, it should still be considered when metabolic, inflammatory or neuropathic myopathies are important considerations within the differential diagnosis.

REFERENCES

1. Kalyan-Raman, UP, Kalyan-Raman, K, Yunus, MB and Masi, AT: Muscle Pathology in Primary Fibromyalgia Syndrome: A Light Microscopic, Histochemical and Ultrastructural Study. J Rheumatol, 11, 1984.

2. Henriksson et al.: Muscle biopsy findings of possible diagnostic importance in primary fibromyalgia (fibrositis, myofascial syndrome). Lancet, December 18: 1982.

3. Drewes, AM, Andreasen, A, Schrøder, HD, Høgsaa, B, Jennum P: Pathology of skeletal muscle in fibromyalgia: A histo-immuno-chemical and ultrastructural study. Br J Rheumatol. in press.

4. Dubowitz, V: Muscle Biopsy. A Practical Approach. Baillière Tindall, 1985, pp 20-40.

5. Bartels, EM, Danneskiold-Samsøe, B: Histological abnormalities in muscle from patients with certain types of fibrositis. Lancet: 155-7, 1986.

6. Bengtsson, A, Henriksson, K-G, and Larsson, J: Muscle Biopsy in Primary Fibromyalgia. Light-microscopical and Histochemical Findings. Scand J Rheumatol 15: 1-6, 1986.

7. Yunus, MB, Kalyan-Raman, UP, Masi, AT and Aldag, JT: Electron Microscopic Studies of Muscle Biopsy in Primary Fibromyalgia Syndrome: A Controlled and Blinded Study. J Rheumatol 16:97-101, 1989.

8. Bartels, EM, Nørregaard, J, Harreby, M, Amris, S, Danneskiold-Samsøe, B: Single cell morphology in fibromyalgia. Scand J Rheumatol suppl 94: 67, 1992.

Changes in Trapezius Muscle Structure in Fibromyalgia and Chronic Trapezius Myalgia

Rolf Lindman
Mats Hagberg
Ann Bengtsson
K-G. Henriksson
Lars-Eric Thornell

SUMMARY. Objectives. To reveal possible changes in muscle structure related to chronic myalgia.

Methods. Muscle biopsies from tender areas of the trapezius muscle, and from corresponding areas of healthy subjects were studied by electron microscopy.

Rolf Lindman, DDS, Mats Hagberg, MD, PhD, Professor, Ann Bengtsson, MD, PhD, Associate Professor, K-G. Henriksson, MD, PhD, Associate Professor, Lars-Eric Thornell, MD, PhD, Professor, are affiliated with the Department of Anatomy, University of Umeå, and the Department of Internal Medicine and the Neuromuscular Unit, University Hospital, Linköping and the National Institute of Occupational Health [NIOH], Division of Work and Environmental Physiology, Solna, Sweden.

Address correspondence to: Rolf Lindman, Department of Anatomy, University of Umeå, S-901 87 Umeå, Sweden.

The present work has been supported by grants from the Swedish Medical Research Council [12X-3934 and 24X-6874 and 02647], the Swedish Work Environment Fund [84-957 and 81-0173], the Swedish Dental Society and the Medical Faculty of Umeå University.

[Haworth co-indexing entry note]: "Changes in Trapezius Muscle Structure in Fibromyalgia and Chronic Trapezius Myalgia." Lindman, Rolf et al. Co-published simultaneously in the *Journal of Musculoskeletal Pain* (The Haworth Press, Inc.) Vol. 1, No. 3/4, 1993, pp. 171-176; and: *Musculoskeletal Pain, Myofascial Pain Syndrome, and the Fibromyalgia Syndrome* (ed: Søren Jacobsen, Bente Danneskiold-Samsøe, and Birger Lund) The Haworth Press, Inc., 1993, pp. 171-176. Multiple copies of this article/chapter may be purchased from The Haworth Document Delivery Center [1-800-3-HAWORTH; 9:00 a.m. - 5:00 p.m. (EST)].

Results. Fibres with an aberrant myofibrillar structure and an altered distribution and structure of the mitochondria and capillaries with altered endothelial structure were observed.

Conclusions. The aberrant myofibrillar structure might correspond to the moth-eaten and the ragged-red fibres seen in light microscopy. The capillary changes could be related to disturbances in muscle microcirculation.

KEYWORDS. Fibromyalgia, chronic trapezius myalgia, ultrastructure

INTRODUCTION

Different models of possible pathophysiological mechanisms of fibromyalgia and chronic neck-shoulder myalgia exist. It is quite possible that chronic myalgia is caused by a combination of activating and modulating peripheral and central factors (1,2). In fibromyalgia and work related neck-shoulder myalgia disturbed muscle microcirculation and/or metabolism are thought to be of importance for the development of myalgia (2-6). Fibres with a special appearance in light microscopy, so called moth-eaten and ragged-red fibres, are found in the trapezius muscle in both disorders and have been proposed to be related to localized hypoxia or ischemia (4,5,7). As ischemia has been reported to cause ultrastructural changes in limb muscles (8) biopsies from the trapezius muscle in patients with fibromyalgia and neck-shoulder myalgia have been analysed by electron microscopy and morphometry. Samples from healthy subjects were also analysed.

MATERIALS AND METHODS

Biopsies from nine patients fulfilling the ACR criteria for fibromyalgia (9) and five patients with established work related trapezius myalgia were studied. All were females and five healthy symptom-free females served as controls.

The *fibromyalgia* patients had a mean age of 41 years and had symptoms for more than 2 years. The patients with *work related neck-shoulder myalgia* had a mean age of 45 years and had symptoms for at least 2 years. The pain was localized to the descending portion of the trapezius muscle. The *healthy females* had a mean age of 39 years and no history of long-lasting musculoskeletal pains.

Muscle biopsies were obtained from tender areas, using an open surgical approach, in the descending portion of the trapezius muscle from the patients and from corresponding areas in the healthy subjects. The samples were processed for electron microscopy according to standardized methods. The muscle fibre and capillary structure were studied on cross-sections.

RESULTS

Capillary structure. Irregularities in the outline of the capillary lumen, electron lucent vacuoles and disrupted mitochondria within the endothelium were randomly present in all three groups. The most prominent abnormal finding was alterations in the endothelium of the capillaries, ranging from an increased cytoplasmic volume and translucency to a complete derangement of the endothelium [Figure 1]. The changes were present in all fibromyalgia patients and all healthy subjects; above 10 per cent in five of the patients whereas none of the healthy subjects had that many deranged capillaries. In the patients with trapezius myalgia three showed no changes, the other two below ten per cent.

Muscle fibre structure. Besides normal sized fibres showing a typical

FIGURE 1. Cross-sections of a capillary from a tender point of the trapezius muscle of patients with fibromyalgia. The capillary endothelium shows a deranged structure with an increased volume and transluscency [arrow]. Note the intact endothelial cell adjacent to the deranged one.

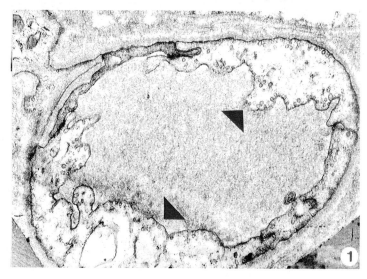

fibrillar pattern of the myofibrils, large fibres with an aberrant myofibrillar structure were observed. Focal streaming of the Z-disc was apparent. The mitochondria were unevenly distributed within the fibre and subsarcolemmal accumulation of mitochondria was frequent [Figure 2]. No mitochondria were found in the area of Z-disc streaming. These fibres were found in both the healthy and myalgic muscles.

Small sized fibres showing aberrant mitochondria with crystalline inclusions were occasionally observed. The mitochondria were often accumulated beneath the sarcolemma or present between myofibrils. Lipofuscin granules were seen and the amount of myofibrillar material seemed to be reduced [Figure 3]. These fibres were only found in the patients.

DISCUSSION

The observed alterations in the capillary endothelium are similar to the observations by Gidlöf et al. (8) in human limb muscles after tourni-

FIGURE 2. Moth-eaten and normal fibres in a cross section of the trapezius muscle showing the aberrant myofibrillar pattern of a moth-eaten fibre (a). In a higher magnification, Z disc streaming is shown (b), and subsarcolemmal accumulation of mitochondria.

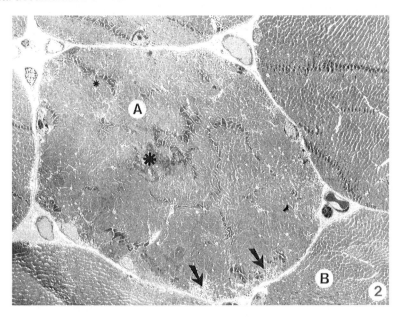

FIGURE 3. A cross section of a ragged-red fibre showing large and abnormal mitochondria in the subsarcolemmal region.

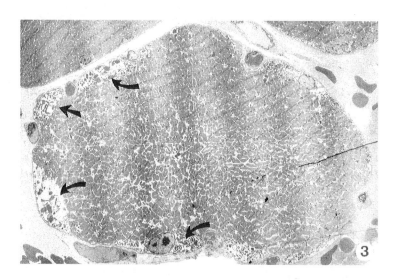

quet induced ischemia. The reason for the architectural derangements of the capillaries in the trapezius muscle is not readily explained but it might be associated with a disturbed microcirculation, localized hypoxia or ischemia.

A relationship between the aberrant myofibrillar pattern, Z-streaming and an abnormal distribution of mitochondria could be the explanation for the moth-eaten appearance of large fibres seen in light microscopy. The small sized fibres with an accumulation of, and abnormal mitochondria, are probably identical to the ragged-red fibres.

Conclusively, the present findings might be a consequence of a disturbed microcirculation and to focal fibre overload in the healthy as well as in the myalgic trapezius muscle. Quantitative analyses of these findings are in progress to determine their possible relation to myalgia.

REFERENCES

1. Edwards RHT: Hypotheses of peripheral and central factors underlying occupational muscle pain and injury. Eur J Appl Physiol 57: 275-281, 1988.

2. Henriksson KG, Bengtsson A: Fibromyalgia–a clinical entity? Can J Physiol Pharmacol 69: 672-677, 1991.

3. Hagberg M: Shoulder Pain–Pathogenesis, Grune Clinical Concepts in Regional Musculoskeletal Illness. Edited by NM Hadler. Statton Inc, New York, 1987, pp. 191-200.

4. Larsson S-E, Bengtsson A, Bodegård L, Henriksson K-G, Larsson J: Muscle changes in work-related chronic myalgia. Acta Orthop Scand 59: 552-556, 1988.

5. Larsson S-E, Bodegård L, Henriksson K-G, Öberg P-A: Chronic trapezius myalgia: morphology and blood flow in 17 patients. Acta Orthop Scand 61: 394-399, 1990.

6. Lindman R, Hagberg M, Ängqvist K-A, Söderlund K, Hultman E, Thornell L-E: Changes in muscle morphology in chronic trapezius myalgia. Scand J Work Environ Health 17: 347-355, 1991.

7. Bengtsson A, Henriksson K-G, Larsson J: Muscle biopsy in primary fibromyalgia. Light microscopical and histochemical findings. Scand J Rheum 15: 1-6, 1986.

8. Gidlöf A, Lewis DH, Hammarsen F: The effect of prolonged ischemia of human skeletal muscle capillaries. A morphometric analysis. Int J Microcirc Clin Exp 7: 67-86, 1987.

9. Wolfe F, Smythe HA, Yunus MB, Bennett RM, Bombardier C, Goldenberg DL, Tugwell P, Campbell SM, Abeles M, Clark P: The American College of Rheumatology 1990 criteria for the classification of fibromyalgia. Report of the Multicenter Criteria Committee. Arthritis Rheum 33: 160-172, 1990.

Cerebral Event Related Potentials
and Heat Pain Thresholds
in Fibromyalgia Syndrome

Gerald Granges
Stephen J. Gibson
Geoffrey O. Littlejohn
Robert D. Helme

SUMMARY. Objectives: To assess the pain threshold to heat and the subsequent event related cerebral evoked potential in patients with fibromyalgia and controls.

Methods: Eleven females with fibromyalgia [mean age 28.3 years] and 11 subjects without symptoms or signs of fibromyalgia

Gerald Granges, MD, Research Fellow in Rheumatology, Rheumatology Unit, Monash Medical Center, Clayton, Victoria 3168, Australia.

Stephen J. Gibson, PhD, is Senior Research Fellow, National Research Institute of Gerontology and Geriatric Medicine, North West Hospital, Mount Royal Campus, Poplar Road, Parkville, Victoria 3052, Australia.

Geoffrey O. Littlejohn, MBBS [Hons], MD, MPH, FRACP, FACRM, is Head of Rheumatology, Monash Medical Center, and Senior Lecturer in Medicine, Monash University, Rheumatology Unit, Monash Medical Center, Clayton, Victoria 3168, Australia.

Robert D. Helme, MBBS, PhD, FRACP, is Professor and Director of National Research Institute of Gerontology and Geriatric Medicine, North West Hospital, Mount Royal Campus, Poplar Road, Parkville, Victoria 3052, Australia.

Address correspondence to: Dr Geoff Littlejohn, Rheumatology Department, Monash Medical Centre, 246 Clayton Road, Clayton, Victoria 3168, Australia.

[Haworth co-indexing entry note]: "Cerebral Event Related Potentials and Heat Pain Thresholds in Fibromyalgia Syndrome." Granges, Gerald et al. Co-published simultaneously in the *Journal of Musculoskeletal Pain* (The Haworth Press, Inc.) Vol. 1, No. 3/4, 1993, pp. 177-184; and: *Musculoskeletal Pain, Myofascial Pain Syndrome, and the Fibromyalgia Syndrome* (ed: Søren Jacobsen, Bente Danneskiold-Samsøe, and Birger Lund) The Haworth Press, Inc., 1993, pp. 177-184. Multiple copies of this article/chapter may be purchased from The Haworth Document Delivery Center [1-800-3-HAWORTH; 9:00 a.m. - 5:00 p.m. (EST)].

177

[mean age 26.6 years] were identified. Using CO_2 laser stimulation on the dorsum of both hands the heat pain threshold was established. Following stimulation with 1 1/2 times of this threshold the event-related electroencephalogram was recorded.

Results: Patients with fibromyalgia [FS] had the same detection threshold using CO_2 laser heat stimulation as controls but pain threshold was significantly reduced. The latency between the onset of the painful heat stimulus and the CNS evoked response was the same in FS subjects and controls, however, FS subjects displayed significant change in peak-to-peak amplitude of the event related CNS evoked response. There was a strong association between neurogenic flare response and the nociceptor evoked cerebral response.

Conclusions: This study provides further evidence of an altered pain threshold to a variety of noxious modalities in FS implying a major role for the polymodal nociceptors in the clinical expression of this syndrome.

KEYWORDS. Fibromyalgia, fibrositis, pain threshold, event related EEG

INTRODUCTION

Fibromyalgia syndrome [FS] has characteristic symptoms and abnormal tenderness in predictable locations. Quantitative studies have shown a lowered pain threshold to mechanical pressure at the tender point sites as well as at other sites (1-4).

Primary afferent C and A-delta fibres with polymodal nociceptors play a major role in the transmission of pain, including mechanically induced pain, to the central nervous system. Stimulation of these fibres also induces neurogenic inflammation, i.e., flare and plasma extravasation in muscle and skin. We have previously shown an increased neurogenic flare response following noxious mechanical and chemical stimulation in FS patients, as well as a reduced chemical threshold for flare induction (5). It was suggested that many of the symptoms of FS, including the pain, local swelling, hyperalgesia and response to modulating factors, may result from a heightened activation of primary afferent fibres with poly modal nociceptors. Such change in the polymodal nociceptor function would be expected to affect response to chemical, mechanical and also thermal modalities to noxious stimulation. However, there has been no previous examination of thermal pain thresholds in fibromyalgia subjects.

Recent evidence indicates that the central nervous system might play an important role in FS. Abnormal sleep, abnormal reaction to stress and abnormalities in the metabolism of various neuropeptides and other transmitters have been noted (6,7). To date there has been no direct investigation of central nervous system processing of nociceptive input in patients with FS. The aim of the present study was to examine heat pain thresholds and nociceptor evoked response following noxious carbon dioxide laser thermal stimulation in control subjects and in patients suffering from FS .

We used cerebral event-related potentials to document their response. This nociceptive evoked response [NER] is thought to reflect secondary processing of noxious input and is thought to be elicited without the need for complex evaluation of attentional, perceptional or cognitive processes. It is generally accepted that the NER represents a physical correlate of the integrated CNS processing which underlies the perception of pain (8). We thus evaluated the severity of FS pain, the number of tender points, the neurogenic flare response and mechanical pain sensitivity and compared these variables to the heat pain threshold and NER responses.

METHODS

Eleven female FS patients fulfilling ACR criteria for fibromyalgia (2) and followed by the same rheumatologist [GL] for at least 12 months were studied. Eleven age and sex matched control volunteers were also examined. All controls were pain free at the time of testing and had no previous history of musculoskeletal pain. The two patients on regular medications [paracetamol and temazepam] ceased these 24 hours prior to study.

All 18 tender points and 4 control points were evaluated by algometry using a 0 to 11 kilogram dolorimeter (9). A painful sensation of pressure of less than 4 kilograms per square centimetre denoted a point to be labelled as a "tender point." A total myalgic score was computed based on the sum of the pressure values at the 18 tender points and 4 control sites. A structured interview was conducted to elicit information on the characteristic symptoms of the FS including evaluation of severity of pain and fatigue [10 cm visual analogue scale], constancy of pain [ordinal scale ranging from "always present" to "less than once a month"], number of painful regions [cervical, thoracic, lumbar, arms, legs], presence or absence of non-restorative sleep, subjective swelling and paraesthesia. Duration and severity of morning stiffness was coded on a 4 point ordinal scale. Grip strength below 300 mm Hg and skin fold tenderness over the mid-dorsal back and both limbs was noted (3). The scores of all of these measures were then combined to provide a pseudo-interval scale of symptom severity, without other weighting of the data. Mechanically-induced neurogenic flares were also evaluated. The latter was induced by firm pressure with a swab stick over the upper thoracic spine with the maximum width at 2 minutes in millimetres being the end point (3).

After obtaining informed consent the subjects were seated in a comfortable chair in a temperature controlled room shielded against electrical and acoustical interference. Closed circuit television monitored the subject and a two way intercom allowed for verbal communication. A CO_2 laser of 10.6 micrometre wave length, situated in an adjoining room, was used to deliver radiant heat pulses 5 millimetres in diameter and of 33 milliseconds duration. This stimulation is believed to be relatively selective for A-delta and C nociceptor fibres. The laser pulse was directed into the subject test room and onto the dorsal surface of either the right or left hand. All subjects were familiarised with the threshold determination procedures and exposed to the thermal stimulus at several intensities prior to formal testing. Detection and pain threshold were determined using the double staircase procedures which are felt to be the most valid for this study design (8).

After threshold determination, a block of 36 stimuli were presented with a randomised interval of between 20 and 40 seconds and at pseudo-random intensities, either at pain or 1.5 times pain threshold. Subjects were instructed to move their hands about 3 seconds after each stimulus in order to minimise habituation or receptor fatigue. Each stimulus was rated on an 8 item word descriptive scale varying from "just noticeable" through "excruciating." Word descriptors included words representing general tactile sensation such as "tingling, touching, warm" and noxious sensation such as "pricking, stinging, burning."

Following each laser stimulation, NER segments of 100 milliseconds were recorded in a modification of standard practice. Measures of heat latency, and peak-to-peak amplitude we calculated for each major wave form component within the average NER. All computer derived calculations were checked visually for accuracy.

Statistical analysis included univariant t-test, MANOVA, univariant ANOVA and Pearson's correlation coefficient (8).

RESULTS

In one control and one FS subject the intensity of stimulation required for threshold report of pain exceeded our safety guidelines which were set at 30 watts. These subjects were excluded from further testing and analysis. Descriptive information on the remaining 20 patients and control

TABLE 1. Descriptive and clinical Information for subjects with fibromyalgia syndrome [n = 10] and pain free control volunteers [n = 10]. Values refer to mean [+/− SEM].

	Fibromyalgia Patients	Control Subjects	p value
Age [years]	28.3 [2.6]	26.6 [2.1]	0.5601
VAS mood [0-10]	3.6 [0.8]	3.8 [0.6]	0.7806
Pain Duration [months]	74.4 [15.4]	0.0 [0.0]	-
Symptom score	10.8 [1.4]	0.2 [0.1]	0.0001
Number Tender Points	13.4 [1.5]	3.6 [1.0]	0.0001
Total Myalgic Score	58.3[5.1]	103.2[6.7]	0.0001
Control Myalgic Score	19.8[2.3]	32.1[2.9]	0.0037
Pain Descriptor	4.3[0.5]	0.0[0.0]	-
VAS[pain]	3.8[0.8]	0.0[0.0]	-

subjects is provided in Table 1. The FS subjects' mean duration of clinical pain was 74 months with a VAS pain score of 3.8 and a corresponding rating of moderate pain on the word descriptor scale. The total myalgic score and the control region myalgic score was significantly lower in the FS patients. After statistical evaluation, no difference was found between right and left side dependent variables and therefore the data from right and left side was combined prior to undertaking analysis of variance.

The mean width of mechanically induced neurogenic flare was significantly increased in FS subjects. The mean detection threshold and pain threshold values in response to CO_2 laser stimulation are shown in Table 2. Detection threshold was similar in both groups but FS subjects exhibited a

TABLE 2. Mean [+/− SEM] detection and pain threshold, flare response and nociceptive evoked response amplitude, latency and percentage of stimuli classified as noxious following 1.5 pain threshold CO_2 laser stimulation, in patients with fibromyalgia syndrome and control volunteers.

	Fibromyalgia Patients [n=20]	Control Subjects [n=20]
Detection Threshold [watts]	5.0 [1.0]	5.1 [2.0]
Pain Threshold [watts]	19.1 [3.0]	12.6 [3.0] *
Neurogenic Flare Response [mms]	16.5 [1.4]	7.2 [0.5] **
Latency N270 [msecs]	267.2 [5.4]	272.5 [6.7]
Latency P370 [msecs]	364.9 [6.6]	368.7 [5.8]
NER Amplitude [volts]	50.5 [3.1]	31.4 [1.8]**
Stimuli rated "pricking" or "stinging"	89.5%	92.1%

**Difference between groups, p < 0.0001

significant reduction in pain threshold intensity when compared to controls.

The NER was characterized by a small negative peak at approximately 270 milliseconds post noxious stimulation and a high amplitude positive peak at 370 milliseconds. There was no difference between the stimulus to onset or stimulus to positive peak between FS subjects and controls. However, the peak-to-peak amplitude of the nociceptor evoked response was significantly increased in subjects with FS. This occurred despite the fact that the intensity of stimulation was actually lower in the FS subjects. Similar numbers of subjects in each group rated the stimulus in descriptive terms as noxious.

Correlation between the clinical characteristics of FS and the NER, the neurogenic flare and threshold measures were examined. The severity of FS, as indexed by the symptom score, visual analogue scale ratings and particularly the mechanical pain increase flare size was also significantly associated with higher amplitude nociceptor evoked responses and a lower thermal pain threshold [P < 0.001]. Finally, as might be expected, the intensity of clinical pain, symptom score and degree of mechanical sensitivity at tender points were significantly inter-related [P < 0.001].

DISCUSSION

This study used heat stimuli delivered in a fashion which was unknown to the examined patient to stimulate poly modal C and A-delta fibres on the back of their hands. The evoked cortical response was evaluated and that component which related to rapid transmission via the A delta fibres alone was analysed. Because latency between stimulus onset and EEG response was the same in FS patients and control subjects we can conclude that the A-delta primary afferent pathways in patients with FS are not structurally altered.

The detection threshold for the thermal stimulus was the same in FS subjects and controls. However, FS subjects had marked lowering of noxious thermal stimulus induced pain threshold and furthermore had markedly significant change in the peak-to-peak amplitude of the CNS evoked response to that stimulus.

There was extremely close association between the clinical features of FS, both symptoms and those which relate to pain threshold to pressure, and the pain threshold to heat and the associated NER response. The phenomenon which is thought to be related to peripheral nociceptor mechanisms, i.e., the neurogenic flare, correlated strongly with the change in thermally induced pain threshold and the NER amplitudes. This is suggestive of pre-existing sensitisation of small peripheral myelinated pain fibres in FS, prior to their stimulation with the thermal stimulus. It is also possible, however, that there is an additional abnormal interpretation of thermal nociceptor stimuli at central levels.

This study provides additional evidence for an altered pain threshold to a variety of noxious sensory stimuli in FS, suggesting sensitization of the poly modal nociceptors as a mediating factor. It is likely that a number of the clinical features of FS relate to heightened activity of peripheral nociceptors. Although the cause for this is not clear, the hypothesis of central pain modulation is consistent with these findings.

REFERENCES

1. Yunus M, Masi AT and Aldag JC: A controlled study of primary fibromyalgia syndrome: Clinical features and association with other functional syndromes. J Rheumatol 16 (supplement 19): 62-71, 1989.

2. Wolfe F, Smythe HA, Yunus MB et al.: The American College of Rheumatology 1990 criteria for the classification of fibromyalgia: Report of the multicenter criteria committee. Arthritis Rheum 33: 160-172, 1990.

3. Granges G, Littlejohn GO: A comparative study of clinical signs in fibromyalgia/fibrositis syndrome, normal and exercising subjects. J Rheumatol 20: 1993 (In press).

4. Quimby LG, Block SR, Gratwick GM: Fibromyalgia; generalised pain intolerance and manifold symptom reporting. J Rheumatol 15: 1264-1270, 1988.

5. Littlejohn GO, Weinstein C, Helme RD: Increased neurogenic inflammation in fibrositis syndrome. J Rheumatol 14: 1022-1025, 1987.

6. Russell IJ, Vipraio GA, Morgan WM, Bowden CL: Is there a metabolic basis for the fibrositis syndrome? Am J Med 81: 50-54, 1986.

7. Vaeroy H, Sakurada T, Forre O, Kass E, Terenius L: Modulation of pain in fibromyalgia: cerebrospinal fluid (CSF) investigation of pain related neuropeptides with special reference to calcitonin gene related peptide (CGRP). J Rheumatol 16: 94-97, 1989.

8. Gibson SJ, Le Vasseur SA, Helme RD: Cerebral event-related responses induced by CO_2 laser stimulation in subjects suffering from cervico-brachial pain syndrome. Pain 47: 173-182, 1991.

9. Fischer AA: Pressure algometry over normal muscles, standard values, validity and reproducibility of pressure threshold. Pain 30: 115-126, 1987.

Psychogenic Motor Unit Activity: A Possible Muscle Injury Mechanism Studied in a Healthy Subject

Morten Wærsted
Torsten Eken
Rolf H. Westgaard

SUMMARY. Objectives: To investigate motor unit firing patterns responsible for prolonged psychogenic muscle activation.

Methods: Integrated surface electromyography [EMG] and single motor unit EMG were recorded from the upper left trapezius muscle of a physically inactive healthy subject solving a reaction time task of 10 min duration.

Results: A stable psychogenic tension representing approximately 0.5% of maximal surface EMG activity was demonstrated, and a single motor unit firing continuously at a median rate of 11 Hz was followed for the full task duration.

Morten Wærsted, MD, is affiliated with the National Institute of Occupational Health, Department of Physiology, Oslo, Norway.

Torsten Eken, MD, is affiliated with the Institute of Neurophysiology, University of Oslo, Oslo, Norway.

Rolf H. Westgaard, PhD, is Professor, Division of Organization and Work Science, The Norwegian Institute of Technology, Trondheim, Norway.

Address correspondence to: Morten Wærsted, National Institute of Occupational Health, Department of Physiology, P.O. Box 8149 Dep, N-0033 Oslo, Norway.

[Haworth co-indexing entry note]: "Psychogenic Motor Unit Activity: A Possible Muscle Injury Mechanism Studied in a Healthy Subject." Wærsted, Morten, Torsten Eken, and Rolf H. Westgaard. Co-published simultaneously in the *Journal of Musculoskeletal Pain* (The Haworth Press, Inc.) Vol. 1, No. 3/4, 1993, pp. 185-190; and: *Musculoskeletal Pain, Myofascial Pain Syndrome, and the Fibromyalgia Syndrome* (ed: Søren Jacobsen, Bente Danneskiold-Samsøe, and Birger Lund) The Haworth Press, Inc., 1993, pp. 185-190. Multiple copies of this article/chapter may be purchased from The Haworth Document Delivery Center [1-800-3-HAWORTH; 9:00 a.m. - 5:00 p.m. (EST)].

185

Conclusions: The observed continuous firing pattern is proposed as a possible injury mechanism in myofascial pain syndrome, if it occurs repeatedly in a small pool of motor units.

KEYWORDS. Electromyography, single motor unit, recruitment

INTRODUCTION

It has long been known that purely psychological influences may provoke muscle activity as identified through surface electromyography [EMG] (1,2). More recently, it has been documented that 'psychogenic' muscle tension provoked in sedentary work tasks with low postural and other physical demands is characterized by a low second-to-second variability in activity level (3,4,5). The activity level is low [typically below 5% of maximal voluntary activity] and may remain stable for several minutes, or only slowly changing, apart from occasional sudden shifts in tension level.

Studies of 'light' mechanical work have documented that continuous muscular activity in the shoulder, neck and upper extremities renders an increased risk of provoking musculoskeletal injuries, even at very low levels of the static load component (6,7). Based on this knowledge, the observed psychogenic muscle tension was hypothesized to be a potential pathway for the often observed link between psychosocial loads and musculoskeletal pain symptoms (8,9,10). The proposed mediating mechanism is repeated prolonged activity in a small pool of low-threshold motor units, where one possible outcome might be an overload of selected muscle fibres. To further investigate this hypothesis, surface gross EMG and single motor unit activity were recorded in parallel in an experimental work task known to readily provoke psychogenic activity in the trapezius muscles. This paper gives preliminary results obtained in one subject with a typical psychogenic tension response. Preliminary results of a pilot study on two other subjects have been presented elsewhere (11).

MATERIALS AND METHODS

One healthy male volunteer [age 22 years] gave an informed consent, and performed a visual display unit-based complex two-choice reaction-time task while sitting comfortably with adjusted chair height, arm rests and back rest. The work task lasted for ten minutes and consisted of single trials where graphical and alphanumerical information were presented simultaneously on the screen. The subject should as fast as possible press a 'yes' button or a 'no' button indicating match or mismatch between the two modes of information. Both buttons were operated by the fingers of the right hand.

Surface EMG and intramuscular EMG were recorded in parallel from the same area of the left upper trapezius muscle. Surface EMG was recorded with two electrodes of a custom made electrode assembly [electrode diameter 6 mm, inter-electrode distance 20 mm]. After amplification and band-pass filtering at 10 Hz and 1 kHz, the EMG signal was stored on a FM tape recorder [Kyowa RTP-600B, frequency response 0-5 kHz], and in the later analysis AD-converted at 2 kHz, rectified and integrated. The integrated EMG was calibrated in percent of EMG activity at maximal voluntary contraction [%MEMG].

Intramuscular EMG was recorded differentially between two 50 μm diameter teflon-coated platinum/iridium wires [A-M Systems, Inc.] twisted tightly together and inserted obliquely through the skin and into the muscle belly leaving the recording surfaces at approximately 10 mm depth. The raw EMG signal was amplified and band-pass filtered at 80 Hz and 32 kHz [Medelec MS6 mainframe with AA6 Mk III and PA 63] and stored on the FM tape recorder. In order to identify a motor unit firing episode the signal was further high-pass or low-pass filtered to increase the signal-to-noise ratio and fed into a spike discriminator [Slope/height Window Discriminator, Frederick Haer & Co.]. All identified spikes were visually controlled without the additional filtering of the signal, to verify that they had similar waveforms throughout the firing sequence and hence probably belonged to the same motor unit. When the discrimination of a motor unit was accepted, the interspike intervals were used to determine the instantaneous motor unit firing rate.

The subject was video filmed during the experiment in order to document movements or other behavior which related to surface or intramuscular EMG activities.

RESULTS

Figure 1 gives time plots of the full 10 min experiment. The upper panel shows integrated surface EMG with 1 s resolution, and the lower panel shows the simultaneous firing frequency of a single motor unit. The surface EMG activity increased from near zero up to approximately 0.5%

Figure 1. Simultaneous time plots of intergrated surface EMG [upper panel] and instantaneous firing frequency of a single motor unit [lower panel]. The reaction time task starts at time 0 s and ends at time 600 s. Surface EMG is calibrated in percent of maximal voluntary activity [%MEMG].

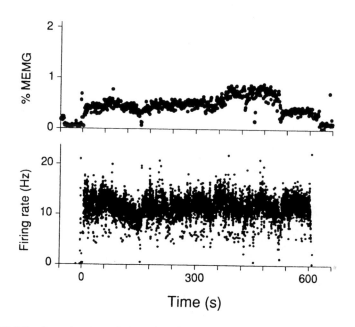

Time (s)

MEMG when the experimental task started, and remained elevated until the end of the task, when the EMG activity soon fell down to a resting level again. The EMG activity showed little second-to-second variability, giving an appearance typical of psychogenic muscle tension. The identified single motor unit [lower panel] started firing at the same time as the surface EMG activity increased at the beginning of the task, and continued firing with a median firing rate of approximately 10-12 Hz for the full duration of the experiment. Then, as the experimental task was finished [time 600 s], the motor unit stopped firing. The video film did not reveal movements which explained the changes in EMG activity.

DISCUSSION

The present results document that psychogenic trapezius muscle tension, characterized in surface EMG by low variability and low amplitude, may be based on prolonged activity in a few motor units, rather than frequent shifts of activity between different units in a large pool of motor units. One motor unit was followed in stable firing for the total duration of the surface EMG tension period. The same observation was made in one out of two subjects in a pilot study (11). In the other subject of the pilot study psychogenic tension was not observed during the experiment. Similar firing behavior with tonic motor unit activity throughout periods with psychogenic tension in surface EMG, is now being confirmed in several subjects in the full study (Wærsted, Eken and Westgaard unpublished).

The low amplitude level of the psychogenic trapezius muscle tension observed in physically inactive subjects (3,4,5) may be conceived as follows: in spite of the low total activity level of the muscle, a small pool of low-threshold motor units may be under a considerable load for prolonged periods of time. Such a recruitment pattern would be in agreement with the size principle, first proposed by Henneman (12), saying that motor units are recruited according to their size. Motor units with type I muscle fibres are predominant among the small, low-threshold units. If tension provoking factors are frequently present and the subject as a result repeatedly recruits the same motor units, the hypothesized overload might follow, possibly resulting in a metabolic crisis (13) and the appearance of type I fibres with abnormally large diameters (14) or "ragged-red fibres" which are interpreted as a sign of mitochondrial overload (15,16,17).

REFERENCES

1. Jacobson E: Action currents from muscular contractions during conscious processes. Science 66: 403, 1927.

2. Malmo RB: Psychological gradients and behavior. Psychol Bull 64: 225-234, 1965.

3. Westgaard RH, Bjørklund R: Generation of muscle tension additional to postural muscle load. Ergonomics 30: 911-923, 1987.

4. Wærsted M, Bjørklund RA, Westgaard RH: Shoulder muscle tension induced by two VDU-based tasks of different complexity. Ergonomics 34: 137-150, 1991.

5. Wærsted M, Bjørklund RA, Westgaard RH: The effect of motivation on shoulder muscle tension in attention-demanding tasks. Ergonomics (in press).

6. Aarås A: Postural load and the development of musculoskeletal illness (Dissertation). Scand J Rehab Med (suppl.18): 1-35, 1989.

7. Westgaard RH: Measurement and evaluation of postural load in occupational work situations. Eur J Appl Physiol 57: 291-304, 1988.

8. Ahles TA, Yunus MB, Riley SD, Bradley JM, Masi AT: Psychological factors associated with primary fibromyalgia syndrome. Arthritis Rheum 27: 1101-1106, 1984.

9. Kamwendo K, Linton SJ, Moritz U: Neck and shoulder disorders in medical secretaries. Part I. Pain prevalence and risk factors. Scand J Rehab Med 23: 127-133, 1991.

10. Westgaard RH, Jansen T: Individual and work related factors associated with symptoms of musculoskeletal complaints. II Different risk factors among sewing machine operators. Br J Ind Med 49: 154-162, 1992.

11. Wærsted M, Eken T, Westgaard RH: Single motor unit activity in psychogenic trapezius muscle tension: a pilot study. Arbete och Hälsa 1992:17: 319-321, 1992.

12. Henneman E: Relation between size of neurons and their susceptibility to discharge. Science 126: 1345-1347, 1957.

13. Edwards RHT: Hypotheses of peripheral and central mechanisms underlying occupational muscle pain and injury. Eur J Appl Physiol 57: 275-281, 1988.

14. Lindman R, Hagberg M, Ängqvist K-A, Söderlund K, Hultman E, Thornell L-E: Changes in muscle morphology in chronic trapezius myalgia. Scand J Work Environ Health 17: 347-355, 1991.

15. Bengtson A, Henriksson KG, Larsson S-E: Muscle biopsy in primary fibromyalgia. Light-microscopical and histochemical findings. Scand J Rheumatol 15: 1-6, 1986.

16. Larsson S-E, Bengtsson A, Bodegård L, Henriksson KG, Larsson J: Muscle changes in work-related chronic myalgia. Acta Orthop Scand 59: 552-556, 1988.

17. Larsson S-E, Bodegård L, Henriksson KG, Öberg PÅ: Chronic trapezius myalgia. Morphology and blood flow studied in 17 patients. Acta Orthop Scand 61: 394-398, 1990.

Fitness Characteristics
and Perceived Exertion
in Women with Fibromyalgia

Sharon R. Clark
Carol S. Burckhardt
Stephen Campbell
Connie O'Reilly
Robert M. Bennett

SUMMARY. Objectives: 1. Determine the aerobic fitness level of women with fibromyalgia; 2. Ascertain current exercise patterns; 3. Evaluate perceived exertion.

Methods: Ninety-five women were tested utilizing modified Balke treadmill protocol and Gould metabolic cart. Ratings of perceived exertion [RPE] were measured [Borg 1982] and weekly Training Index [TI] calculated [Hagberg 1986].

Results: 1. 78 [83%] were not engaging in regular exercise; 2. 61 [65%] were below average aerobic fitness; 3. 48 [51%] perceived themselves to be working at the expected intensity; 4. 28 [29%] were

---

Sharon R. Clark, PhD, Associate Professor of Nursing, and Assistant Professor of Medicine [Research], Carol S. Burckhardt, PhD, Associate Professor of Nursing, and Assistant Professor of Medicine [Research], Stephen Campbell, MD, Associate Professor of Medicine, Connie O'Reilly, PhD, Assistant Professor of Medicine [Research], Robert M. Bennett, MD, Professor of Medicine and Chairman, are all affiliated with the Division of Arthritis and Rheumatic Diseases, Oregon Health Sciences University, Portland, OR.

Address correspondence to: Dr. Sharon R. Clark, SN/AHI, Oregon Health Sciences University, Portland, OR 97201.

[Haworth co-indexing entry note]: "Fitness Characteristics and Perceived Exertion in Women with Fibromyalgia." Clark, Sharon R. et al. Co-published simultaneously in the *Journal of Musculoskeletal Pain* (The Haworth Press, Inc.) Vol. 1, No. 3/4, 1993, pp. 191-197; and: *Musculoskeletal Pain, Myofascial Pain Syndrome, and the Fibromyalgia Syndrome* (ed: Søren Jacobsen, Bente Danneskiold-Samsøe, and Birger Lund) The Haworth Press, Inc., 1993, pp. 191-197. Multiple copies of this article/chapter may be purchased from The Haworth Document Delivery Center [1-800-3-HAWORTH; 9:00 a.m. - 5:00 p.m. (EST)].

unable to reach anaerobic threshold but perceived themselves to be working at a higher than expected intensity.

Conclusions: 1. Most fibromyalgia patients are unfit and not engaging in regular exercise; 2. RPE is an appropriate method for monitoring intensity for only 50% of patients tested.

KEYWORDS. Fibromyalgia, fitness, perceived exertion

INTRODUCTION

Since the earlier work of Moldofsky (1) it has been recognized that endurance fitness is an important factor in ameliorating the symptoms of fibromyalgia. Despite this recognition, there remains a paucity of literature substantiating the fitness level or current exercise habits of patients with fibromyalgia. Additionally, it remains unknown whether patients with fibromyalgia perceive themselves to be working at an expected level of intensity when performing endurance exercise.

METHODS

We evaluated the current level of endurance ["aerobic"] fitness of 95 women with fibromyalgia by directly measuring oxygen consumption and carbon dioxide production while they exercised on a treadmill utilizing a modified Balke protocol [3.0 mph, grade increased 2.5% every 2 minutes]; a method previously determined appropriate for evaluating women with fibromyalgia (2). All women had been referred to a comprehensive fibromyalgia treatment program by a health care provider. All were evaluated by a board certified rheumatologist and found to meet the criteria of generalized aching with pain in all four quadrants; on examination they had at least 11 of 18 fibromyalgia tender points (3).

Endurance capacity was measured in a Human Performance Laboratory utilizing a Gould 9000 metabolic cart. Each subject was able to terminate the test at any time although was encouraged to continue as long as able; thus the test was a symptom limited exercise test to tolerance. Breath to breath analysis of oxygen consumption and carbon dioxide production was monitored as well as heart rate, workload, minutes of exercise and rating of perceived exertion. The maximum oxygen consumption [VO_2 max] was expressed as ml/kg/min.

The subject's rating of perceived exertion (4) was asked at the beginning of each new workload and at the end of testing. Functional and psychological evaluations were obtained using the Fibromyalgia Impact Questionnaire (5), Cornell Medical Index, MMPI, Diagnostic Interview schedule and Beck anxiety and depression inventories.

A current exercise pattern was determined by calculating a weekly training index [T.I.]: the product of *Intensity* [percent maximum heart rate] × *Duration* in minutes/sessions × *Frequency* [Number of exercise sessions/ week] (6). The recommended training index to attain health-related benefits is 42 (7).

The ventilatory flexion point also called the "anaerobic threshold" was evaluated by determining the point at which the workload and ventilation rate became nonlinear. Since this corresponded to the point at which CO_2/O_2, i.e., Respiratory Quotient [RQ], was greater than 1.0, the latter calculation was used.

RESULTS

All participants are women, age 20-70 years [$\bar{x}$ = 43.2]; the average number of years of symptoms was 9 and time since initial diagnosis of fibromyalgia 2.7 years.

Forty-six [48%] of the subjects reached an RER [analogous to the RQ] of at least 1.1 and thus met the criteria for a maximal test (8). Fitness categories were expressed as levels of poor, fair, average, good or excellent based on data from the American Heart Association (9); 61 [64%] were below average when compared to other women their age [see Figure 1].

The VO_2 max achieved ranged from 10.56 to 37.74 ml/kg/min, [$\bar{x}$ = 22.23]. The maximum workload achieved showed a wide range of variability [21-283] as did the number of minutes of exercise [2.2-27.4].

Sixty-one [64%] were not engaging in any form of regular exercise; seventeen [18%] were exercising occasionally but at a weekly training index < 42 thus inadequate to produce health related benefits. Only ten [11%] were exercising at a level considered adequate for endurance benefits.

Most [74%] exercised to a level at or above the ventilatory flexion point [A.T. group] and 47 [70%] reported an RPE consistent with sedentary women utilizing the modified Balke protocol in the same human performance laboratory. Sixteen [24%] reported working at an intensity less than expected while only 4 [0.6%] reported working at a higher than expected intensity. In contrast 28 women, [29%] were unable to reach A.T. [non A.T.

FIGURE 1. Exercise Testing on Apparently Healthy Individuals. Source: A Handbook for Physicians. American Heart Association [1975]

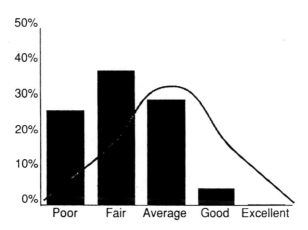

group] and 27 [96%] of this group perceived themselves to be working at a higher than expected intensity.

While there was no difference in the percentage from each group who were exercising, none of the non A.T. group were exercising at a sufficient intensity. While the two groups did not differ significantly in their VO_2 max, the A.T. group achieved a higher workload and were able to exercise for a longer period of time. The A.T. group had slightly more fibromyalgia tender points than the non A.T. group [16 of 18 vs. 14]. However the total myalgic score was not significantly different [see Table 1]. The groups did not differ on the fibromyalgia impact questionnaire or any of the psychological variables.

DISCUSSION

This work adds a large sample size to the current literature regarding the physical fitness and exercise habits of patients with fibromyalgia. Forty-eight percent of the women tested were able to reach an RER of at least 1.1, criteria for a maximal test, and thus afford confidence in the ability to evaluate fitness levels. The findings support previous work demonstrating that women with fibromyalgia are physically unfit (10,11) and not engaging in regular endurance exercise (12). Our finding that only 11% were currently exercising at a level sufficient to improve/sustain endurance is consistent with data for the general United States adult popu-

Table 1. Exercise and Pain Characteristics of Women with Fibromyalgia

Variable		Reached anaerobic threshold	Did not reach anaerobic threshold	p
Training Index	x̄	18.197	7.815	0.06
	SD	39.178	11.553	
VO2 max	x̄	21.655	23.86	0.12
	SD	5.286	6.34	
Workload	x̄	119.667	83.44	0.002
	SD	55.420	45.99	
Number of	x̄	16.17	14.6	0.03
Tender Points	SD	2.27	3.2	
Myalgic Score	x̄	36.69	32.75	0.12
	SD	9.55	11.53	

lation (13). Since endurance exercise is an important factor in the reduction of limitations associated with fibromyalgia, this finding should be considered unacceptable.

It has been proposed that women with fibromyalgia have an altered pain perception (14); a factor which would produce proneness to overestimate the peripheral sensations. We evaluated whether patients with fibromyalgia were able to perceive themselves to be working at an intensity consistent with their physiological exertion. The 12 point Borg RPE scale (4) [Table 2] has simple to understand verbal expressions that describe peripheral sensations, is commonly used, and has been shown to correlate perceived and physiologic exertion (15). We found that 50% of the women with fibromyalgia appropriately reported their exertion when compared to data from a population of normal, sedentary women; 34% overestimated their exertion. This finding supports work by Campbell et al. (16) that most fibromyalgia patients do not have altered peripheral sensations outside the tender point area.

Drop out from exercise in any population is high, often the result of doing "too much too soon" (17). Discovering a method for patients to self-monitor appropriate work intensity may reduce this rate. While our data support that most [66%] patients perceived their exertion below or within the range of sedentary normal women, they were working at 78% of maximum heart rate when they achieved A.T. While this level may be appropriate for persons with no adverse health problems, it is above that recommended for persons with underlying health conditions who desire

Table 2. Rating of Perceived Exertion

Rating	Description
0	Nothing
0.5	Very, very light (just noticeable)
1	Very light
2	Light (weak)
3	Moderate
4	Somewhat hard
5	Heavy (strong)
6	
7	Very heavy
8	
8	
10	Very, very heavy (almost max)

*modified from "Psychological bases of physical exertion" by G.A.V. Borg, 1982, *Medicine and Science in Sport and Exercise*, 14(5).

health benefits from exercise while simultaneously reducing the risk of adverse effects.

Despite the commonality of practice, comparisons with normal populations may not be appropriate for establishing criteria in *exercise prescriptions* for groups suffering from painful conditions. In order to apply the RPE for exercise prescription to patients with fibromyalgia, it is imperative that we establish normative data for this population.

REFERENCES

1. Moldofsky H, Scarisbrick P: Induction of neurasthenic musculoskeletal pain syndrome by selective sleep stage deprivation. Psychosom Med 38: 35-44, 1976.

2. Burckhardt CS, Clark SR, Padrick KP: Use of the modified Balke treadmill protocol for determining the aerobic capacity of women with fibromyalgia. Arthritis Care Res 2: 165-167, 1989.

3. Wolfe F, Smythe HA, Yunus MB, Bennett RM, Bombardier C, Goldenberg DL, Tugwell P, Campbell SM, Abeles M, Clark P, Fam AG, Farber SJ, Fiechtner JJ, Franklin CM, Gatter RA, Hamaty D, Lessard J, Lichtbroun AS, Masi AT, McCain GA, Reynolds WJ, Romano TJ, Russell IJ, Sheon RP: The American College of Rheumatology 1990 criteria for the classification of fibromyalgia: Report of the Multicenter Criteria Committee. Arthritis Rheum 33: 160-172, 1990.

4. Borg GAV: Psychophysical bases of perceived exertion. Medicine and Science in Sports and Exercise 14: 377-381, 1980.

5. Burckhardt CS, Clark SR, Bennett RM: The fibromyalgia impact questionnaire: development and validation. J Rheumatol 18: 728-733, 1991.

6. Hagberg JM: Central and peripheral adaptations to training in patients with coronary artery disease. in Biochemistry of Exercise VI 16: 267-277, 1986.

7. American College of Sports Medicine: The recommended quantity and quality of exercise for developing and maintaining cardiorespiratory and muscular fitness in healthy adults. Medicine and Science in Sports and Exercise 22: 265-274, 1990.

8. Astrand PO, Rodahl K: Textbook of Work Physiology: Physiological Bases for Exercise. McGraw-Hill, New York, 1986.

9. American Heart Association: Exercise Testing on Apparently Healthy Individuals: A Handbook for Physicians, 1975.

10. Bennett RM, Clark SR, Goldberg L, Nelson D, Bonafede RP, Porter J, Specht D: Aerobic fitness in the fibrositis syndrome: A controlled study of respiratory gas exchange and [133]xenon clearance from exercising muscle. Arthritis Rheum 32: 454-460, 1989.

11. Klug GA, McAuley E, Clark SR: Factors influencing the development and maintenance of aerobic fitness: lessons applicable to the fibrositis syndrome. J Rheumatol 16 (Suppl 19: 30-39), 1989.

12. McCain GA, Bell DA, Mai FM: A controlled study of the effects of a supervised cardiovascular fitness training program on the manifestations of primary fibromyalgia. Arthritis Rheum 31: 1135-1141, 1988.

13. Center for Disease Control: Progress toward achieving the 1990 national objectives for physical fitness and exercise. Morbidity and Mortality Weekly Report 38: 451-453, 1989.

14. Scudds RA, Rollman GB, Harth M, McCain GA: Pain perception and personality measures as discriminators in the classification of fibrositis. J Rheumatol 14: 563-569, 1987.

15. Birk TJ, Birk CA: Use of ratings or perceived exertion for exercise prescription. Sports Medicine 4: 1-8, 1987.

16. Campbell SM, Clark S, Tindall EA, Forehand ME, Bennett RM: Clinical characteristics of fibrositis. I. A "blinded," controlled study of symptoms and tender points. Arthritis Rheum 25: 817-824, 1983.

17. Dishman RK: Compliance/adherence in health-related exercise. Health Psychol 1: 237-267, 1982.

CLINICAL STUDIES–MYOFASCIAL PAIN AND FIBROMYALGIA

Quality of Life of Swedish Women with Fibromyalgia Syndrome, Rheumatoid Arthritis or Systemic Lupus Erythematosus

Carol S. Burckhardt
Birgitha Archenholtz
Kaisa Mannerkorpi
Anders Bjelle

SUMMARY. Objectives: This study sought to: 1. compare life quality of Swedish women with either fibromyalgia [FMS], rheumatoid arthritis [RA] or systemic lupus erythematosus [SLE] and 2. determine factors that predict life quality.

Methods: One hundred fifty age-matched women who met criteria for the above conditions filled out the following questionnaires: Quality of Life Scale [QOLS-S], McGill Pain Questionnaire-Short

[Haworth co-indexing entry note]: "Quality of Life of Swedish Women with Fibromyalgia Syndrome, Rheumatoid Arthritis or Systemic Lupus Erythematosus." Burckhardt, Carol S. et al. Co-published simultaneously in the *Journal of Musculoskeletal Pain* (The Haworth Press, Inc.) Vol. 1, No. 3/4, 1993, pp. 199-207; and: *Musculoskeletal Pain, Myofascial Pain Syndrome, and the Fibromyalgia Syndrome* (ed: Søren Jacobsen, Bente Danneskiold-Samsøe, and Birger Lund) The Haworth Press, Inc., 1993, pp. 199-207. Multiple copies of this article/chapter may be purchased from The Haworth Document Delivery Center [1-800-3-HAWORTH; 9:00 a.m. - 5:00 p.m. (EST)].

199

Form [MPQ-S], Rheumatology Attitudes Index [RAI], and the Arthritis Impact Measurement Scales [AIMS].

Results: The FMS group's mean on the QOLS-S total score and on individual items measuring health, relationships, and recreation were significantly lower. Depression and anxiety were the most significant predictors of quality of life in all groups.

Conclusions: Treatment of psychological distress has potential to impact life quality in all groups.

KEYWORDS. Quality of life, fibromyalgia, lupus, rheumatoid arthritis

Quality of life encompasses a broad spectrum of domains that includes health status, environment, economic resources, relationships, work, self enhancement, and leisure activities (1). In the rheumatology literature, quality of life instrumentation tends to be limited to the measurement of specific signs, symptoms and functional status. For example, the Auranofin Cooperating Group used the Health Assessment Questionnaire, Keitel Functional Test and Quality of Well-being Questionnaire; whereas, Morgan and his colleagues used the Arthritis Impact Measurement Scales [AIMS] (2-4).

Evidence exists, however, that persons with chronic diseases evaluate the quality of their lives on a much wider spectrum. Positive relationships, work, a sense of security, leisure activities and meaning in life are all important factors along with health and independence (5-7). So far few studies in rheumatology have focussed on measuring quality of life from this broader perspective. One, conducted in the United States, showed that women with fibromyalgia [FMS] perceived the quality of their lives to be lower than those with other rheumatic and non-rheumatic chronic diseases, including severe systemic diseases such as rheumatoid arthritis [RA], diabetes mellitus and chronic obstructive pulmonary disease (8).

The purposes of this study were to replicate the USA study with Swedish women with RA and FMS, to include a group of women with systemic lupus erythematosus [SLE] since this group was not included in the USA study, and to describe factors that predict quality of life in each of the groups.

PATIENTS AND METHODS

All participants were inpatients or outpatients who had been seen in a Swedish university-based rheumatology department during 1990-91. Criteria for selection included: a. female gender; b. age between 20 and 70 years; c. duration of disease longer than one year; and d. diagnostic criteria for the disease fulfilled (9-11).

The study design was descriptive and correlational. Patients were contacted by telephone and given information about the study. If they expressed interest, an appointment was made for them to come into the rheumatology clinic where one of the researchers administered a battery of tests including the following self-report instruments:

Quality of Life Scale [QOLS-S]. This questionnaire asks patients to rate their level of satisfaction on 16 items using a 7-point scale with higher being more satisfied. Derived originally from a scale developed by Flanagan, the scale has undergone extensive testing in chronic illness populations and has been translated and validated in a Swedish version (12-14).

Arthritis Impact Measurement Scales [AIMS]. The original version of this well-known instrument was used. Consisting of 9 subscales that can be further reduced to five components of lower extremity, upper extremity, social, psychological function and pain, each subscale can range from 0-10, with 10 meaning higher impact. Demographic characteristics of the participants were also obtained from the AIMS (1,15).

Rheumatology Attitudes Index [RAI]. This 15-item scale measures the patient's sense of control over the condition and feelings of helplessness that may result from the unpredictable nature of the rheumatic diseases (16,17). A higher score indicates a greater sense of control.

Short Form McGill Pain Questionnaire [SF-MPQ]. This instrument consists of 15 adjectives [11 sensory, 4 affective] taken from the large MPQ. These are rated on a scale from 0 = none to 3 = severe pain. The Present Pain Intensity Index [PPI] and the visual analog scale [VAS] are also included. Melzack's work indicates that the short form is as sensitive to differences due to treatment as the longer form and takes much less time to administer (18).

RESULTS

Characteristics of the sample are shown in Table 1. There were no significant differences between the groups on any of the demographic variables. The FMS group's mean disease duration was significantly lower. The means and standard deviations of the self-report questionnaires by patient group are shown in Table 2. There were no significant differences between the groups on the AIMS global impact score. However, RA group's AIMS lower extremity and upper extremity scores were significantly higher than the other two groups. The FMS group had significantly higher scores on AIMS pain, social, and psychological subscales as well as the SF-MPQ total score. Their

TABLE 1. Descriptive Characteristics of the Sample by Patient Group.

Variable	SLE	RA	FMS
Age (years)	43.5 (± 12.7)	44.9 (± 10.3)	45.7 (± 10.8)
Disease duration (years)	13.9 (± 10.2)	15.2 (± 7.7)	8.0 (± 6.5)*
Marital Status (% married)	48%	60%	60%
Education (% > 9 years)	68%	72%	56%
Income (% > $33,000)	45%	42%	58%
Employment (% employed at least part time)	48%	58%	64%

* $p < .05$

TABLE 2. Means and Standard Deviations of the Instruments.

Instrument	SLE	RA	FMS
RAI	48.2 (± 6.7)	49.9 (± 6.1)	44.8 (± 7.2)*
SF-MPQ	6.8 (± 6.5)	9.6 (± 8.3)	20.8 (± 10.1)*
AIMS - Lower	7.1 (± 6.4)	11.5 (± 6.3)*	8.0 (± 6.0)
AIMS - Upper	3.3 (± 3.0)	7.1 (± 2.5)**	4.7 (± 3.4)
AIMS - Social	3.8 (± 1.7)	3.7 (± 1.5)	5.2 (± 2.0)*
AIMS - Pain	4.2 (± 4.5)	6.0 (± 2.3)*	7.2 (± 1.9)*
AIMS - Psych	6.5 (± 4.5)	5.7 (± 3.0)	9.6 (± 4.1)*
AIMS - Global	3.9 (± 2.5)	4.7 (± 2.0)	5.6 (± 2.3)*
QOLS-S	86.0 (± 13.6)	83.4 (± 9.6)	77.6 (± 14.2)*

*$p < .05$ & **$p < .01$ indicate that the group was significantly different from at least one other group using the Tukey method of multiple comparison.

RAI score was significantly lower. The FMS group had a significantly lower QOLS-S total score and as shown in Figure 1 lower individual scores on health, interactions with relatives and close friends, participating in organizations, continuing to learn, socializing, and passive recreation. There were no significant differences between the RA and SLE patients. There were no significant associations between any of the demographic variables and the QOLS-S. Correlations between the RAI, SF-MPQ, AIMS and the QOLS-S are shown in Table 3. All variables with the exceptions of the SF-MPQ and AIMS upper extremity were correlated significantly with the QOLS-S at the .01 level or less. These variables along with disease duration were entered into a step-wise regression analysis. Four separate analyses were performed [Table 4]. In all four analyses, the AIMS psychological function subscale score was the best predictor of quality of life followed by the AIMS social and global impact subscales in the total sample, AIMS global impact and AIMS other [social and pain subscales] in the lupus group, AIMS social and lower extremity subscales in the RA group, and AIMS social, global impact, and pain in the FMS group.

CONCLUSIONS

Although all three groups were less than satisfied with their health and ability to engage in active recreation, in the other domains measured, the

FIGURE 1. Quality of Life Scale Item Means.

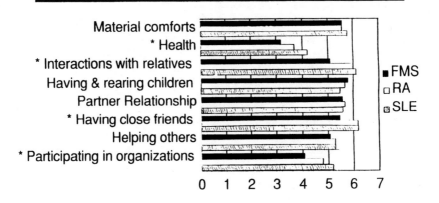

Quality of Life Scale Items

TABLE 3. Correlations Between the RAI, SF-MPQ, AIMS and QOLS-S.

Instrument	Total Sample	SLE	RA	FMS
RAI	.31***	.29*	.20	.28*
SF-MPQ	-.22	-.01	-.13	-.12
AIMS - Lower	-.22**	-.08	-.24	-.41**
AIMS - Upper	-.12	-.01	-.18	-.22
AIMS - Social	-.43***	-.25	-.39**	-.49***
AIMS - Pain	-.25**	-.21	-.08	-.14
AIMS - Psych	-.61***	-.63***	-.46***	-.58***
AIMS - Global	-.40***	-.41**	-.23	-.35**

* p < .05
** p < .01
*** p < .001

Swedish RA and SLE groups were at least somewhat satisfied. Their scores on the QOLS-S compare favorably with previous evidence from research on women with RA in the United States (8). The Swedish FMS group, on the other hand, was more dissatisfied on a wider range of quality of life domains, especially satisfaction with their health, relationships, and ability to participate in activities.

The strength of the AIMS psychological variable, a composite of depression and anxiety, to predict quality of life was striking. It is important to note that depression and anxiety were not limited to FMS patients. In fact, psychological distress was most predictive of quality of life in the SLE group. Further analysis of the correlations between the psychological variable and individual QOLS items showed that high psychological distress was strongly correlated with dissatisfaction with health, ability to socialize, and understanding self in all three groups. These findings are highly comparable to the earlier USA work. The strong negative relationship between psychological distress and quality of life points to the importance of treating depression and anxiety in Swedish patients with all three conditions if quality of life is to be enhanced.

TABLE 4. Stepwise Regression of Arthritis Impact Measurement Scales (AIMS), Rheumatology Attitudes Index (RAI), and Short Form McGill Pain Questionnaire (SF-MPQ) on the Quality of Life Scale (QOLS-S).

	R^2	F	p
Total Sample			
AIMS psychological	.31	43.34	.0000
AIMS global impact	.35	4.98	.0281
AIMS social	.36	1.94	.1673
Full Model	.38	5.28	.0000
FMS group			
AIMS psychological	.33	21.44	.0001
AIMS social	.47	8.38	.0070
AIMS global impact	.51	1.31	.2606
AIMS pain	.53	1.21	.2796
Full Model	.53	5.44	.0007
SLE group			
AIMS psychological	.42	29.41	.0000
AIMS global impact	.44	2.02	.1638
Full Model	.48	3.37	.0033
RA group			
AIMS psychological	.21	13.80	.0007
AIMS social	.32	6.86	.0125
AIMS lower extremity	.36	2.26	.1405
Full model	.39	2.54	.0182

AUTHOR NOTE

Carol S. Burckhardt, PhD, is Associate Professor of Mental Health Nursing, School of Nursing and Assistant Professor [Research], Division of Arthritis and Rheumatic Diseases, School of Medicine, Oregon Health Sciences University, Portland, OR, USA.

Birgitha Archenholtz is Occupational Therapist, Department of Rheumatology, Sahlgren University Hospital, Gothenburg University, Gothenburg, Sweden.

Kaisa Mannerkorpi is Physical Therapist, Department of Physiotherapy, Sahlgren University Hospital, Gothenburg University, Gothenburg, Sweden.

Anders Bjelle, MD, PhD, is Professor, Department of Rheumatology, Sahlgren University Hospital, Gothenburg University, Gothenburg, Sweden.

Address correspondence to: Carol S. Burckhardt, PhD, Department of Mental Health Nursing, Mail Code SNMH, Oregon Health Sciences University, Portland, OR 97201 USA.

The study was supported by the Swedish Society against Rheumatism and the Ragnar and Lisa Stensberg Fund.

REFERENCES

1. Mason JH, Anderson JJ, Meenan RF: A model of health status for rheumatoid arthritis. Arthritis Rheum 31:714-720, 1988.

2. Bell MJ, Bombardier C, Tugwell P: Measurement of functional status, quality of life, and utility in rheumatoid arthritis. Arthritis Rheum 33:591-601, 1990.

3. Bombardier C, Ware J, Russell IJ, Larson M, Chalmers A, Read JL: Auranofin therapy and quality of life in patients with rheumatoid arthritis: Results of a multicenter trial. Am J Med 81:565-578, 1986.

4. Morgan GJ: Quality of life in patients receiving auranofin therapy: Confirmation of efficacy using nontraditional health status measures. Scand J Rheumatol 63(suppl):29-35, 1986.

5. Burckhardt CS: The impact of arthritis on quality of life. Nurs Res 34:11-16, 1985.

6. Burckhardt CS: Quality of life for women with arthritis. Health Care Women Internat 9:229-238, 1988.

7. Hollandsworth JG: Evaluating the impact of medical treatment on the quality of life: a 5-year update. Sac Sc Med 26:425-434, 1988.

8. Burckhardt CS, Clark SK, Bennett RM: Fibromyalgia and quality of life: A comparative analysis. J Rheumatol (in press).

9. Arnett FC, Edworthy SM, Block DA et al.: The American Rheumatism Association 1987 revised criteria for the classification of rheumatoid arthritis. Arthritis Rheum 31:315-324, 1988.

10. Wolfe F, Smythe HA, Yunus MB et al.: The American College of Rheumatology 1990 criteria for the classification of fibromyalgia. Arthritis Rheum 33:160-172, 1990.

11. Tan EM, Chen AS, Fries JF et al.: The 1982 revised criteria for the classification of systemic lupus erythematosus. Arthritis Rheum 25:1271-1277, 1982.

12. Flanagan JC: A research approach to improving our quality of life. Am Psychol 33:138-147, 1978.

13. Burckhardt CS, Woods SL, Schultz AA, Ziebarth DM: Quality of life of adults with chronic illness: A psychometric study. Res Nur Health 12:347-354, 1989.

14. Burckhardt CS, Archenholtz B, Bjelle A: Measuring the quality of life of women with rheumatoid arthritis or systemic lupus erythematosus: A Swedish version of the Quality of Life Scale (QOLS). Scand J Rheumatol 21:190-195, 1992.

15. Meenan RF, Gertman PM, Mason JH: Measuring health status in arthritis: The arthritis impact measurement scales. Arthritis Rheum 23:146-152, 1980.

16. Nicassio PM, Wallston KA, Callahan LF, Herbert M, Pincus T: The measurement of helplessness in rheumatoid arthritis: the development of the Arthritis Helplessness Index. J Rheumatol 12:462-467, 1985.

17. Callahan L, Brooks RH, Pincus T: Further analysis of learned helplessness in rheumatoid arthritis using a "Rheumatology Attitudes Index." J Rheumatol 15:418-426, 1988.

18. Melzack R: The short-form McGill Pain Questionnaire. Pain 30:191-197, 1987.

Pain Experience, Psychological Functioning and Self-Reported Disability in Chronic Myofascial Pain and Fibromyalgia

Randy S. Roth
Jan E. Bachman

SUMMARY. Objectives: Psychological studies of myofascial pain and fibromyalgia typically compare these syndromes with other chronic pain conditions or combine them to ascertain psychopathological correlates. To determine differences between these groups, this study compared pain experience, disability and psychological functioning in myofascial pain and fibromyalgia.

Methods: Consecutive female patients, who presented to a university pain clinic and who were diagnosed with myofascial pain [N = 34] or fibromyalgia [N = 21], were assessed by psychometric testing before intervention.

Results: Myofascial pain was associated with traumatic onset and greater trait anxiety. Fibromyalgia patients reported greater severity

Randy S. Roth, PhD, is Lecturer, Departments of Anesthesiology and Physical Medicine and Rehabilitation, University of Michigan Medical Center.

Jan E. Bachman, PhD, is Staff Psychologist, Department of Anesthesiology, University of Michigan Medical Center.

Address correspondence to: Randy S. Roth, PhD, University of Michigan, Medical Center, Coordinated Chronic Pain Program, C233 Med Inn Building, Ann Arbor, MI 48109-0824.

[Haworth co-indexing entry note]: "Pain Experience, Psychological Functioning and Self-Reported Disability in Chronic Myofascial Pain and Fibromyalgia." Roth, Randy S., and Jan E. Bachman. Co-published simultaneously in the *Journal of Musculoskeletal Pain* (The Haworth Press, Inc.) Vol. 1, No. 3/4, 1993, pp. 209-216; and: *Musculoskeletal Pain, Myofascial Pain Syndrome, and the Fibromyalgia Syndrome* (ed: Søren Jacobsen, Bente Danneskiold-Samsøe, and Birger Lund) The Haworth Press, Inc., 1993, pp. 209-216. Multiple copies of this article/chapter may be purchased from The Haworth Document Delivery Center [1-800-3-HAWORTH; 9:00 a.m. - 5:00 p.m. (EST)].

of pain, more occupational disability and lower educational achievement. No differences were obtained on measures of sleep, fatigue, depression or personality functioning.

Conclusions: Myofascial pain and fibromyalgia patients are similar on most measures of psychological functioning although fibromyalgia appears to be more severe and disabling. Trauma may be particularly important in understanding the chronicity of myofascial pain.

KEYWORDS. Fibromyalgia, myofascial pain, psychology

INTRODUCTION

Interest in the contribution of psychological factors to myofascial pain and fibromyalgia has been long-standing and controversial (1). Early investigations of the "fibrositis syndrome," with which myofascial pain and fibromyalgia have been historically linked, ascribed causality to psychological processes by attributing fibrositis to psychogenic rheumatism (2) or hysteria (3). However, these studies failed to distinguish between myofascial pain and fibromyalgia patients, thus obscuring possible psychological correlates unique to each syndrome (4). Recently, diagnostic criteria have been established which differentiate the diffuse myalgias of fibromyalgia with their related tender points from the regional myofascial syndromes, that are characterized by the presence of trigger points which give rise to patterns of referred pain (5).

This new taxonomy has produced renewed interest in psychological contributions to the etiology and maintenance of chronic muscle pain (6,7). There are several reasons that explain the trend to associate musculoskeletal pain with emotional and behavioral disturbance. The pathophysiologic mechanisms that underlie chronic muscle pain remain obscure (8). In addition, the absence of positive radiographic and serologic findings to confirm a diagnosis makes clinical decision-making more difficult and the inference of physiologic impairment more suspect (1). The common belief in a stress-tension model of muscle pain (9), while still to be validated empirically (10), further strengthens the association of psychological processes with muscle pain. Finally, the psychological impairment described among chronic musculoskeletal pain patients may represent referral bias as most published accounts derive from tertiary care or specialty clinics that are likely to see a more chronic, disabled and psychologically complex population (11).

Recent studies go beyond notions of hysteria to reflect a more diverse view of psychological correlates of fibromyalgia and myofascial pain. For example, a psychophysiologic model has been proposed for both fibromyalgia (12) and myofascial pain (9) in which response to life stress results in sustained muscle tension leading to intractable pain. Consistent with this conceptualization has been evidence for the co-occurrence of these pain disorders with various psychosomatic illnesses (9,13). For myofascial pain an alternative perspective identifies psychological factors such as anxiety, depression or secondary gain as perpetuating factors that contribute to the maintenance of pain complaints rather than their cause (14). Concerning fibromyalgia, considerable controversy surrounds the contention that fibromyalgia be included within a spectrum of affective disorders (15). Empirical support of this view has been both favorable (16,17) and unfavorable (18,19). In contrast, it has been suggested that psychological factors play a limited role in understanding fibromyalgia pain, particularly for those patients with a premorbid psychiatric history (20).

Typically, psychological studies of fibromyalgia and myofascial pain compare these groups with other chronic pain conditions such as rheumatoid arthritis (20) and temporomandibular joint syndrome (21) or combine them to assess the incidence of psychopathology (22). No studies have directly compared fibromyalgia with myofascial pain patients to determine differences in pain experience and psychological functioning between these groups. Such data would be important for ascertaining psychological factors that may be particularly relevant to each of these chronic musculoskeletal disorders. To this end, the present study assessed pain experience, mood and personality factors, and self-reported disability for patients with these diagnoses.

MATERIALS AND METHODS

The subject pool consisted of consecutive female patients [with a primary complaint of intractable musculoskeletal pain] who were referred to a university hospital pain clinic over a one year period. Female patients were selected in order to control for gender effects in view of the high prevalence of females among fibromyalgia patients (5). Prior to initial evaluation and intervention, each subject completed the following psychometric battery: McGill Pain Questionnaire (23), Beck Depression Inventory (24), Spielberger State-Trait Anxiety Inventory (25), Brief Symptom Inventory (26), Profile of Mood States (27), Pain Disability Index (28) and a pain questionnaire assessing medical history and sociodemographic information. These data served as dependent measures for the statistical analyses.

Each subject underwent a multidisciplinary assessment by a staff anesthesiologist, psychologist and physical therapist. Subjects were diagnosed with either myofascial pain [N = 34] or fibromyalgia [N = 21] according to the diagnostic guidelines described by Travell and Simons (29) and Wolfe et al. (30), respectively. The groups did not differ for age [x̄ = 37.2 years] or duration of pain [x̄ = 56.9 months].

RESULTS

A series of one-way ANOVAs across groups [Myofascial × Fibromyalgia] was computed for each of the dependent measures. Myofascial patients reported that the onset of pain was more likely to be associated with trauma [P < .05] and scored higher on a measure of trait [but not state] anxiety [P = .06]. While they were more likely to be receiving compensation for their pain [P < .10] myofascial patients tended to report less occupational disability [P < .10]. Fibromyalgia patients reported lower educational achievement [P < .05] and greater pain severity as measured by the sensory [P = .05] and affective [P = .05] dimensions of the McGill Pain Questionnaire. No group differences were obtained for measures of sleep disturbance, fatigue, depression, personality functioning, personal or familial alcoholism or marital satisfaction.

DISCUSSION

The results of the present study suggest that patients suffering chronic myofascial pain and fibromyalgia report similar levels of psychological distress. These data are consistent with previous studies that found no differences between fibromyalgia and other chronic pain syndromes in measures of psychopathology (31,32). Further, the failure to obtain group differences in the incidence of personal or familial alcoholism and depression supports earlier reports (18) and contrasts with studies identifying fibromyalgia as a primary depressive disorder (16). In a related finding, the depressive somatic complaints of fatigue and sleep disturbance, previously considered to be major diagnostic features of fibromyalgia (33), appear equally prevalent among sufferers of myofascial pain at least based on their self-report. These data discourage a psychopathology model specific to the genesis of fibromyalgia and support the view that the psychological disturbances observed in fibromyalgia and myofascial pain patients represent the effects of persistent pain, disability and suffering (21,34).

The finding that fibromyalgia patients report significantly greater pain severity supports previous studies that compared these patients with other chronic pain syndromes (20,35). Fibromyalgia appears to be a particularly painful disorder (36) that may be best understood as a disorder of pain modulation (37). Given the severity of their pain complaints it is not surprising that there was a trend for the fibromyalgia group in this study to perceive themselves as less able to work despite the relative absence of financial incentive to remain disabled. In contrast, Cathey et al. (36) noted relatively small disability rates among their fibromyalgia population. This discrepancy may represent sampling bias, as their patients derived from a rural primary care rheumatologic practice, while the present study examined patients attending a university pain clinic, the former of which would be expected to display more severe and disabling symptoms (34). It is not surprising that myofascial pain patients report trauma as the triggering event for their pain (11). Unfortunately, the role of trauma in understanding the psychological profile of chronic pain patients has received only scarce consideration (38). Fishbain et al. (22) speculate that a history of trauma may account for observed differences between fibromyalgia and myofascial pain groups. Among the mood measures administered in this study only trait anxiety distinguished the groups, with myofascial patients reporting greater distress. The association of trait anxiety and myofascial pain raises the possibility that individuals who premorbidly experience elevated levels of trait anxiety may be predisposed to chronic musculoskeletal pain, particularly following a traumatic injury. An alternative explanation, which places primary emphasis on the traumatic event, would view trait anxiety as a hidden sequela of traumatically-induced pain and within a broader context of post-traumatic stress disorder (39).

Finally, fibromyalgia and myofascial patients differed significantly in their levels of educational achievement. Previous fibromyalgia studies have observed an inverse correlation between level of education and both pain and disability (40). These observations raise questions regarding the contribution of sociodemographic factors to fibromyalgia pain. As the treatment for chronic musculoskeletal pain typically includes an emphasis on patient education to facilitate self-management skills, the design of future intervention studies for fibromyalgia patients may need to consider educational achievement as an important patient variable.

REFERENCES

1. Merskey H: Psychosocial factors and muscular pain. Edited by JR Fricton and E Awad. Advances in Pain Research and Therapy. Vol 17. Raven Press, New York, 1990, pp. 213-225.

2. Boland EW: Psychogenic rheumatism: The musculoskeletal expression of psychoneurosis. Ann Rheumatol Dis 6: 195, 1947.

3. Ellman P, Savage DA, Wittkower E, Rodger TF: "Fibrositis"–a biographical study of fifty civilian and military cases. Ann Rheum Dis 3: 56-76, 1942.

4. Wolfe F: Methodological and statistical problems in the epidemiology of fibromyalgia. Edited by JR Fricton and E Awad. Advances in Pain Research and Therapy. Vol 17: Raven Press, New York, 1990, pp. 147-163.

5. Wolfe F: Fibrositis, fibromyalgia, and musculoskeletal disease: The current status of the fibrositis syndrome. Arch Phys Med Rehab 69: 527-531, 1988.

6. Goldenberg DL: Psychiatric and psychologic aspects of fibromyalgia syndrome. Rheum Dis Clin North Am 15: 105-114, 1989.

7. Boissevain MD, McCain GA: Toward an integrated understanding of fibromyalgia syndrome II. Psychological and phenomenological aspects. Pain 45: 239-248, 1991.

8. Simons DG: Myofascial trigger points: A need for understanding. Arch Phys Med Rehab 62: 97-99, 1981.

9. Sarno JE: Etiology of neck and back pain: An autonomic myoneuralgia. J Nerv Ment Dis 169: 55-59, 1981.

10. Dolce JJ, Raczynski JM: Neuromuscular activity and electromyography in painful backs: Psychological and biomechanical models in assessment and treatment. Psych Bull 97: 502-520, 1985.

11. Yunus MB: Research in fibromyalgia and myofascial pain syndromes: Current status, problems and future directions. J. Musculoskel Pain 1: 23-41, 1993.

12. Yunus MB, Masi AT: Association of primary fibromyalgia syndrome with stress-related syndromes. Clin Res 33: 923A, 1985.

13. Yunus M, Masi AT, Calabro JJ, Miller KA, Feigenbaum SL: Primary fibromyalgia [fibrositis]: Clinical study of 50 patients with matched normal controls. Semin Arthritis Rheum 11: 151-171, 1981.

14. Fricton JR: Management of myofascial pain syndrome. Edited by JR Fricton and E Awad. Advances in Pain Research and Therapy. Vol 17: Raven Press, New York, 1990, pp. 325-346.

15. Hudson JI, Pope HG: Fibromyalgia and psychopathology: Is fibromyalgia a form of "affective spectrum disorder?" J Rheumatol 16 (suppl 19): 15-22, 1989.

16. Hudson JI, Hudson MS, Pliner LF, Goldenberg DL, Pope HG: Fibromyalgia and major affective disorder: A controlled phenomenology and family history study. Am J Psychiat 142: 441-446, 1985.

17. Goldenberg DI: Psychologic studies in fibrositis. Am J Med 81 (suppl 3A): 67-72, 1986.

18. Ahles TA, Yunus MB, Masi AT: Is chronic pain a variant of depressive disease? The case of fibromyalgia syndrome. Pain 29: 105-111, 1987.

19. Kirmayer LJ, Robbins JM, Kapusta MA: Somatization and depression in fibromyalgia syndrome. Am J Psychiat 145: 950-954, 1988.

20. Leavitt HF, Katz RS, Golden HE, Glickman PB, Layfer LF: Comparison of pain properties in fibromyalgia patients and rheumatoid arthritis patients. Arthritis Rheum 29: 775-781, 1986.

21. Marbach JJ, Richlin DM, Lipton JA: Illness behavior, depression and anhedonia in myofascial face and back pain patients, Psychother Psychosom 39: 47-54, 1983.

22. Fishbain DA, Goldberg M, Steele R, Rosomoff H: DSM-III diagnoses of patients with myofascial pain syndrome [Fibrositis]. Arch Phys Med Rehab 70: 433-438, 1989.

23. Melzack R: The McGill Pain Questionnaire: Major properties and scoring methods. Pain 1: 277-299, 1975.

24. Beck AT, Ward CH, Mendelson M, Mock J, Erbaugh J: An inventory measuring depression. Arch Gen Psychiat 4: 561-571, 1961.

25. Spielberger CD, Gorsuch RL, Lushene RE: State-Trait Anxiety Inventory. Consulting Psychologists Press, Palo Alto, 1970.

26. Derogatis LR, Spencer PM: Brief Symptom Inventory. Clinical Psychometric Research, Baltimore, 1982.

27. McNair JM, Lorr M, Droppleman LF: Profile of Mood States. San Diego: Educational and Industrial Testing Service, 1971/81.

28. Tait RC, Chibnall JT, Drause S: The pain disability index: Psychometric properties. Pain 40: 171-182, 1990.

29. Travell JG, Simons DG: Myofascial Pain and Dysfunction: The Trigger Point Manual. Williams & Wilkins, Baltimore, 1983.

30. Wolfe F, Smythe HA, Yunus MB, Bennett RM, Bombardier C, Goldenberg DL, Tugwell P, Campbell SM, Abeles M, Clark P, Fam AG, Farber SJ, Fiechtner JJ, Franklin CM, Gatter RA, Hamaty D, Lessard J, Lichtbroun AS, Masi AT, McCain GA, Reynolds WJ, Romano TJ, Russell IJ, Sheon RP: The American College of Rheumatology 1990 Criteria for the Classification of Fibromyalgia: Report of the Multicenter Criteria Committee. Arthritis Rheum 33: 160-172, 1990.

31. Clark S, Campbell SM, Forehand ME, Tindall EA, Bennett RM: Clinical characteristics of fibrositis II. A "blinded," controlled study using standard psychological tests. Arthritis Rheum 28: 132-137, 1985.

32. Birnie DJ, Knipping AA, vanGrijswijk MH, deBlecourt C, deVoogd: Psychological aspects of fibromyalgia compared with chronic and nonchronic pain. J Rheumatol 18: 1845-1848, 1991.

33. Smythe HA, Moldofsky H: Two contributions to the understanding of the fibrositis syndrome. Bull Rheum Dis 28: 928-931, 1978.

34. Merskey H: Physical and psychological considerations in the classification of fibromyalgia. J Rheumatol 16 (suppl 19): 72-79, 1989.

35. Nolli M, Ghirell L, Ferraccioli GF: Pain language in fibromyalgia, rheumatoid arthritis and osteoarthritis. Clin Exp Rheumatol 6: 27-33, 1988.

36. Cathey MA, Wolfe F, Kleinheksel SM: Functional ability and work status in patients with fibromyalgia. Arthritis Care Res 1: 85-98, 1988.

37. Smythe HA: Fibrositis as a disorder of pain modulation. Clin Rheum Dis 5: 823-832, 1979.

38. Muse M: Stress-related, posttraumatic chronic pain syndrome: Criteria for diagnosis, and preliminary report on prevalence. Pain 23: 295-300, 1985.

39. Scrignar CB: Post-traumatic stress disorder. Bruno Press, New Orleans, 1988.

40. Hawley DJ, Wolfe F: Pain, disability and pain/disability relationships in seven rheumatic disorders: A study of 1,522 patients. J Rheumatol 18: 1552-1557, 1991.

Evidence for Neuroendocrine Disturbance Following Physical Exercise in Primary Fibromyalgia Syndrome

Eduard N. Griep
Johannes W. Boersma
E. Ronald de Kloet

SUMMARY. Objective: To test pituitary-adrenal responses to physical exercise in patients with primary fibromyalgia syndrome [PFS].

Methods: Eighteen female PFS patients [1981 Yunus criteria] and 18 matched, healthy but strictly sedentary controls performed a bicycle ergometer test with stepwise increasing workload. The first 10 couples did submaximal exercise; the next 8 couples continued until volitional exhaustion. During and after the test measurement of ACTH and cortisol was done at intervals.

Eduard N. Griep, MD, is Rheumatologist, Departments of Rheumatology, Rijnstate Hospital, Arnhem, and Jan van Breemen Institute, Amsterdam.

Johannes W. Boersma, MD, is Rheumatologist, Department of Rheumatology, Rijnstate Hospital, Arnhem.

E. Ronald de Kloet, PhD, is Professor of Medical Pharmacology, Division of Medical Pharmacology, Center for Bio-Pharmaceutical Sciences, Leiden University, Leiden, the Netherlands.

Address correspondence and reprint requests to: Dr. E. N. Griep, Scientific Division/Department of Rheumatology, Jan van Breemen Institute, Dr Jan van Breemenstraat 2, 1056 AB Amsterdam, the Netherlands.

This study was supported by a grant from the "Het Nationaal Reumafonds" of the Netherlands.

[Haworth co-indexing entry note]: "Evidence for Neuroendocrine Disturbance Following Physical Exercise in Primary Fibromyalgia Syndrome." Griep, Eduard N., Johannes W. Boersma, and E. Ronald de Kloet. Co-published simultaneously in the *Journal of Musculoskeletal Pain* (The Haworth Press, Inc.) Vol. 1, No. 3/4, 1993, pp. 217-222; and: *Musculoskeletal Pain, Myofascial Pain Syndrome, and the Fibromyalgia Syndrome* (ed: Søren Jacobsen, Bente Danneskiold-Samsøe, and Birger Lund) The Haworth Press, Inc., 1993, pp. 217-222. Multiple copies of this article/chapter may be purchased from The Haworth Document Delivery Center [1-800-3-HAWORTH; 9:00 a.m. - 5:00 p.m. (EST)].

Results: During submaximal exercise the PFS patients, compared to the controls, displayed a [very early] significantly augmented ACTH release without a corresponding cortisol response. Within the group that performed exhaustive exercise, the 8 PFS patients achieved a lower [mean] maximum workload. At exhaustion and during early recovery ACTH and cortisol reached maximum values, which tended to be higher in PFS patients.

Conclusion: PFS patients show altered pituitary-adrenal responses to physical exercise, which supports the clinical significance of the disturbance following neuroendocrine challenge tests in these patients.

KEYWORDS. Fibromyalgia, neuroendocrinology, physical exercise

INTRODUCTION

Primary fibromyalgia syndrome [PFS] is a nonarticular rheumatic disorder without underlying conditions, characterized by chronic widespread musculoskeletal aching with multiple tender points upon examination. The syndrome is often accompanied by fatigue, anxiety, poor sleep, headache, irritable bowel complaints and numbness (1). However, distinct morphological and/or pathological features are lacking.

The pathophysiology of PFS remains unknown (2). There is growing awareness, however, that central mechanisms have to be involved (3). In this respect, some reports suggest neuroendocrine dysfunction (4-6), which in our view could well be stress-related. Recently, we demonstrated in PFS patients enhanced pituitary adrenocorticotropic hormone [ACTH] release in response to a corticotropin-releasing hormone [CRH] test and to insulin-induced hypoglycemia [IH] (7,8). Since adrenocortical secretion following these neuroendocrine challenge tests did not differ from controls, this suggested an [primary] adrenocortical insufficiency.

Here, we report pituitary-adrenal responses of fibromyalgia patients following physical exercise.

MATERIALS AND METHODS

Eighteen female PFS patients fulfilling the 1981 Yunus criteria (1) were compared to 18 matched, healthy control persons who did not have any complaint of pain or fatigue. Moreover, attempting to avoid a difference in aerobic capacity, these controls had to have a strictly sedentary style of living. Furthermore, criteria of inclusion were: age 18-50 years; no medication, [suspected] pregnancy, concomitant disease, signs of adrenal disorder or obesity; secondary fibromyalgia was excluded.

All persons were subjected to physical exercise by means of a bicycle ergometer test under guidance of an exercise technician 'blinded' to diagnosis, to avoid bias in test performance. The first 10 patient/control couples performed submaximal exercise. The next 8 couples did the same exercise, but continued until volitional exhaustion. The bicycle ergometer test consisted of stepwise increasing workload, implying a start at 50 watts with an increase of 30 watts every 5 minutes. During and after the test the heart rate [HR] was recorded continuously, while blood samples for measurement of ACTH and cortisol were obtained during the test at the end of each workload and during recovery at 2 fixed time-points.

RESULTS

As shown in Table 1, demographic and basal characteristics of the PFS patients and controls did not differ. In addition, these variables were essentially equal in the first and second group of patient/control couples [10 vs. 8 - submaximal vs. maximal exercise].

In the submaximal exercise period the whole group of 18 PFS patients displayed a very early and highly significant [P < 0.001] augmented

Table 1. Demographic and basal characteristics of the fibromyalgia patients and controls[*]

	Patients [N=18]	Controls [N=18][†]
Age [years]	38.3 ± 7.8	36.8 ± 7.6
Sex [female/male]	18/0	18/0
Quetelet index [kg/m^2]	23.5 ± 2.4	23.3 ± 2.8
Heart rate at rest [bpm]	75.6 ± 12.9	71.7 ± 11.6
Mean arterial pressure [mmHg]	99.4 ± 7.1	99.3 ± 9.0
Tender point number[‡]	12.5 ± 2.4	NP
Tender point score[‡]	1.8 ± 0.6	NP

[*] Data, except sex, given as mean ± SD
[†] NP = not present
[‡] Assessment according to Smythe (9) with a maximum of 14 tender points, evaluated by digital palpation with an approximate pressure of 4 kg; scoring system: 0 = no pain, 1 = pain without grimas or withdrawal, 2 = pain and grimas, 3 = pain plus grimas plus withdrawal; tender point score is computed mean of the score on the 14 tender points

ACTH release without a rise in cortisol levels. In contrast, the controls did not show any ACTH response.

Within the group that performed exhaustive exercise, the 8 PFS patients achieved a lower [mean] maximum workload. Only one of them was able to maintain a 5-minute period of 140 watts completely and not one could exceed the 140 watts in contrast to all controls. ACTH and cortisol reached maximum values at exhaustion and during early recovery, and tended to be higher in the patients. Also, the cortisol response in patients appeared more prolonged.

The HR of all patients and controls was not significantly different before [see Table 1], during or after exercise.

DISCUSSION

From recent literature (10) it is concluded that PFS patients have reduced aerobic fitness. Research data therefore must be judged on the possibility of detraining effects. At study entry we did attempt to overcome the problem of differential physical fitness by recruiting only strictly sedentary, healthy control persons. Nevertheless, our patients probably had lower fitness than our controls, as those patients who performed volitional exhaustive exercise achieved a lower maximum workload than controls.

In that respect, it is quite surprising that during the whole test the HR did not show any differences, as in PFS patients, a higher HR at rest and upon exercise would be expected. Perhaps, this indicates a sympathetic dysfunction, i.e., too low activity upon challenge, as was suggested previously (11).

During submaximal exercise, there was in PFS patients an inappropriate, very early and significantly augmented ACTH release while no rise in cortisol levels occurred. Normally, an exercise of as low as 50-80 watts does not result in any rise in ACTH [or cortisol] levels (12). Our healthy, though strictly sedentary controls reacted this way. Hence, in accordance with the response to CRH and to IH (7,8), there also seems to be ACTH hyperreactivity to submaximal physical exercise in PFS patients.

Following exhaustive exercise, despite the lower maximum workload achieved by the 8 PFS patients, they displayed a tendency to a higher ACTH and a higher and possibly more prolonged cortisol response versus the controls. This seems at first at some variance with the neuroendocrine challenge tests in which there was ACTH hyperreactivity, but no difference in cortisol response. However, the strenuous exercise, besides being an effort, also caused marked distress in our patients as it worsened their complaints, mainly pain and fatigue. In the controls there was no apparent distress following the exhaustive physical exercise. The neuroendocrine response after the challenge tests, particularly after CRH, is concerned with one specific step in the cascade of events occurring after stress. Other studies have pointed out that it is stress or distress rather than an effort per se that activates the hypothalamic-pituitary-adrenal axis (13). It cannot be excluded, therefore, that in the case of the fibromyalgia patients the enhanced neuroendocrine response following the exhaustive physical exercise is [mainly] due to discomfort.

In conclusion, the bicycle ergometer test shows altered pituitary-adrenal responses to physical exercise in fibromyalgia, which in our view supports the clinical significance of the disturbance found with the neuroendocrine challenge tests. Taken together, our data underscore the hypothesis on neuroendocrine dysfunction in PFS patients, which could explain at least some of their symptoms. We have planned further studies to elucidate the exact nature and specificity of this disturbance.

REFERENCES

1. Yunus MB, Masi AT, Calabro JJ, Miller KA, Feigenbaum SL: Primary fibromyalgia (fibrositis): clinical study of 50 patients with matched normal controls. Semin Arthritis Rheum 11: 151-171, 1981.

2. Goldenberg DL: Fibromyalgia, chronic fatigue syndrome and myofascial pain syndrome. Curr Opin Rheumatol 3: 247-258, 1991.

3. Yunus MB: Towards a model of pathophysiology of fibromyalgia: aberrant central pain mechanisms with peripheral modulation [editorial]. J Rheumatol 19: 846-850, 1992.

4. Russell IJ: Neurohormonal aspects of fibromyalgia syndrome. Rheum Dis Clin North Am 15: 149-168, 1989.

5. McCain GA, Tilbe KS: Diurnal hormone variation in fibromyalgia syndrome: a comparison with rheumatoid arthritis. J Rheumatol 16 (Suppl 19): 154-157, 1989.

6. Ferraccioli G, Cavalieri F, Salaffi F, Fontana S, Scita F, Nolli M, Maestri D: Neuroendocrinologic findings in primary fibromyalgia (soft tissue chronic pain syndrome) and in other chronic rheumatic conditions (rheumatoid arthritis, low back pain) [editorial]. J Rheumatol 17: 869-873, 1990.

7. Griep EN, Boersma JW, De Kloet ER: Disturbed neuroendocrine reactivity in the primary fibromyalgia syndrome (PFS) [abstract]. Hung Rheumatol 32 (Suppl): 25, 1991.

8. Griep EN, Boersma JW, De Kloet ER: Altered reactivity of the hypothalamic-pituitary-adrenal axis in the primary fibromyalgia syndrome. J Rheumatol (in press).

9. Smythe H: "Fibrositis" and other diffuse musculoskeletal syndromes, Textbook of rheumatology. Edited by WN Kelley et al. WB Saunders Company, Philadelphia, 1985, pp. 481-489.

10. Bennett RM, Clark SR, Goldberg L, Nelson D, Bonafede RP, Porter J, Specht D: Aerobic fitness in patients with fibrositis: a controlled study of respiratory gas exchange and ^{133}Xenon clearance from exercising muscle. Arthritis Rheum 32: 454-460, 1989.

11. Van Denderen JC, Boersma JW, Zeinstra P, Hollander AP, Van Neerbos BR: Physiological effects of exhaustive physical exercise in primary fibromyalgia syndrome (PFS): is PFS a disorder of neuroendocrine reactivity? Scand J Rheumatol 21: 35-37, 1992.

12. Few JD: Effect of exercise on the secretion and metabolism of cortisol in man. J Endocr 62: 341-353, 1974.

13. Lundberg U, Frankenhaeuser M: Pituitary-adrenal and sympathetic-adrenal correlates of distress and effort. J Psychosom Res 24: 125-130, 1980.

Alpha Intrusion in Fibromyalgia

Asbjørn Mohr Drewes
Kim Dremstrup Nielsen
Poul Jennum
Arne Andreasen

SUMMARY. Objectives: It has been proposed that the alpha sleep anomaly plays a pathogenic role in fibromyalgia [F]. We have reexamined this question using digitized sleep recording to quantify the alpha EEG-band in the various stages of sleep.

Methods: Sleep recordings from 20 women with F and 10 age matched normals [N] were used. All epochs without arousals generated by movements, apnoea, etc., were subjected to automatic frequency analysis and the relative power of the alpha band was estimated.

Results: The power in the alpha EEG-band was relatively constant [22.0-27.8] in all sleep stages, and there were no differences between F and N.

Asbjørn Mohr Drewes, MD, is affiliated with the Department of Rheumatology, Aalborg Hospital, Denmark, and the Department of Rheumatology, Viborg Hospital, Denmark.

Kim Dremstrup Nielsen, MSc, is affiliated with the Department of Medical Informatics, Institute of Electronic Systems, University of Aalborg, Denmark.

Poul Jennum, MD, is affiliated with the Department of Clinical Neurophysiology, Hvidovre Hospital, University of Copenhagen, Denmark.

Arne Andreasen, MD, is affiliated with the Department of Rheumatology, Viborg Hospital, Denmark.

Address correspondence and reprint requests to: Asbjørn Mohr Drewes, MD, Department of Rheumatology, Aalborg Hospital, DK-9000 Aalborg, Denmark.

[Haworth co-indexing entry note]: "Alpha Intrusion in Fibromyalgia." Drewes, Asbjørn Mohr et al. Co-published simultaneously in the *Journal of Musculoskeletal Pain* (The Haworth Press, Inc.) Vol. 1, No. 3/4, 1993, pp. 223-228; and: *Musculoskeletal Pain, Myofascial Pain Syndrome, and the Fibromyalgia Syndrome* (ed: Søren Jacobsen, Bente Danneskiold-Samsøe, and Birger Lund) The Haworth Press, Inc., 1993, pp. 223-228. Multiple copies of this article/chapter may be purchased from The Haworth Document Delivery Center [1-800-3-HAWORTH; 9:00 a.m. - 5:00 p.m. (EST)].

Conclusion: No significant differences were found in the alpha EEG patterns of patients with fibromyalgia relative to the normal controls.

KEYWORDS. Sleep, fibromyalgia, atypical polysomnographic features, automatic sleep analysis

INTRODUCTION

Several studies (1,2) have provided evidence for disturbance of sleep in patients with F. As sleep seems to be a process necessary for bodily restoration (3) it could be hypothesized that disordered sleep may play a pathogenetic role in F. One of several sleep disorders is the alpha sleep anomaly (2), but a valid estimation of the alpha-EEG has been difficult. In this preliminary report a model for quantification of various EEG bands is described.

MATERIAL AND METHODS

Twenty women with F and 10 normal subjects entered the study. The median age for F was 45.6 years [35-58] and for N 42.8 years [41-59]. The median duration of the disease in F was 7.25 years [1-25]. All F fulfilled the Yunus-criteria. All subjects had 2 full-night sleep recordings, but only the second record was analyzed, to avoid the "first night effect." The sleep staging was accomplished manually by 2 independent, "blinded" physicians. Epochs with disagreement were reevaluated by one of the authors [AMD], supported by the frequency analysis of the EEG [see below], and a final staging was then reached.

As the main object of this study was to quantify the "endogenous" alpha, as an "internal arousal mechanism," all epochs [30 s segments of the EEG] with movement-arousals [epochs in which the EEG and EOG tracings are obscured in more than half the epoch by muscle tension/artifacts due to movements] and movement-time [an increase in EMG accompanied by EEG arousal activity and many artifacts–Figure 1] were excluded. In this way artifacts and "natural occurring" alpha-like activity in the EEG were omitted from the analysis. The number of epochs excluded according to the above procedure were median 29.5 [19-50] in N and 26.5 [21-61] in F [NS]. Many of the subjects [12 F and 2 N] had slight evidence

FIGURE 1. A movement arousal [increase in EMG of both legs and chin, large arrow] accompanied by alpha-EEG [small arrow]. Resolution in the figure is limited by the PC-screen [VGA resolution].

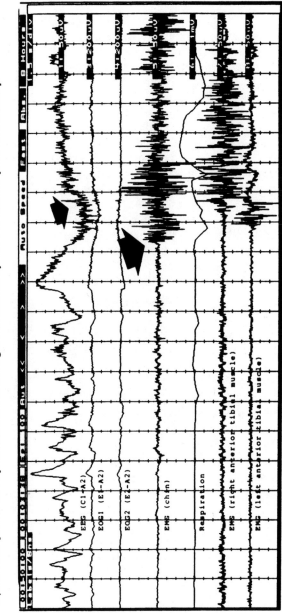

of apnoea [apnoea-hypopnoea index > 5/h]. As patients with apnoea have a lot of alpha-activity during and after resumption of ventilation–Figure 2, these subjects were excluded. Otherwise apnoea-related alpha might bias the frequency analysis. Moreover, some of the symptoms could be related to the apnoea and these patients may not be "genuine" fibromyalgics. One N was excluded because of artifacts in the EEG. The excluded patients did not differ from the others in respect to age, duration of disease, subjective sleep disturbances [scale 1-5] or pain [scale 1-5]. Moreover, epochs with stage W and NREM1 were not analyzed.

The recordings were digitized with a sampling rate of 100 Hz. In every 30 second epoch the power spectrum was calculated using autoregressive modelling based on the autocorrelation coefficients from fifteen 2 second segments (4). The power in all EEG bands [delta [0.5-3.5 Hz], theta [3.5-8 Hz], alpha [8-12 Hz], sigma [12-14.5 Hz], beta [14.5-25 Hz] and total [0.5-25 Hz]] was calculated and the alpha-power in percentage of the power in the delta band and the total EEG-power was calculated for all selected epochs. This relative energy should be regarded the best biological measure of the alpha-intrusion.

RESULTS

The results are shown in Table 1. According to the above exclusion criteria, the material was reduced to 8F and 7N. In total 8269 epochs [248,070 2 second segments] were analyzed. The power of the alpha-band was very constant in all sleep stages, and there were no differences between the two groups. The alpha in percentage of the power in the delta band decreased with increasing sleep depth.

DISCUSSION

The systematic quantification of the alpha-band showed no differences in F and N, when patients with evidence of primary sleep disorders were excluded. As the sleep is fragmented and disturbed in F, and the alpha-EEG is represented in arousals, we expected to find more alpha-activity in F. This means that an increased background of alpha-activity should be detected in the sleep-EEG, as a kind of "carry-over effect" from the arousals, even when alpha-activity directly related to arousals were excluded. We believe, however, that the epochs with arousals should be excluded as this alpha-activity represents naturaly occurring awakenings, and the object of the study was to measure the endogenous generated alpha-activity, as an internal arousal mechanism, disturbing the normal sleep architecture.

FIGURE 2. The patient hyperventilates following apnoea [respiration determined using a strain gauge] and alpha-EEG is seen [arrow]. Resolution in the figure is limited by the PC-screen [VGA resolution].

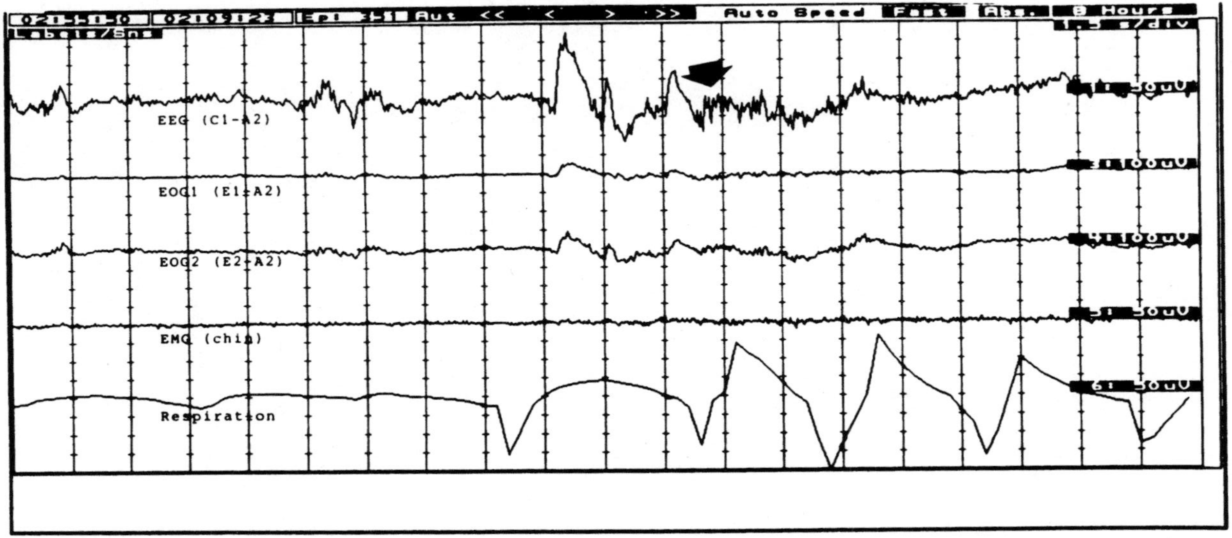

227

TABLE 1

Sleep stage		Epochs analyzed	alpha/total %	alpha/delta %
NREM2	F	1094	22.8 [17.7-32.5]	584.9 [318.2-903.6]
	N	909	22.8 [19.6-32.9]	485.7 [305.7-1012.6]
NREM3	F	579	25.2 [18.0-33.3]	332.2 [234.5-693.7]
	N	744	27.8 [20.4-34.8]	425.5 [289.4-1002.0]
NREM4	F	741	22.1 [17.9-27.8]	218.0 [162.3-376.1]
	N	721	23.9 [21.6-34.9]	223.6 [146.0-591.0]
REM	F	1094	22.0 [11.7-29.5]	555.0 [249.5-1144.0]
	N	909	25.6 [14.4-32.0]	687.8 [254.0-1211.6]

Relative power, median and [range] in the alpha EEG-band [8-12 Hz] compared to the total power [0.5-25 Hz] and the power in the delta [0.5-3.5 Hz] band. No significant differences were found between fibromyalgics [F] and normals [N].

The reason for our findings may partly be due to the fact that all subjects [including N] reported that they slept poorly in the sleep laboratory, and an experimental light sleep with relatively much alpha-activity in the EEG might have been generated in both groups. Future studies on discrete EEG phenomenons should rely on ambulatory monitoring, which probably gives a more normal, undisturbed sleep.

REFERENCES

1. Moldofsky H, Scarisbrick P, England R, Smythe H. Musculoskeletal symptoms and non-REM sleep disturbance in patients with "fibrositis syndrome" and healthy subjects. Psychosomatic Medicine 37: 341-351, 1975.

2. Moldofsky H. Sleep and fibrositis syndrome. Rheumatic Disease Clinics of North America 15: 91-103, 1989.

3. Adam K. Sleep as a restorative process and a theory to explain why. Process on Brain Research 53: 289-305, 1980.

4. Nielsen K D, Drewes A M, Andreasen A, Jennum P. Computer analysis of sleep in fibromyalgia. Sleep Research 20A: 506, 1991.

Psychosomatic Aspects
of Primary Fibromyalgia Syndrome [PFS]

Gerhard Schuessler
Juergen Konermann

SUMMARY. **Objectives:** The importance of psychosomatic factors in Primary Fibromyalgia Syndrome [PFS] is discussed with regard to the controversy about the prevalence of psychiatric disorders and psychological dysfunction.

Methods: In a multicenter controlled study we investigated the psychological and organic factors of 65 patients with PFS and 53 patients with rheumatoid arthritis.

Results: Pain behavior, psychological distress and psychiatric disorders differed significantly between PFS and RA patients. PFS patients were generally more disturbed and had more developmental risk factors [for example loss of parents or family violence] in their childhood.

Conclusions: Nevertheless, PFS does not seem to be a psychogenic disease. According to a bio-psychosocial model, psychosomatic factors play a different etiological role within the different subgroups. This prospective investigation was designed to better elucidate these interconnections.

Gerhard Schuessler, MD, University Lecturer, and Juergen Konermann, Psychologist, are both affiliated with the Department of Psychosomatics and Psychotherapy, University of Göttingen.

Address correspondence to: Dr. G. Schuessler, Department of Psychosomatics and Psychotherapy, Von-Siebold-Str. 5, D-3400 Göttingen, Germany.

This study was supported by grants from the BMFT [07 016 467].

[Haworth co-indexing entry note]: "Psychosomatic Aspects of Primary Fibromyalgia Syndrome [PFS]." Schuessler, Gerhard, and Juergen Konermann. Co-published simultaneously in the *Journal of Musculoskeletal Pain* (The Haworth Press, Inc.) Vol. 1, No. 3/4, 1993, pp. 229-236; and: *Musculoskeletal Pain, Myofascial Pain Syndrome, and the Fibromyalgia Syndrome* (ed: Søren Jacobsen, Bente Danneskiold-Samsøe, and Birger Lund) The Haworth Press, Inc., 1993, pp. 229-236. Multiple copies of this article/chapter may be purchased from The Haworth Document Delivery Center [1-800-3-HAWORTH; 9:00 a.m. - 5:00 p.m. (EST)].

KEYWORDS. Fibromyalgia, rheumatoid arthritis, psychosomatic aspects

INTRODUCTION

In the past years, fibromyalgia has been differentiated from other soft tissue rheumatic diseases. The present investigation employs the American College of Rheumatology [ACR] criteria prepared for classification of primary fibromyalgia (1): generalized pain associated with evidence of tenderness to pressure in the area of at least 11 of 18 specifically described pressure points.

Based on the unclear etiology and the lack of a specific pathophysiology, fibromyalgia was frequently regarded either as a purely psychogenic disease or as physical expression of a psychiatric illness, usually of depression.

Disregarding a few exceptions (2), it has been only recently that controlled studies have been conducted to investigate the psychiatric and psychosomatic aspects of PFS. To date, these studies have not produced any unified picture (3). Psychological and psychiatric anomalies, however, do manifest themselves more frequently in PFS. The research results of the last two decades prove that pain diseases do not involve a causal "and/or" [either somatic or psychogenic], but a procedural "not only/but also." Complex reasoning is required.

The present paper examines the question of the extent to which patients with PFS and rheumatoid arthritis differ from each other in the areas of functional disability, pain, psychological distress and psychiatric disorders. This investigation is part of a prospective multicenter study on illness coping mechanisms and psychotherapeutic treatment of patients with PFS.

MATERIAL AND METHODS

Within the framework of a research project conducted in the rheumatology policlinic of the University of Göttingen and the Medical School of Hannover, 65 patients with PFS and 53 patients with RA have been enrolled and intensively examined to date. These patients will be followed for 1 year, and some will take part in a psychotherapeutic program. Patients with RA met the ARA criteria (4), individuals with fibromyalgia satisfied the current diagnostic criteria (1). At each clinic visit, in addition to the standard rheumatological examination, all patients completed self-administered questionnaires and underwent psychosomatic interviews with specially trained psychologists. The semi-standardized interview focused on pain behaviour, coping and psychopathological disorders. The life-situation during childhood and adolescence was explored and rated in three domains: the financial situation of parents and their living conditions, traumas and characteristics of the important relationships. The developmental conditions were evaluated individually, but also were combined for statistical comparisons [0 = no risk factor, 6 = severe risk factors in three domains]. We summarized the complex interplay of all these different levels as psychosomatic factors, they completed the traditional organic-rheumatological findings. Psychiatric diagnosis was performed according to the research criteria of the International Classification of Diseases (5). Pain was rated on visual analogue scales [VAS], self-rating of general symptoms, thinking of pain and global rating of severity were questioned and ranked from 0 to 4. The impairment of sleep, concentration, mobility or daily planning was assessed by a Likert self-rating scale ranking from 0 to 4 (6). Anxiety was measured with the State-Trait-Anxiety-Inventory, [STAI] (7) and depression with the Depression Scale, [DS] (8). We used the German version of the MPQ (9) for pain description. The FFBH-K (10), a German instrument comparable to the HAQ, was used to assess functional disabilities [0-24, 24 = 100% functional ability].

The following statistical procedures were used: chi-square tests, adjusted t-tests and wilcoxon tests. The fibromyalgia patients had been ill for 9.5 years [SD = 8.1] and the arthritis patients had been ill for 7.9 years [SD = 6.4]. There was no significant difference in the duration of illness between the two groups. There were more females in both groups. The mean age was 51.7 years for the PFS patients and 50.5 years for the RA patients. There were no statistically significant differences in the main social and demographic parameters such as marital status, school graduates and occupational status.

RESULTS

Pain: Variables of interest are described in Table 1. Intensity of pain [VAS] and thinking of pain were significantly higher in the PFS group. Pain description in a modified German version of the MPQ yielded higher values in the area of number of words used, affect score and sensory score for the PFS group [Table 1].

Functional disability: The FFBH assesses functional disability on the basis of 8 questions [e.g., walking, grip strength, dressing; 24 points

Table 1: Study variables comparing FMS-Patients and RA-Patients. As statistical tests are used Wilcoxon-, T-Test and chi^2 (n.s = p > .05)

	FMS-Patients (n = 65)	RA-Patients (n = 53)	statistical-test
sex (female in %)	87,6%	73,6%	n.s.
age (in years)	51,7 (6,5)	50,5 (11,6)	n.s.
disease duration (in years)	9,5 (8,1)	7,9 (6,4)	n.s.
pain intensity (VAS 0 -100)	60,5 (21,7)	45,0 (22,0)	.0001
thinking of pain (1 - 5)	3,2 (0,8)	2,8 (0,7)	.0098
global severity (1 - 5)	3,5 (0,8)	3,1 (0,7)	.0027
pain description (modified german MPQ):			
number of words (0 - 49)	36,1 (9,8)	28,5 (12,6)	.0011
affect score (0 - 48)	25,3 (10,6)	17,9 (11,5)	.0006
sensory score (0 - 144)	67,2 (24,2)	45,0 (24,7)	.0001
functional ability (FFbH-score in %)	75,8 %	74,6 %	n.s.
subjective disturbance (1 - 4) of:			
sleep	2,8 (0,9)	2,3 (1,0)	.0088
concentration	2,5 (0,9)	1,9 (0,8)	.0005
daily planning	2,6 (0,8)	2,0 (0,9)	.0006
mobility	3,0 (0,8)	2,7 (0,8)	.0205
trait-anxiety (STAI)	47,2 (11,1)	40,5 (9,7)	.0021
depression (D-S)	15,2 (8,4)	10,0 (6,3)	.0006
psychosomatic symptoms (BL)	39,1 (12,0)	30,0 (11,9)	.0000
ICD-10 disorders (in %)	53,8%	26,4%	.0010
risk factors in childhood (0 - 6)	2,5 (1,9)	1,3 (1,5)	.0010

means hundred percent ability]. It is comparable to the Stanford Health Assessment Questionnaire. Table 1 shows no significant differences.

Global severity: PFS patients perceived their condition as being significantly worse than did RA patients [Table 1]. General symptoms such as sleep disorders, concentration disorders, limitation of mobility and disruption of daily schedule contributed to this subjective impression. The PFS patients proved to be more limited than the RA patients in all of these areas [Table 1].

Self-rating of psychiatric symptoms: In two different questionnaires employed, the PFS patients had higher scores: trait anxiety [STAI] and current symptoms of depression [DS]. If we take the adjusted t-values of both tests and setting a cut-off point at 60 for STAI-values [meaning plus one standard deviation] and at 65 for DS-values [meaning plus one and a half standard deviations] 67.5% of the PFS-patients had clear symptoms of depression and/or anxiety. Using the same criteria only 40% of the RA-patients showed signs of depression and/or anxiety.

Prevalence of mental and behavioral disorders: Table 1 describes the frequency of psychiatric diagnoses. Chi-square analysis shows significant differences among the two groups with a higher prevalence in the PFS group. Regarding the different psychiatric disorders 24% of PFS patients had [according to ICD-10] a depressive disorder [RA patients only 6%], 10% an adjustment disorder [depressive reaction, RA patients 4%] and 17% of the PFS patients had anxiety disorders [RA patients 8%]. In all of them, this involved current psychiatric disorders. PFS patients also had more stress factors in their childhood or youth, e.g., separation, loss of parents, family violence or bad living conditions. Patients with a psychiatric diagnosis had had clearly less favorable developmental conditions [P = .001]. PFS patients with psychiatric disorders have significantly higher self-ratings of depression [P = .002] and anxiety [P. = .01].

DISCUSSION

These are the initial preliminary results of a prospective multicenter study on RA and PFS patients. The objective of this survey was to develop multidimensional models for fibromyalgia which encompass physiological, affective, cognitive, behavioral and social components. Our procedure is oriented along the biopsychosocial model of Engel (11).

Our investigation comprises patients of a university rheumatological policlinic. The present results therefore are only transferable to a limited degree to patients in other treatment conditions–or even untreated patients. However, from our daily experience almost all PFS patients from general practitioners or other doctors in private practice are referred to our policlinics. Our results show no demographic or social differences in the two patient groups. With regard to patient age, sex distribution and the duration of illness, our findings are also for the most part consistent with the comparative collectives in the literature.

In virtually all parameters which involve the subjective appraisal of the illness [pain, general symptoms, global severity], the PFS patients rate themselves as more seriously impaired than the RA patients. This correlates with the results of Hawley and Wolfe (12). In the PFS patients, a more pronounced affective pain component was evident and more adjectives were used to describe the pain which was also elaborated with more sensory terminology. This suggests a tendency in PFS patients to perceive more pain and portray it more dramatically; they are also more involved with it, a fact indicated by the finding of higher thinking of pain. Clear statements about any causalities [greater pain leads to more thinking about pain or vice versa] cannot be made at this moment.

In a differentiated survey of functional disability, on the other hand, there are no major differences between RA and fibromyalgia. Here as well, our findings mostly correspond to those of Hawley and Wolfe (12). Although PFS patients can perform everyday tasks [movement, personal hygiene] to the same extent as RA patients, they experience themselves as being more severely ill and more markedly impaired.

In the literature as well, PFS patients are mostly shown with higher levels of psychological distress (13,14), however, some studies show no higher incidence of depression and anxiety (15). Our results of increased manifestation of anxiety and depression in the self appraisal of PFS patients is, to this extent, consistent with most of the findings of the previous investigations. The anxiety and depression values for PFS patients are borderline to the means of psychiatric populations, whereas the RA patients showed normal means or slightly elevated means compared to the normal collectives.

This elevated incidence in the self-rating of anxiety and depression is expressed in a greater prevalence of mental and behavioral disorders in the PFS patients. These prevalences are clearly higher than those of Ahles et al. (15) who conducted a blind comparative study and found no difference between fibromyalgia and RA patients in the life-time psychiatric diagnoses. Our findings appear to be validated in that the diagnosis of depression or anxiety corresponds with clearly higher values in the depression and anxiety scales filled out by the patient themselves. The frequency of psychiatric diagnoses in RA patients, however, is comparable with similar prevalence rates in other patient groups of the chronically ill (16).

The diversity of the psychiatric diagnoses does not support the hypothesis that fibromyalgia is a variant of psychiatric disorders such as depression. The majority of disorders are also not to be understood as reactive adjustment phenomena to the enhanced perception of pain and helplessness. Rather, the psychiatric anomalies are closely associated with a life history, childhood or youth, characterized by risk factors such as separation, family violence or poor living conditions.

The present results speak for the fact that psychopathological anomalies and a predisposing life history exist in a major percentage of PFS patients: taking in account the different levels of self-rating and interview results about 50% of the PFS are really psychologically disturbed. In contrast to these findings RA patients show a prevalence of psychogenic disorders comparable to other chronic diseases and only slightly higher than the general prevalence found in epidemiologic studies (17).

Not all PFS-patients show psychological anomalies (14). It is thus necessary to compile individual and intra-group differences in order to illustrate a different significance of psychosomatic factors in the development and clinical course of PFS. We hope that the ongoing evaluations of our research project may clarify these questions.

REFERENCES

1. Wolfe F, Smythe HA, Yunus MB et al.: The American college of rheumatology 1990 criteria for the classification of fibromyalgia. Arthritis and Rheumatism 33: 160-172, 1990.

2. Payne TC, Leavit F, Garron DC, Katz RS, Goden HE, Glickman PB, Vanderplate C: Fibrositis and psychological disturbances. Arthritis Rheum. 25: 213-217, 1982.

3. Boisseveain MD, McCain GA: Toward an integrated understanding of fibromyalgia syndrome. Pain: 239-248, 1991.

4. Arnett FC, Edworthy SM, Block DA et al.: The American Rheumatism Association 1987 revised criteria for the classification of rheumatic arthritis. Arthritis Rheum 31: 315-324, 1988.

5. Dilling H, Mombour W, Schmidt MH: Internationale Klassifikation psychischer Störungen, ICD-10. Bern: Huber, 1991. WHO: Tenth Revision of the International Classification of Diseases, Chapter V. Geneva, 1991.

6. Schade FD: Die Wirksamkeit eines ambulanten Schmerzbewältigungstrainings für Rheumakranke im Rahmen einer Felderprobung. Zschr. Klin. Psychol 20: 115-127, 1991.

7. Laux L, Glanzmann P, Schaffner P, Spielberger CD: Das Trait-State-Angstinventar. Weinheim: Beltz, 1981.

8. Zerssen v. D: Depressivitäts-Skala [DS]. Beltz, Weinheim, 1976.

9. Eggebrecht D, Hildebrandt J, Franz C: Die Göttinger Schmerzskala [modified version of the MPQ]. Göttingen: manuscript, 1987.

10. Raspe HH, Hagedorn U, Kohlmann TH, Mattusek S: Der Funktionsfragebogen Hannover [FFbH]: Ein Instrument zur Funktionsdiagnostik bei polyartikulären Erkrankungen. In: J. Siegrist [ed]: Wohnortnahe Betreuung Rheumakranker. Ergebnisse einer sozialwissenschaftlichen Evaluation eines Modellversuchs. Stuttgart: Schatthauer, S. 164-182, 1990.

11. Engel GL: The need for a new medical model: a challenge for biomedicine. Science 196: 129-135, 1977.

12. Hawley DJ, Wolfe F: Pain, disability, and pain/disability relationship in seven rheumatic disorders: A Study of 1,522 Patients. J Rheumatol 18: 1552-1557, 1991.

13. Uveges JM, Parker JC, Smarr JF et al.: Psychological symptoms in primary fibromyalgia syndrome: relationship to pain, life stress, and sleep disturbance. Arthritis and Rheumatism 33: 1279-1283, 1990.

14. Goldenberg DC: Psychiatric and psychology aspects of Fibromyalgia Syndrome. Rheum. Dis. Clin. North America 15: 105-114, 1989.

15. Ahles TA, Khan SH, Yunus MB, Spiegel DA, Masi AT: Psychiatric status of patients with primary fibromyalgia, patients with rheumatoid arthritis, and subjects without pain. Am J Psychiat 148: 1721-1726, 1991.

16. Schuessler G: Bewältigung chronischer Erkrankungen. Vandenhoeck, Göttingen, 1993.

17. Schepank H: Epidemiology of psychogenic disorders. Berlin: Springer, 1987.

Diurnal Variation
in the Symptoms and Signs
of the Fibromyalgia Syndrome [FS]

Paul A. Reilly
Geoffrey O. Littlejohn

SUMMARY. Objectives: To document possible diurnal variation in the severity of symptoms [pain, fatigue, stiffness and global sense of well-being] and signs [tender point count and sensitivity to pressure] in fibromyalgia.

Methods: Seventeen females with fibromyalgia [mean age 49.6 years] were seen in their own homes at 9.00 a.m. and again at 7.00 p.m. Symptoms were assessed using 100 mm VAS scales. All 18 tender points of the 1990 ACR criteria for fibromyalgia were examined using a 0-11 kg/cm^2 dolorimeter. Pain elicited at pressures < 4 kg/cm^2 denoted a tender point.

Paul A. Reilly, MB ChB, MRCP, is Research Fellow in Rheumatology, Rheumatology Unit, Monash Medical Centre, Clayton, Victoria 3168, Australia.

Geoffrey O. Littlejohn, MB BS[Hons], MD, FRACP, FACRM, is Head of Rheumatology, Monash Medical Centre, and Senior Lecturer in Medicine, Monash University, Rheumatology Unit, Monash Medical Centre, Clayton, Victoria 3168, Australia.

Address correspondence to: Dr. Reilly, Consultant Rheumatologist, Frimley Park NHS Trust Hospital, Portsmouth Road, Frimley, Surrey, GU16 5UJ, England, U.K.

Dr. Reilly was supported by the Michael Mason Fellowship of the Arthritis and Rheumatism Council of Great Britain.

[Haworth co-indexing entry note]: "Diurnal Variation in the Symptoms and Signs of the Fibromyalgia Syndrome [FS]." Reilly, Paul A., and Geoffrey O. Littlejohn. Co-published simultaneously in the *Journal of Musculoskeletal Pain* (The Haworth Press, Inc.) Vol. 1, No. 3/4, 1993, pp. 237-243; and: *Musculoskeletal Pain, Myofascial Pain Syndrome, and the Fibromyalgia Syndrome* (ed: Søren Jacobsen, Bente Danneskiold-Samsøe, and Birger Lund) The Haworth Press, Inc., 1993, pp. 237-243. Multiple copies of this article/chapter may be purchased from The Haworth Document Delivery Center [1-800-3-HAWORTH; 9:00 a.m. - 5:00 p.m. (EST)].

237

Results: Pain, fatigue and global score were worse in the evening in the majority of patients, while a similar proportion felt as stiff in the morning as in the evening. Tender points tended to be more numerous and more sensitive by evening. Most patients said they felt at their best around mid-day.

Conclusions: The features of fibromyalgia are more pronounced later in the day. Fatigue and pain contribute more to this deterioration than does stiffness. This diurnal variation should be considered when evaluating results of treatment.

KEYWORDS. Soft tissue, rheumatism, fibrositis, fibromyalgia

INTRODUCTION

Prominent among the many non-specific symptoms of fibromyalgia syndrome [FS] are pain, stiffness and fatigue (1). The pain is widely distributed in the neck, shoulders, low back, upper and lower limbs, and is often of a nagging, aching quality. Morning stiffness may be prolonged, lasting several hours, while fatigue may be severe enough to interfere with domestic, occupational and recreational activities.

Also prominent is a non-restorative sleep disturbance, with frequent waking and feeling unrefreshed in the morning. Moldofsky et al. have demonstrated a relationship between this sleep disturbance and an overnight increase in musculoskeletal pain and tender point [TeP] sensitivity (2). In a comparative study between two groups of patients with FS, one elderly [> 60 years], the other younger [< 60 years] Yunus et al. recorded that approximately half of the patients experienced pain mainly in the morning or evening, or both. One third had no such diurnal variation. Stiffness was predominant in the morning in 55% of both patient groups (3). However, there are no formal studies of diurnal variation in the symptoms and signs of FS, and such variation may be important when assessing the results of treatment regimes.

The purpose of this study was: 1. to document possible diurnal variation in subjective and objective features of FS, and 2. to assess whether the subjective severity of symptoms is matched by an appropriate change in the sensitivity of tender points.

METHODS

Seventeen female patients with FS [mean age 49.6 years, illness duration 2-25 years], diagnosed in the previous 12 months using the 1981 criteria of Yunus et al. (3), were recruited from the rheumatology out-patient practice of GOL, and all gave informed consent for the study. Patients were selected on their willingness to participate in, and availability for, the study and on the basis of reasonable geographic proximity to Monash Medical Center [essentially the eastern suburbs of metropolitan Melbourne]. Each patient was seen in their own home by PAR on two occasions on the same day at 9.00 a.m. and again at 7.00 p.m. Between these visits patients were asked to perform the routine of their normal day. Two were full-time students in further education, two worked full-time and one part-time. The others were either full-time housewives or had retired on medical grounds. At the first visit each was asked what was normally their best time of the day ["When would you choose to attend an important appointment so as to be at your best?"]. On both visits they filled in 100 mm visual analogue scales [VAS] for pain, stiffness, fatigue and global well-being. The global scale was marked "best" on the left and "worst possible" on the right. Therefore on all scales any shift to the right denoted deterioration and to the left an improvement in symptoms.

The 18 TePs [9 symmetrical sites] of the 1990 ACR criteria for FS (4) were pressed using a 0-11 kg dolorimeter surmounted by a circular, flat rubber tip of area 1.0 cm^2 [Pain Diagnostics and Thermography, Great Neck, NY] in the manner described by Fischer (5). As each TeP was pressed patients were asked to "Tell me when this begins to feel painful," thus giving a measure of pain threshold at that site.

The pressure in kg/cm^2 was then recorded. To prevent manipulation of results patients were not allowed in the evening to review the results from the morning assessment, nor were they reminded how severe or mild their symptoms had been.

For purposes of comparison only VAS changes of 5 mm or more were considered significant and only pressure gauge differences of more than 0.2 kg/cm^2, both arbitrarily decided upon before the study. Similarly a TeP was considered to be present only if pain was produced at pressures $< 4.0 \text{ kg/cm}^2$. This value has been used in other studies (4), and approximates to digital pressure sufficient to blanch the fingernail.

Because of the highly subjective nature of the data recorded, reflecting the subjective nature of the illness, no detailed statistical analysis has been applied, and the findings remain descriptive only.

RESULTS

Table 1 gives the numbers of patients who felt better, worse or unchanged in their symptoms and signs of FS in the evening compared to

Table 1: A summary of the diurnal variation in symptoms and signs of fibromyalgia in 17 female patients.

	WORSE MORNING	SAME	WORSE EVENING
Pain	1	4	12
Stiffness	6	4	7
Fatigue	2	2	13
Global	2	0	15
Tender Points	5	2	10

morning. The actual values [means and ranges] for the whole group were given in Table 2 together with median change in VAS scores and tender point count and sensitivity.

Best time of day: Fourteen of the 17 patients usually felt at their best around mid-day, between 11.00 a.m. and 2.00 p.m., while 3 felt best on rising in the morning. None felt better at the end of the day than at the beginning.

1. *Pain:* The median increase in VAS score for pain was 28 mm by evening. In 12 patients pain was more intense by evening, in 4 it was of similar intensity morning and evening, and in one it was less severe by evening.
2. *Stiffness:* The group as a whole showed little difference between morning and evening. Seven patients were more stiff and 6 less stiff by evening, while in four it was equally severe.
3. *Fatigue:* The majority of patients [13 of 17] were more fatigued later in the day than in the morning. The median change in VAS score was +39 mm for the group as a whole.
4. *Global well-being:* Most patients [15 of 17] felt worse overall by evening, and the median increase was +35 mm on VAS scores. Only 2 patients felt better by evening. Of the 15 patients who were globally worse by evening, 13 also had worse fatigue and 12 an increase in pain, but only 7 greater stiffness. The 2 patients who felt better in the evening had either less or no change in fatigue, pain and stiffness compared to the morning.

Tender points: All 17 patients had 11 or more TePs on at least one of the two visits, but in only 2 cases did the number of TePs fall below the 11 needed to satisfy ACR criteria. One lady had 7 TePs in the morning, rising to 11 by evening, while the other increased from 10 to 12 TePs. The range

Table 2: The median values recorded on the VAS scales are shown, together with the ranges. A +ve change indicates more severe symptoms in the evening for pain, stiffness, fatigue and global well–being. The –ve value for tender point measurements by dolorimetry [the charge in total delorimetry measurements for all 18 tender points listed in the ACR criteria] indicates a greater degree of sensitivity.

	9 a.m.	7 p.m.	Change
Pain	28(6–68)	66(2–94)	+28(–10–+75)
Stiffness	53(0–82)	46(9–92)	+3 (–63–+51)
Fatigue	7(0–82)	74(0–99)	+39(–21–+92)
Global	28(6–61)	67(2–98)	+35(–10–+74)
TePs [count]	16(6–18)	16(10–18)	+1(–3–+4)
TePs [dolorimeter]	49.6(37.2–85)	46.3(34.9–74.7)	–2.9(–14.2–+15.8)

in the change of TeP count was between a reduction of 3 TePs to an increase of 4 during the day, with the median change of plus 1. Thirteen of 17 patients had an increase or decrease of TeP count of plus or minus 2 TePs.

A pressure pain threshold was available for all 18 TePs in the 17 patients, giving a total of 306 measurements at each assessment time. A greater proportion of these became more sensitive by evening than less sensitive [160 vs. 123, with 23 unchanged]. For each patient the sum of the change for each individual TeP was calculated, using negative values for those more sensitive and positive values for those less so [i.e., a positive value indicated higher pressure pain threshold]. Ten patients had a total increase and 5 a total decrease in TeP sensitivity by evening, with a median difference of -2.9 kg/cm^2 for the group as a whole. Therefore the tendency was for TePs to become rather more numerous and more tender by evening in the majority of patients.

DISCUSSION

This study is a clinical observation of what changes occur in the main complaints of patients with FS during their normal day. It indicates that most feel at their best in the middle of the day, and feel worse by evening than they had felt in the morning. This is in contrast to the hospital out patient-based study of 50 patients by Yunus et al. (3), 28% of whom had symptoms predominantly in the morning, compared to only 14% who were worse in the evening.

The majority [15/17] of patients in this study had a worse global assessment of their condition by evening, as measured on a VAS scale. This was usually accompanied by concomitant deterioration in what may be the main contributors to that global assessment, i.e., pain and fatigue, while many felt that stiffness eased as the day progressed. Worse subjective measures tended to be reflected in the overall sensitivity of tender points, which increased even in the absence of any major change in the actual tender point count. It seems logical that the follow-up of patients with FS should be at a similar time of day to the initial evaluation, to minimise the possible confounding effect of diurnal variation when evaluating the outcome of therapeutic intervention.

We accept that our study raises questions about flaws in methodology. We have no data on the intra-observer reliability of dolorimeter readings, nor do we know if the results on the day of assessment were a true reflection of what occurs on other days. Although most patients declared themselves to be at their best around mid-day, it would have been more satisfactory to have confirmed this using VAS scales and tender point examination as described above. The sprawling geography of Melbourne made this impractical in our study, however.

Fibromyalgia is, like many other chronic pain syndromes, almost entirely subjective, without confirmatory laboratory or radiologic tests. The "softness" of the data recorded in studies limits the firmness of conclusions to be drawn, but a trend is apparent; that FS is bad on rising in the morning, then begins to ease by the middle of the day [perhaps as stiffness diminishes], and then becomes particularly bad in the evening with the onset of fatigue and an increase in locomotor pain. All 17 patients in our study had chronic non-restorative sleep, but its influence on the overall clinical picture of FS may have been over-emphasized. It is now recognised that patients with FS score highly on the Daily Hassles Scale (6), and perhaps daytime stresses, physical or psychological, are just as important as poor sleep in influencing diurnal variation in the features of fibromyalgia.

REFERENCES

1. Wolfe F: Fibromyalgia: the clinical syndrome. Rheum Dis Cin North Am 15(1): 1-18, 1989.

2. Moldofsky H: Sleep and fibrositis syndrome. Rheum Dis Clin North Am 15(1): 91-103, 1989.

3. Yunus MB, Holt GS, Masi AT, Aldag JC: Fibromyalgia syndrome among the elderly. Comparison with younger patients. J AM Geriatr Soc 36: 987-995, 1988.

4. Yunus M, Masi AT, Calabro JJ, Miller KA, Feigenbaum SL: Primary fibromyalgia [fibrositis]: clinical study of 50 patients with matched normal controls. Semin Arthritis Rheum 11(1): 151-171, 1981.

5. Wolfe F, Smythe HA, Yunus MB et al.: The American College of Rheumatology 1990 criteria for the classification of fibromyalgia. Report of the multicenter criteria committee. Arthritis Rheum 33: 160-172, 1990.

6. Fischer AA: Pressure threshold meter: its use for quantification of tender spots. Arch Phys Med Rehabil 67: 836-838, 1986.

7. Dailey PA, Bishop GD, Russell IJ, Fletcher EM: Psychological stress and the fibrositis/fibromyalgia syndrome. J Rheumatol 17: 1380-1385, 1990.

Does a Fibromyalgia Personality Exist?

Valur Johannsson

SUMMARY. Objectives: To compare a computerized version of a personality test with the traditional method and to investigate if specific traits of fibromyalgia personality do exist.

Methods: One hundred and ten females with fibromyalgia syndrome performed a computer-administrated version of the Cesarec Marke Personality Schedule [CMPS]. The scores were compared to a group of female fibromyalgia patients performing the traditional paper and pen method of CMPS.

Results: There were no differences between the results of the computer tested and conventional tested groups in personality profile. Compared to a normative Swedish female population significant differences were found.

Conclusions: The computer version of the CMPS can be used equivalent to the traditional method. Female fibromyalgia patients have a great need for Order but low needs for Exhibition, Autonomy and Aggressive non-conformance but other-wise only showed modest or no differences from a normative Swedish female population.

KEYWORDS. Fibromyalgia syndrome, personality, CMPS, computer test

Valur Johannsson, MD, is Medical Director, The Hospital of National Social Insurance, Tranås, Sweden.

Address correspondence to: Valur Johannsson, MD, The Hospital of National Social Insurance, S-573 81 Tranås, Sweden.

The author would like to acknowledge Psychologist Lars Isberg.

[Haworth co-indexing entry note]: "Does a Fibromyalgia Personality Exist?" Johannsson, Valur. Co-published simultaneously in the *Journal of Musculoskeletal Pain* (The Haworth Press, Inc.) Vol. 1, No. 3/4, 1993, pp. 245-252; and: *Musculoskeletal Pain, Myofascial Pain Syndrome, and the Fibromyalgia Syndrome* (ed: Søren Jacobsen, Bente Danneskiold-Samsøe, and Birger Lund) The Haworth Press, Inc., 1993, pp. 245-252. Multiple copies of this article/chapter may be purchased from The Haworth Document Delivery Center [1-800-3-HAWORTH; 9:00 a.m. - 5:00 p.m. (EST)].

245

INTRODUCTION

The purpose of this study was to evaluate if a computerized version of the Cesarec Marke Personality Schedule [CMPS] (1) was equivalent to the conventional CMPS and to examine if the personalities of female fibromyalgia [FMS] patients differed from a normative Swedish female population.

Much research has been done to find a relationship between FMS and various forms of psychopathology (2). Many studies have found elevated rates of specific psychiatric disorders. Particularly depression, hypochondriasis, and hysteria. Most used psychological scales and instruments, however, have the drawback that patients with chronic pain or medical illness automatically get high scores (3).

Holmlund (4) found that by using the CMPS test when following 15 year old females over a ten year period that all personality traits were moderately stable over time. The needs expressing aggression, extraversion, and neuroticism [Aggression, Dominance, Defence of Status and Guilt Feelings] showed the highest correlation coefficients, rs ranging from 0.3 to 0.4. This was in concordance with several other studies. She also found that at the age of 25, the needs Defence of Status, Guilt Feelings and Succourance were positively related to symptoms of depression and anxiety, while the need Dominance showed a negative relation. Earlier research had shown that unipolar depressive patients during remission differed from normal controls in higher scores of needs Defence of Status and Guilt Feelings, and lower score of need Dominance (5).

Personality traits can be characterized in terms of stability and change. Some aspects of the personality structure change over time. Maturation, environmental changes and medical illness can affect some personality traits and thus influence the scores of the tests (6,7).

The CMPS was chosen for this study because the test was validated and normative on a Swedish female population and has been widely used in Sweden. The CMPS and the internationally recognized Edvards Personal Preference Schedule have been examined and the results suggested that the two tests can be used as parallel tests (1). The CMPS is a Swedish personality inventory based on Murray's [1938] theory of needs. It consists of 11 subscales and five factor indices derived from factor analysis of the subscales. The subscales are:

1. *Achievement* (ach): A need to accomplish something important and difficult, and to compete with and surpass others.
2. *Affiliation* (aff): A need and ability to form close emotional relations.

3. *Aggression* (agg): A need to take revenge, to tease others and enjoy doing so, irritability, impulsive aggression.
4. *Defence of Status* (dst): Sensitivity to the opinion of others, tendency to refrain from actions in order to avoid failures, and a need to explain and defend mistakes.
5. *Guilt Feelings* (gui): A strict conscience with a strong sense of duty, and a need to reform oneself.
6. *Dominance* (dom): A need to take the lead, to assert oneself and do succeed in doing so.
7. *Exhibition* (exh): A need to be in the centre, to be noticed, to dramatize.
8. *Autonomy* (aut): A need to be independent, to disregard the opinion of others, to oppose others, and to avoid responsibilities.
9. *Nurturance* (nur): A need to help and defend others.
10. *Order* (ord): A need for order, punctuality, cleanliness and planning.
11. *Succourance* (suc): A need to be taken care of and to be helped both emotionally and practically, difficulties in managing solely.

The CMPS has a response set scale *Acquiescence* (acq): the tendency to answer yes or no irrespective of content. The factor indices consists of the weighed sums of the subscales.

I. *Neurotic Self-Assertiveness,* consists of the sum: Achievement × 6, Guilt Feelings × 5, Defence of Status × 5, and Aggression × 4.
II. *Rational Dominance,* the sum: Dominance × 7, Exhibition × 7, Defence of Status × −5, Guilt Feelings × −5.
III. *Aggressive Non-Conformance,* the sum: Order × −5, Autonomy × 5, and Aggression × 4.
IV. *Passive Dependency,* the sum: Succourance × 6, Affiliation × 5, Defence of Status × 3.
V. *Sociability,* the sum: Nurturance × 5, Affiliation × 3, and Aggression × −3.

MATERIALS AND METHODS

One hundred and ten female inpatients at the Hospital of National Social Insurance in Tranås, Sweden with fibromyalgia syndrome [FMS] according to the ACR-90 criteria (8) performed a computerized version of CMPS with a "Touch–screenfunction" [Hardware Hewlett-Packard PC, software Vicsoft]. Their average age was 43 years [range 21-59]. The duration of disease was average 14 years [range 1-37].

The significance was calculated from the average raw-points compared to the norm for Swedish female population. The raw-points were then changed to Stanine-points from 1-9 which represents the normal distribution. Statistical analysis was accomplished by Statgraphic ver. 5. 0. One sample analysis, t-test. Confidence interval 95%. [Table 1].

A comparison of scores was made to a study (9) with the traditional

TABLE 1. Statistical evaluation of computerized CMPS test performed by 110 female FMS patients.

	Testaverage Rawpoints	Normated average Rawpoints	Standard devation	T-value	P-value
1. (Ach:)	6,97	8,15	2,93	-4,22	<0,001
2. (Aff:)	10,05	9,8	2,03	1,32	N.S
3. (Agg:)	5,55	7,0	2,71	-5,6	<0,001
4. (Dst:)	7,35	6,9	3,22	1,48	N.S
5. (Gui:)	7,74	6,8	3,49	2,81	<0,01
6. (Dom:)	6,7	8,0	3,2	-4,26	<0,001
7. (Exh:)	5,6	8,2	3,52	-7,14	<0,001
8. (Ant:)	6,94	8,4	2,09	-7,36	<0,001
9. (Nur:)	12	11,6	2,12	1,98	N.S
10. (Ord:)	10,99	8,1	2,84	10,68	<0,001
11. (Suc:)	9,19	9,2	2,72	-0,04	N.S
(Acq:)	46,43	47	7,57	-0,8	N.S
I. (Neur:)	139,5	145,2	42,37	-1,41	N.S
II. (R Domin:)	18,38	51,1	60,42	-5,68	<0,001
III. (Agg. N. Conf):	1,95	29,1	24,3	-11,72	<0,001
IV. (D.Dep:)	127,49	124,4	25,42	1,27	N.S
V. (Soc:)	73,5	67,3	16,83	3,86	<0,001

paper and pen method of CMPS performed by 45 female FMS inpatients at the same hospital and according to Yunus criteria (10).

RESULTS

The scores of the two FMS groups were practically identical [Figure 1, Table 2]. The need Order got high scores. The needs Autonomy, Dominance and Exhibition and the index Aggressive Non-Conformance had the lowest scores. In other needs they showed modest or no differences from a normative Swedish female population. Only the computer tested group had significant differences from the norm because of the greater material with exception of the need Order which was significant in both patient groups.

DISCUSSION

The study has shown that computerized CMPS gives extremely equivalent scores compared to the conventional CMPS, although the criteria was according to ACR-90 in the first case and to Yunus in the second case.

To be able to collect large amounts of data computer-aided questionnaires [CAQ] become more important. It is therefore of great importance that the methods of CAQ are reliable and valid.

The results also confirm the common clinical impression that the FMS patients are pedantic and have great needs for order, perfectionism, planning and cleanliness. You may speculate if this character of personality make them prone to be more attentive, watchful and demanding towards their somatic functions and dysfunctions? The low scores in index III Aggressive Non-Conformance indicate a rather low self-confidence. The modest tendency to have slight elevated scores of Defence of Status, Guilt Feelings and low scores of Dominance doesn't confirm that FMS patients are more prone to develop depression. It may indicate that a subgroup of FMS patients are more vulnerable in this aspect but this hypothesis needs further investigation.

The index I Neurotic Self-Assertiveness scores were slightly lower compared to a normative Swedish female population and thus contradict that the FMS patients should be neurotic in this aspect. The low scores on Achievement can seem to be surprising but Achievement means that the person always want to compete with and surpass others. But FMS patients don't seem to be ambitious in that manner. Anyhow it must again be empha-

FIGURE 1. The scores of the conventional CMPS with patients tested according to Yunus criteria are shown by a diamond [N = 45]. Stanine point 5 is the normative average for Swedish females and is shown by a line. The computerized CMPS scores with patients tested according to ACR-90 criteria are shown by staples [N = 110]. N.S. = not significant.

Results of CMPS test.

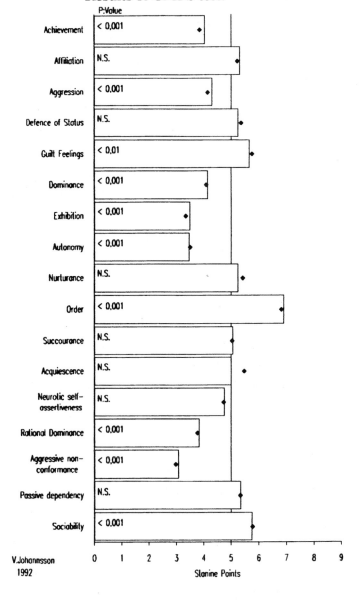

TABLE 2. Comparison of Average Stanine Points and S.D. by computerized versus conventional CMPS test.

	Computer version CMPS N=110 FMS females Stanine points	Conventional version CMPS N = 45 FMS females Stanine points	Computer version CMPS N=110 FMS females Standard deviation	Conventional version CMPS N=45 FMS females Standard deviation
1. (Ach:)	4,02	3,84	2,13	2,14
2. (Aff:)	5,31	5,22	1,71	1,92
3. (Agg:)	4,29	4,13	1,64	2,3
4. (Det:)	5,25	5,36	2,01	2,3
5. (Gui:)	5,65	5,76	1,97	1,97
6. (Dom:)	4,13	4,09	1,65	1,86
7. (Exh:)	3,48	3,83	1,87	1,73
8. (Ant:)	3,45	3,49	1,59	1,74
9. (Nur:)	5,25	5,42	1,96	2,31
10. (Ord:)	6,9	6,82	1,46	1,61
11. (Suc:)	5,06	5,04	2,02	1,98
(Acq:)	5,0	5,47	2,18	2,46
I. (Neur:)	4,75	4,73	2,13	2,52
II. (R Domin:)	3,83	3,76	1,92	1,96
III. (Agg. N. Conf):	3,07	2,98	1,41	1,7
IV. (D.Dep:)	5,35	5,33	1,89	2,09
V. (Soc:)	5,75	5,70	1,69	1,76

sized that personality traits change during maturation and by environmental influences. The impact of a longterm disease must also be considered.

A Note on Type II Errors and the Interpretation of Non-Significant Differences

While our interpretation of the statistically significant differences obtained between average test scores and the norm group is fairly straightforward, some caution is well advised when it comes to the acceptance of non-significant differences: Does the lack of a difference great enough for statistical significance really mean that there is truly no difference between experimental and norm group on these variables? It is our view that these cases should be interpreted with caution in order not to make unnecessary Type II errors.

Specifically, in cases where the mean test score of the experimental group is greater–albeit non significantly so–that the normative score, rejection of H1 [that the true score of the experimental group is greater than that of the norm group] should be seen rather as provisional, awaiting further confirmation. This being said, however, we feel that the proposed interpretations in many of these cases are supported by what seems reasonable, and even probable, from the point of view of our general clinical experience.

REFERENCES

1. Cesarec Z, Marke S: Mätning av psykogena behov med frågeformulärsteknik (Manual of CMPS) Skandinaviska testförlaget, Stockholm, Sweden, 1968.

2. Hudson JI, Pope HG, Jr.: Fibromyalgia and psychopathology: Is fibromyalgia a form of "Affective Spectrum Disorder?" J Rheumatol 16 (Suppl 19): 16-22, 1989.

3. Goldenburg DL: An overview of psychologic studies in fibromyalgia. J Rheumatol 16 (Suppl 19): 12-4, 1989.

4. Holmlund U: Change and stability of needs from middle adolescence to young adulthood in Swedish females. European Journal of Personality "(in press)."

5. Strandman E: Psychogenic needs in patients with affective disorders. Actapsychiathrica Scandinavica 58: 16-29, 1978.

6. Costa PT, Jr. et al.: Enduring dispositions in adult males. Journal of Personality and Social Psychology 38: 793-800, 1980.

7. Moss HA, Susman EJ: Longitudinal study of personality development. Constancy and change in human development, Howard University Press, Cambridge, USA, 190: 130-595.

8. Wolfe F, Smythe HA, Yunus MB et al.: The American College of Rheumatology 1990 criteria for the classification of fibromyalgia. Arthritis Rheum 33: 160-72, 1990.

9. Hultén Bo, Wiik Eva-Maria: What have fibromyalgia-patients in common, Psychological institution, University of Gothenburg, Sweden, 1992.

10. Yunus MB, Masi AT, Callabro JJ, Miller KA, Feigenbaum SL: Primary fibromyalgia (fibrositis): Clinical study of 50 patients with matched normal controls. Semin Arthritis Rheum 11: 151-71, 1981.

TREATMENT OF MYOFASCIAL PAIN AND FIBROMYALGIA

Effects of Amitriptyline and Cardiovascular Fitness Training on Pain in Patients with Primary Fibromyalgia

Risto Isomeri
Marja Mikkelsson
Pirjo Latikka
Kerttu Kammonen

SUMMARY. Objectives: The aim of the study was to compare the value of amitriptyline [AT] and cardiovascular fitness training [CFT] in the treatment of pain in patients with primary fibromyalgia syndrome [PFS].

Risto Isomeri, MD, Chief, Marja Mikkelsson, MD, Assistant Physician, Pirjo Latikka, MD, Assistant Physician, and Kerttu Kammonen, Senior Ward Physician, are all affiliated with the Rehabilitation Department of the Rheumatism Foundation Hospital [RFH].

[Haworth co-indexing entry note]: "Effects of Amitriptyline and Cardiovascular Fitness Training on Pain in Patients with Primary Fibromyalgia." Isomeri, Risto et al. Co-published simultaneously in the *Journal of Musculoskeletal Pain* (The Haworth Press, Inc.) Vol. 1, No. 3/4, 1993, pp. 253-260; and: *Musculoskeletal Pain, Myofascial Pain Syndrome, and the Fibromyalgia Syndrome* (ed: Søren Jacobsen, Bente Danneskiold-Samsøe, and Birger Lund) The Haworth Press, Inc., 1993, pp. 253-260. Multiple copies of this article/chapter may be purchased from The Haworth Document Delivery Center [1-800-3-HAWORTH; 9:00 a.m. - 5:00 p.m. (EST)].

Methods: A total of 45 patients [39 ♀, 6 ♂, mean age 43.7, range 24-55 years] with PFS were randomized into three treatment groups: A. Sixteen patients who received AT 25 mg at 9 p.m. daily; B. Fifteen patients with heavy CFT; and C. Fourteen patients who received AT 25 mg at 9 p.m. daily and who had heavy CFT. The duration of treatment was 15 weeks.

Results: Pain measured as the pressure pain threshold and tolerance on muscle and bone control points and as the pain threshold on tender points and on a visual analogue scale [VAS] were similar in all three groups at the start of the trial. After 15 weeks all measurements showed less pain experience in patients treated with both AT and CFT [group C] than in patients treated with AT alone [group A]. The effect of CFT alone [group B] was better than that of AT alone, but not as good as that of the combination. General pain as measured by VAS only declined in patients treated with both AT and CFT.

Conclusions: A combination of AT and CFT is more effective in the treatment of PFS than either of these alone.

KEYWORDS. Amitriptyline, cardiovascular fitness training, fibromyalgia

INTRODUCTION

Treatment of patients with PFS is difficult. Complete and long-lasting cure of symptoms has not been reported with any of the therapies used, although some benefits have been achieved with tricyclic antidepressive drugs (1,2), analgetic drugs (3), biofeedback (4), hypnosis (5), and physical fitness training strenuous enough to increase oxygen intake capacity (6,7). Experience of combinations of these therapies is limited (2).

Because the therapeutic effects of low-dose tricyclic antidepressive drugs and of physical training have been favourable, we carried out a study to establish whether a combination of these two therapies would produce better results than either of them alone.

PATIENTS AND METHODS

A total of 51 patients fulfilling the diagnostic criteria of Yunus et al. (8) and of Wolfe et al. (9) for PFS were randomized into three treatment groups of 17 patients each. Other diseases causing pain were excluded in a thorough medical examination that included a wide range of laboratory tests and X rays. Patients unable to participate in the heavy physical training because of other diseases or drug therapy were excluded. Six patients discontinued the trial. There were no significant differences between the treatment groups in age, sex, duration of symptoms, physical disability index (10) or depression index (11) [Table 1].

The first group of patients [A] was treated with conventional physiotherapy consisting of light muscle stretching exercises only. Amitriptyline 25 mg was given in the evenings. The second group of patients [B] underwent physical fitness training of increasing strenuousness. The third group of patients [C] followed the same physical training programme as group B and received the same dose of amitriptyline in the evenings as group A. The treatment programme for all patients was started in the hospital during a three-week rehabilitation course, and was continued at home during the next 12 weeks. At home, the patients had to keep a diary of the exercise programme.

Pain was evaluated at the beginning of the trial and after 15 weeks, on a 100 mm VAS and by measuring the pain threshold and pain tolerance with a pressure dolorimeter [FS Products] on the deltoid muscle and the tibial bone [control points]. Pressure pain thresholds were also measured from approximately 15 tender points in each patient. Pressure pain measurements were carried out by two physicians [MM, PL], who had standardized their procedures.

TABLE 1

Background of 45 PFS patients

GROUP	A (N 16)	B (N 15)	C (N 14)
Age (mean, SD)	45.9 (7.9)	40.5 (8.7)	44.6 (6.2)
Sex female	13	12	14
male	3	3	0
Years at work	28.3 (9.6)	23.8 (9.3)	26.9 (6.9)
HAQ-disability (10)	0.44(0.26)	0.39(0.40)	0.36(0.33)
Depression index(11)*	12.8 (5.0)	9.4 (5.0)	12.2 (4.8)
Duration of symptoms (years)	10.2 (7.0)	6.6 (6.3)	7.0 (4.9)
Age at onset	35.7 (9.1)	33.8 (10.0)	37.5 (6.4)

* Depression index (11) 0-6 no depression, 7-11 light, 12-16 moderate and 17-21 severe depression.

RESULTS

Figure 1 shows that the pressure pain experience at the beginning of the trial was similar in all three groups. After 15 weeks of therapy all the pressure pain measurements showed similar differences between the groups: the patients in most pain were those receiving amitriptyline only, those in least pain were receiving the combination therapy, and those between these two were receiving CFT only [Figures 2 and 3]. General pain on VAS only decreased in the patients receiving the combination therapy [Figure 4]. One-way analysis of variance was used to compare the

FIGURE 1. Pressure pain threshold [left] and tolerance [right] from control points of deltoid muscle and tibial bone [mean, SEM] at the beginning of the trial. A amitriptyline alone, B CFT alone, C amitriptyline and CFT.

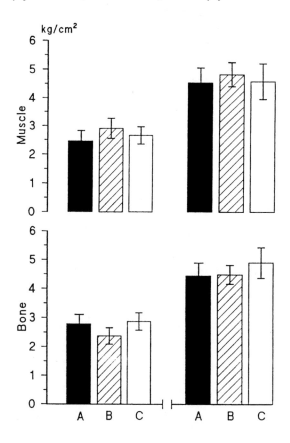

FIGURE 2. Pressure pain threshold [left] and tolerance [right] from control points of deltoid muscle and tibial bone [mean, SEM] at the end of the trial. A amitriptyline alone, B CFT alone, C both amitriptyline and CFT.

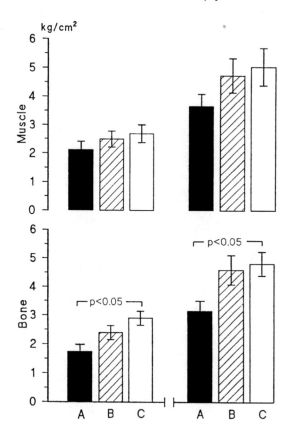

means of the different groups. The P-values of the statistical differences were corrected for multiple comparisons.

DISCUSSION

The therapeutic result of this study was disappointing, because pressure pain experience did not decrease during the therapy. On the contrary, the pressure pain threshold and tolerance deteriorated in patients receiving AT treatment alone [group A], and an improvement was seen only in patients

FIGURE 3. Pressure pain threshold from tender points [mean from 15 points] at the beginning and at the end of the trial. A amitriptyline alone, B CFT alone, C both amitriptyline and CFT.

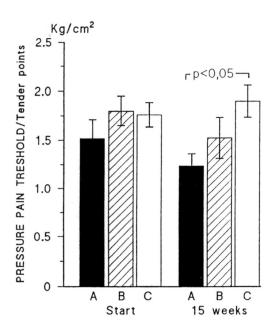

receiving the combination therapy. The similarity in the differences between the treatment groups after the trial indicates a true therapeutic effect by the combination. Despite the small number of patients, we found statistically significant differences [P < 0.05] at the end of the study between groups A and C in the tender point measurements and in the bone control point measurements. It is possible that quantification of pain using the pressure dolorimeter is not possible, and that the therapeutic effect is masked by measurement error. The only clear improvement was seen in the general pain measured by VAS in patients receiving combination therapy.

The depression levels were rather high in all treatment groups [Table 1]. Although a low dose of AT has only minor antidepressive effects, it may improve the quality of sleep and correct aberrations of serotonin in the brain stem (2,12). This may raise the spirits, as does physical training, by causing post exercise hypoalgesia through increased endogenous opioids in the brain (6,7). It is known that physical training is able to alleviate depression (13) and to improve the quality of sleep (14).

FIGURE 4. General pain on visual analogue scale at the beginning and at the end of the trial. A amitriptyline alone, B CFT alone, C both AT and CFT.

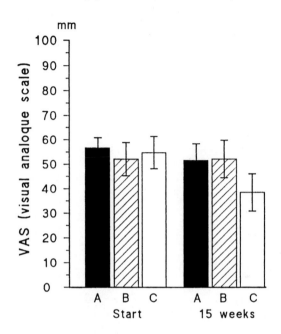

In conclusion, a combination of AT and CFT seems to be more effective in the treatment of pain in patients with PFS than either of these alone.

AUTHOR NOTE

Address reprint requests to: Risto Isomeri, Rheumatism Foundation Hospital, SF-18120 Heinola, Finland.

The valuable help of Mr Hannu Kautiainen, who carried out the statistical analyses of the results, is gratefully acknowledged.

This study was supported by grants from the Rheumatism Research Foundation.

REFERENCES

1. Carette S, McCain GA, Bell DA, Fam AG: Evaluation of amitriptyline in primary fibrositis. Arthritis Rheum 29: 655-659, 1986.

2. Goldenberg DL, Felson DT, Dinerman H: Randomized, controlled trial of amitriptyline and naproxen in the treatment of patients with fibromyalgia. Arthritis Rheum 29: 1371-1377, 1986.

3. Vaerøy H, Abrahamsen A, Førre Ø, Kåss E: Treatment of fibromyalgia (fibrositis syndrome): A parallel double blind trial with carisoprodol, paracetamol and caffeine (Somadril comp[R]) versus placebo. Clinical Rheum 8, No 2: 245-250, 1989.

4. Furaccioli G, Chirelli L, Scita F, Nolli M, Mozzani M, Fontana S, Scorsonelli M, Tridenti A, De Risio C: EMG-biofeedback training in fibromyalgia syndr. J Rheumatol 14: 820-825, 1987.

5. Haanen HCM, Hoenderdos HTW, van Romunde LKJ, Hop WCJ, Mallee C, Terwiel JP, Hekster GB: Controlled trial of hypnotherapy in the treatment of refractory fibromyalgia. J Rheumatol 18: 1, 72-75, 1991.

6. McCain GA: Role of physical fitness training in the fibrositis/fibromyalgia syndrome. Am J Med Vol. 81 (suppl 3A): 73-77, 1986.

7. McCain GA, Bell DA, Mai FM, Halliday PD: A controlled study of the effects of a supervised cardiovascular fitness training program on the manifestations of primary fibromyalgia. Arthritis Rheum Vol. 31, No 9: 1135-1141, 1988.

8. Yunus MB, Masi AT, Calabro JJ, Miller KA, Feigenbaum SL: Primary fibromyalgia (fibrositis): clinical study of 50 patients with matched normal controls. Semin Arthritis Rheum 11: 151-171, 1981.

9. Wolfe F, Hawley DJ, Cathey MA, Caro X, Russell IJ: Fibrositis: symptom frequency and criteria for diagnosis: An evaluation of 291 rheumatic disease patients and 58 normal individuals. J Rheumatol 12: 1159-1163, 1985.

10. Fries JF, Spitz P, Kraines RG, Holman HR: Measurement of patients outcome in arthritis. Arthritis Rheum, Vol. 23, No 2: 137-145, 1980.

11. Rimon R et al.: Psychiatrica Fennica, No 59, pp. 1-16, 1984.

12. Rice JR: "Fibrositis" syndrome. Med Clin North Am Vol. 70 (2): 455-468, 1986.

13. McCann IL, Holmes DS: Influence of aerobic exercise on depression. J. Personal and Social Psychol Vol. 46, No 5, 1142-1147, 1984.

14. Torsvall L, Akestedt T, Lindbeck G: Effects on sleep stages and EEG power density on different degrees of exercise in fit subjects. Electroencephalogr Clin Neuropshysiol 57: 347-353, 1984.

Patients with Fibromyalgia in Pain School

Odd Kogstad
Franz Hintringer

SUMMARY. Methods: Seventy-one patients with fibromyalgia according to Yunus 1981 criteria were compared with 71 controls matched with age, sex and total pain score (VAS) in a one-year period. The study group had pain school as the only therapy intervention. The pain school consisted of education, group therapy and psychomotoric physiotherapy.

Results: The pupils' overall assessment showed a significant improvement compared with the controls [P = 0.01]. Some pain consequences, psychosocial factors and quality of life also improved significantly.

Conclusions: A structured pain school is a useful supplement to other treatments of fibromyalgia.

KEYWORDS. Fibromyalgia treatment, pain school, chronic pain treatment

Patients with chronic muscular pain syndromes are a daily and difficult challenge in medicine. As we don't have a single cause to treat, our main task will be to activate patients' own positive powers in fighting the pain, managing chronic pain consequences and improving life quality.

Odd Kogstad, MD, Head of the Department, and Franz Hintringer, MD, are both affiliated with the Department of Physical Medicine and Rehabilitation, Aust-Agder County Hospital, Arendal, Norway.

Address correspondence to: Odd Kogstad, MD, Department of Physical Medicine and Rehabilitation, Aust-Agder Central Hospital, 4800 Arendal, Norway.

[Haworth co-indexing entry note]: "Patients with Fibromyalgia in Pain School." Kogstad, Odd, and Franz Hintringer. Co-published simultaneously in the *Journal of Musculoskeletal Pain* (The Haworth Press, Inc.) Vol. 1, No. 3/4, 1993, pp. 261-265; and: *Musculoskeletal Pain, Myofascial Pain Syndrome, and the Fibromyalgia Syndrome* (ed: Søren Jacobsen, Bente Danneskiold-Samsøe, and Birger Lund) The Haworth Press, Inc., 1993, pp. 261-265. Multiple copies of this article/chapter may be purchased from The Haworth Document Delivery Center [1-800-3-HAWORTH; 9:00 a.m. - 5:00 p.m. (EST)].

METHODS

Seventy-one consecutive patients were referred from general practitioners. They had clinical examinations with relevant laboratory tests and X ray. All fulfilled the Yunus 1981 criteria of fibromyalgia (1). They were compared with a control group consisting of 71 consecutive patients from a study the previous year (2). They were matched in pairs with age, sex and total pain score [VAS]. Total pain score was pain intensity graded 1-10 with visual analogue scale [VAS] in seven different body parts. The patients' self-estimation of total health was also graded 1-10 with VAS. Fatigue and sleep disturbances were recorded present/not present. Pain was evaluated with a modified McGill Pain Questionnaire (3). A Norwegian version of the Sickness Impact Profile (4) together with the other questionnaires were evaluated at start, after three months and 12 months. Tender points were recorded diagnostically on 18 localizations only at baseline. No differences were found between the groups in the use of analgesics, tricyclic antidepressants or conventional physiotherapy. The pain school was the only different treatment intervention between the groups.

The classes had weekly two hour lessons six times. The topics were education, exercises/physical training, demonstration of relaxation techniques and group discussion. The goal of the education was mainly to teach the pupils self-help principles and how to cope with chronic pain (5). Communication and problem solving were also important parts of the discussions. Family members were invited to one of the lessons.

A physiotherapist specially trained in psychomotoric physiotherapy, which is a subspecialty in the Norwegian physiotherapy education, trained the participants in relaxation techniques, guided imagery, vivid imagery, self-talk and distraction. The statistical analyses were done by paired T-test on a 5% significance level. Each compared pair accepted in the analysis had observations at start and after one year.

RESULTS

Table 1 shows insignificant differences between the groups as to duration of disease and total pain score [VAS] and were otherwise comparable.

The patients' overall assessment after one year follow-up is shown in Table 2. The pupils had significantly better global outcome than the controls. Some pain consequences also showed significant differences between pupils and controls [Table 3]. However, there were no significant

TABLE 1

GROUP DIFFERENCES

	Pupils	Controls
Age	43 (23-69)	43 (22-67)
Sex	49 female	49 female
	22 male	22 male
Average duration	9,6	6,3
Total pain score (VAS)	3,7	2,4
Health evaluation (VAS)	3,1	3,3
Fatigue	27	24
Sleep disturbance	32	28
Tender points	10,5	9,8

TABLE 2

RESULTS ONE YEAR FOLLOW-UP

Per cent (N= 71)

	Pain school	Controls
Better	28	15
Unchanged	54	39
Worse	18	46

P= 0,01 (chi-square test)

differences between pupils and controls as to depression, physical activity, medication, sleep disturbances and fatigue.

The statistical analyses of total pain score, physical SIP, psychological SIP and total SIP showed no significant differences. The pupils evaluated the group therapy part of the programme as more important than the psychomotoric physiotherapy and the theoretical part of the education.

TABLE 3

PAIN CONSEQUENCES AFTER ONE YEAR

	Per cent			
	Pain school		Controls	
Less social withdrawal	42/57	74	40	P=0,004
More satisfied with life	36/51	71	50	P=0,03
Less family problems	36/56	64	43	P=0,03
Easier contact with others	35/57	61	28	P=0,004
More relaxed	27/56	48	28	P=0,04

Fischer's exact test (significance 0,05)

TABLE 4

WORK - SOCIAL SUPPORT

	Pupils		Controls	
	Start/1 year		Start/1 year	
Paid job	5	13	23	12
Home working	3	4	3	4
Social security	1	0	0	4
Sick leave	19	2	25	4
Rehabilitation	19	24	14	23
Disability pension	23	27	6	24

The average use of health services were reduced 10% among the pupils compared with the controls. This is not statistically significant. Table 4 shows increase in paid jobs from 5-13 among the pupils while it was a decrease from 23-12 among the controls. The figures are difficult to evaluate because of differences in disease duration, sick leave and disability pension at start.

CONCLUSIONS

A structural pain school is a supplement to other treatments of chronic, non-malignant muscular pain as in this controlled study with 71 fibromyalgia patients. Some pain consequences and life quality were improved significantly in a one-year period for the pain school participants. Group therapy in pain school models may give additional beneficial results in chronic pain patients and further clinic trials are recommended to find the best components in a structured educational programme.

REFERENCES

1. Yunus M, Masi AT, Calabro JJ et al.: Primary fibromyalgia (fibrositis). Arthritis Rheum 11: 151-71, 1981.

2. Kogstad O: Fibromyalgia (fibrositt). Tidsskr Nor Lægeforen nr. 32, 108: 2997-3000, 1988.

3. Kogstad O, Ljunggren E: Low-back pain. Pain description as a diagnostic aid. Scand J Rehab Med 22: 77-82, 1988.

4. Bergner M, Babitt RA, Carter WB, Gilson BS: The Sickness Impact Profile. Med Care 19: 787-805, 1981.

5. Lorig K, Gonzales V: The integration of theory with practice: A 12-year case study. Health Education Quarterly 19(3): 355-68, 1992.

Physical Fitness Training
in Patients with Fibromyalgia

Anne Marit Mengshoel
Øystein Førre

SUMMARY. Objectives: The aim of this study was to examine whether participation in low-intensity endurance training influenced pain and fatigue symptoms of fibromyalgia.

Methods: A training group [n = 11] exercised one hour twice a week for twenty weeks, while a control group [n = 14] did not change their physical activity level.

Results: During the twenty weeks no statistically significant changes in symptoms were observed in the training group compared with their baseline recordings, or any differences compared with the outcomes of the control group.

Conclusion: Patients with fibromyalgia might perform low-intensity endurance training without exacerbation of pain and fatigue.

KEYWORDS. Fibromyalgia, exercise, pain

Anne Marit Mengshoel, Physiotherapist and Research Fellow, and Øystein Førre, MD, PhD, Professor, are both affiliated with Oslo Sanitetsforening Rheumatism Hospital, Akersbakken 27, 0172 Oslo, Norway.

Address reprint requests to: Anne Marit Mengshoel, Oslo Sanitetsforenings Rheumatism Hospital, Akersbakken 27, 0172 Oslo.

This study was supported by grants from the Norwegian Fund for Postgraduate Training in Physiotherapy, the Olga Immerslund Legacy for Rheumatological Research and Hafslund-Nycomed.

[Haworth co-indexing entry note]: "Physical Fitness Training in Patients with Fibromyalgia." Mengshoel, Anne Marit, and Øystein Førre. Co-published simultaneously in the *Journal of Musculoskeletal Pain* (The Haworth Press, Inc.) Vol. 1, No. 3/4, 1993, pp. 267-272; and: *Musculoskeletal Pain, Myofascial Pain Syndrome, and the Fibromyalgia Syndrome* (ed: Søren Jacobsen, Bente Danneskiold-Samsøe, and Birger Lund) The Haworth Press, Inc., 1993, pp. 267-272. Multiple copies of this article/chapter may be purchased from The Haworth Document Delivery Center [1-800-3-HAWORTH; 9:00 a.m. - 5:00 p.m. (EST)].

INTRODUCTION

Fibromyalgia is a chronic pain syndrome. The patients claim that physical activity can be a pain modulating as well as a pain aggravating factor (1). Previously it has been shown that fibromyalgia patients have a reduced aerobic capacity (2). Improved aerobic capacity and some pain reduction were obtained after exercising on a cycle ergometer (3). Pain has been found to be induced by dynamic and static endurance work in the upper extremities (4).

The aim of the present study was to determine whether patients with fibromyalgia can perform low intensity dynamic endurance training without exacerbation of general pain and fatigue.

MATERIAL AND METHODS

Subjects

Twenty-five female patients with fibromyalgia according to the criteria of the ACR 1990 (5) were included in this study. Patients with co-existing diseases were excluded. All patients were outpatients, and their characteristics are presented in Table 1.

Study Design

The study had an experimental parallel group test design. The patients were assigned at random to a training group [n = 11] and a control group [n = 14]. The training group participated in an exercise program for twenty weeks. The control group kept their habits regarding physical activities during the same period. The study was approved by the Regional Ethical Committee for Medical Research.

The Exercise Protocol

A modified low-impact aerobic dance program was undertaken in groups twice a week for twenty weeks. Continuous dynamic exercises activating large muscle groups were performed for 60 minutes. The training intensity was kept at a heart rate level not exceeding 150 beats per minute.

Pain and Fatigue

The pain was recorded in both groups at weeks 0, 10 and 20 by the McGill Pain Questionnaire (6,7). According to the method different scores

Table 1.Characteristics of twenty-five female fibromyalgia
patients completing a twenty week study.

	Training group (N = 11)		Control group (N = 14)	
	Median (range)	Percent	Median (range)	Percent
Age (yrs)	30 (21-42)		34.5 (25-37)	
Duration of symptoms (yrs)	9 (4-20)		9 (3-21)	
Number of tenderpoints	16 (11-18)		16 (11-18)	
Pain during last week (mm VAS)*	51 (4-78)		59 (33-85)	
Fatigue during last week (mm VAS)*	67 (32-93)		69.5 (33-93)	
Sleep during last week (mm VAS)*	60 (2-90)		51.5 (0-100)	
Full or partly employment (%)		54.5		36.4
Weekly exercising >30min causing sweating (%)		27.3		35.7

* measured on a 100mm visual analogue scale

corresponding to pain intensity were assigned to the qualitative pain descriptive words. The pain descriptors were classified as sensory [PRIS], affective [PRIA] and evaluative words [PRIE]. The total sum of scores [PRIT] and the number of words chosen [NWCH] were also given (8). In addition, the training group recorded general pain and fatigue intensity during the last seven days on 100 mm visual analogue scales [VAS] at weeks 0, 2, 5, 8, 10, 15 and 20.

Statistics

Changes within the groups were analyzed by Wilcoxon Sign Rank Test and the differences between the groups by Wilcoxon Sum Rank Test. These methods were chosen as the problem of type-2 error was considered as a greater problem than the type-1 error problem. Two-tailed tests were applied. P-values at 5% level were considered as statistically significant.

RESULTS

General Pain and Fatigue

All the patients in the training group showed a general feeling of well-being after exercising. Furthermore, nine patients reported a reduced feeling of muscle tension. There were no statistically significant changes in pain and fatigue recordings during the 20 week period for the training group [Figure 1] and no significant differences between the two groups at any testpoint [Table 2].

DISCUSSION

Our data showed that general pain and fatigue intensity did not change significantly during a period of low-intensity training. An improved dynamic endurance capacity and reduced exercise-induced pain in the upper extremities were demonstrated in the training group (8).

FIGURE 1. General fatigue and pain during a twenty week period of training in eleven fibromyalgia patients.

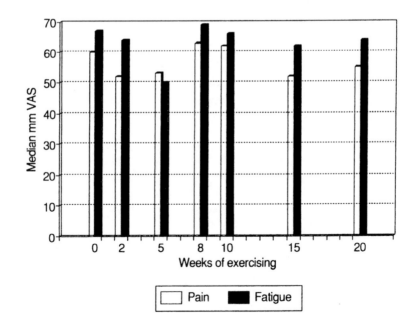

Table 2. The result of the McGill Pain Questionnaire in two
groups of female fibromyalgia patients during a
period of 20 weeks.

	Training group n=11			Control group n=14		
	0 week Median range	10 week Median range	20 week Median range	0 week Median range	10 week Median range	20 week Median range
PRIT	58 15-78	50 10-77	50 10-91	69 14-93	71 24-98	51* 13-88
PRIS	37 15-49	36 10-48	36 10-57	42 6-57	47 16-57	27 12-58
PRIA	17 0-27	13 0-25	10 0-30	22 4-32	17 4-33	17 0-29
PRIE	4 0- 9	4 0- 9	4 0- 9	4 0- 9	4 3- 9	4 0- 9
NWCH	11 3-16	11 2-15	11 2-18	13 3-18	14 5-17	11 3-16

* Statistically significant change (p=0.02) between week 0
and week 20.

The small sample size makes it impossible to draw definite conclusions. There was no statistically significant difference initially between the groups with respect to aerobic capacity, dynamic and static endurance capacity [data not shown]. We thus regarded the groups as comparable.

In conclusion, one might say that fibromyalgia patients can perform low-intensity endurance training without experiencing exacerbation of pain and fatigue symptoms.

REFERENCES

1. Yunus M, Masi AT, Calabro JJ, Miller KA, Feigenbaum SL: Primary fibromyalgia (fibrositis): Clinical study of 50 patients with matched normal controls. Semin Arthr Rheum 11: 1: 151-171, 1981.

2. Bennett RM, Clark SR, Goldberg L, Nelson D, Bonafede RP, Porter J, Specht D: Aerobic fitness in patients with fibrositis. A controlled study of respiratory gas exchange and xenon clearance from exercising muscles. Arthr Rheum 32: 4: 454-460, 1989.

3. McCain GA, Bell DA, Mai FM, Halliday PD: A controlled study of the effects of a supervised cardiovascular fitness training program on the manifestation of primary fibromyalgia. Arthr Rheum 31: 9: 1135-1141, 1988.

4. Mengshoel AM, Førre Ø, Komnæs HB: Muscle strength and aerobic capacity in primary fibromyalgia. Clin Exp Rheumatol 8: 475-479, 1990.

5. Wolfe F, Smythe HA, Yunus MB, Bennet RM, Bombardier C, Goldenberg DL et al.: The American College of Rheumatology 1990. Criteria for the classification of fibromyalgia. Report of the Multicenter Criteria Committee. Arthr Rheum 33: 2: 160-172, 1990.

6. Dubuisson D, Melzack R: Classification of clinical pain descriptions by multiple group discriminant analysis. Exp Neurol 51: 480-7, 1976.

7. Strand LI, Wisnes A: The development of a Norwegian pain questionnaire. Pain 46: 61-66, 1991.

8. Mengshoel AM, Komnæs HB, Førre Ø: The effects of twenty weeks of physical fitness training in female patients with fibromyalgia. Clin Exp Rheumatol 10: 345-49, 1992.

Treatment of Fibromyalgia Syndrome with Psychomotor Therapy and Marital Counselling

J. N. de Voogd
A. A. Knipping
A. C. E. de Blécourt
M. H. van Rijswijk

SUMMARY. Objectives: In this study we tried to determine if a combined treatment of psychomotor therapy and marital counselling was suitable for treatment of the fibromyalgia syndrome.

Methods: Fifty fibromyalgia patients were treated, after psychological and medical screening, with group psychomotor therapy combined with marital counselling for couples. Fifty fibromyalgia patients participated as non-treatment controls. The treatment goal was to help the patient learn to cope with the disabilities of the syn-

---

J. N. de Voogd, MA, Psychologist, A. A. Knipping, MA, Psychologist, and A. C. E. de Blécourt, MD, Physician, all are affiliated with the Department of Rehabilitation, University Hospital Groningen, the Netherlands.

M. H. van Rijswijk, MD, is Professor of Medicine and Chief of the Department of Rheumatology, University Hospital Groningen, the Netherlands.

Address correspondence to: Mr. J. N. de Voogd, Department of Rehabilitation, University Hospital Groningen, P.O. Box 30.001, 9700 RB Groningen, the Netherlands.

This study was granted by "het Nationaal Reumafonds."

[Haworth co-indexing entry note]: "Treatment of Fibromyalgia Syndrome with Psychomotor Therapy and Marital Counseling." de Voogd, J. N. et al. Co-published simultaneously in the *Journal of Musculoskeletal Pain* (The Haworth Press, Inc.) Vol. 1, No. 3/4, 1993, pp. 273-281; and: *Musculoskeletal Pain, Myofascial Pain Syndrome, and the Fibromyalgia Syndrome* (ed: Søren Jacobsen, Bente Danneskiold-Samsøe, and Birger Lund) The Haworth Press, Inc., 1993, pp. 273-281. Multiple copies of this article/chapter may be purchased from The Haworth Document Delivery Center [1-800-3-HAWORTH; 9:00 a.m. - 5:00 p.m. (EST)].

273

drome. The therapy consisted of psychomotor and behavioral therapy techniques to enhance relaxation, assertiveness and learning to differentiate between the complaints of the syndrome and other bodily and emotional sensations.

Results: The patients [70%] reported to be satisfied with regard to self-confidence and methods to enhance relaxation. Many patients [66%] reported improvement in their ability to deal with the disabilities. The drop-out percentage was rather high; [33%]. These data were not confirmed by the assessment material [SCL-90R and UCL], which were applied prior to directly after, and 6 months after treatment. There were no significant differences compared to the non-treatment controls.

Conclusions: The current treatment program was not sufficient to enhance significant and durable changes in fibromyalgia patients. Further modification of the treatment program and research seems to be necessary.

KEYWORDS. Fibromyalgia, psychomotor therapy, psychological therapy

INTRODUCTION

In 1950, the main event for cycling, the Tour de France was won by Ferdi Kubler, a Swiss cyclist. One year later he became World Champion. He had a remarkable way of going downhill and of going after an opponent. He had a lump of sugar between his teeth. Whenever his performance was good he swallowed the lump as a reward for his effort. This anecdote shows one of the most important principles of behavior therapy: Reinforcement. By rewarding, [the sugar lump] or reinforcing a certain behavior [a fast ride downhill], that behavior might occur more often.

This was one of the basic idea's behind our treatment program for fibromyalgia. During the last 3 years, a research project was conducted at the University Hospital of Groningen, the Netherlands, to examine this hypothesis in fibromyalgia.

MATERIALS AND METHODS

As a part of this research project, fifty fibromyalgia patients were treated with group psychomotor therapy and marital counselling for couples. The mean age was 41.9 years [range 22-59 years], mean duration of complaints 102.7 months [range 23.1-230.5 months]. The group consisted mostly of women [90%]. Fifty patients participated as non-treatment controls after being matched on gender and age. Each patient underwent psychological and medical screening, prior to, directly after, and 6 months after therapy.

The groups were compared using the Student's t test, where a parametric test was appropriate (1). Applying the Bonferroni procedure (2) [with type-I error for each comparison set to 0.05], significance was set to 0.006 for the SCL-90R, 0.007 for the UCL and 0.02 for the MMQ. Pooled variance estimates were used if the standard deviations did not differ significantly, otherwise separate variance estimates were used. The F-value was used as a criterion for difference in standard deviation [$P < 0.05$, 2 tailed]. All analyses were performed using SPSSX on the CYBER 962 computer of the University of Groningen.

The therapy goal was to help the patient learn to cope with the disabilities of fibromyalgia [pain, fatigue, stiffness and depression] on a personal level and in relations towards others, first with their spouses and then with significant others [family/friends].

Prior to and throughout the therapy-program the patients were, explicitly, told that pain reduction was not a goal of the program.

Psychomotor therapy, as we used it, is a behavioral therapy oriented approach which refers to body-experience and awareness. It consists of relaxation techniques, visualisation techniques, stimulation of social activities and aims to break through the preoccupation circle with pain and other physical complaints. The fibromyalgia patients were offered 10 group sessions of one hour and a half each over a period of 9 months. The groups consisted of 8 or 9 patients.

The group therapy was combined with 10 one hour sessions of marital counselling for the patients and their spouses. These counselling sessions were based on directive therapeutic techniques. The focus was on improving the communication between the patient and their spouse and/or their direct environment [significant others].

RESULTS

The first task of the treatment was to break through the preoccupation with the physical complaints. Relaxation techniques focused the attention of the patient on their body. Most of the patients were afraid to concentrate on their bodily sensations for fear of making their pain more severe.

Slowly they learned to relax more fully, go to sleep more easily and began to feel better. They learned to shift their attention to other bodily sensations which were more pleasant to them compared with the complaints of fibromyalgia. This was a reward in itself and the patients were also praised for their efforts and achievements by the therapists.

Also in this part of the treatment the patients were advised to balance their activities. Being more aware of their physical state and being able to relax, the patients were able to dose their activity level. Some patients chose not to; they only relaxed when the complaints were at a level that completely forced them to do nothing.

The second part of the treatment was to change the avoidance behavior. Most patients avoided certain activities, e.g., social activities out of fear of having to experience a lot of pain or other complaints during or after such activities. This could deprive them of meeting others and receiving social reinforcement. The patients were feeling helpless and powerless by this and these feelings contributed to their depression. By way of structured homework assignments the patients were stimulated to engage in certain activities that were pleasing to them. They were instructed to reward themselves directly after the effort. Some of them bought flowers or a magazine or did a relaxation exercise. Many of them found that engaging in the activity was satisfying enough and did not need extra reinforcement.

Many patients were becoming aware, during this phase of the treatment, that they could influence the impact of the complaints of fibromyalgia on their lives. For some of them this was a real eye-opener, others resisted this idea. They were not able to give up their powerlessness.

The third and last part of the treatment was learn to cope with the disabilities of the syndrome in relation towards others. By way of role play and homework assignments, the patients developed their assertiveness and social skills. Learning to say "no" to others when they are asked to do things that were physically too much for them was very hard. Knowing that they would pay a price, most patients chose to do others a favour anyway.

The therapy was ended with an evaluation session.

In the same period the patients and their partners went to see a social worker for marital counselling. The marital counselling was partly a back-up for the psychomotor treatment and partly to improve the partner relationship with relation to coping with the syndrome. Sometimes a sidestep was necessary when unsolved problems came up.

Unfortunately 17 [34%] of the 50 patients dropped out before the end of the program for several reasons; 7 relating to the program, 10 not relating directly to the program.

Directly after treatment the patients were asked to fill out an open questioned treatment evaluation form. Seventy percent [23/33] reported to be satisfied with regard to self-confidence and methods to enhance relaxation. Two thirds [22/33][66%] of the patients reported to have improved their ability to deal with the disabilities. Some patients [8/33][24%] asked for a more structured approach.

These data were not confirmed by the assessment material [Symptom Checklist 90R [SCL-90R], validated for the Dutch population (3), and the Utrechtse Copinglijst [UCL]; a coping style inventory (4). There were no significant differences compared to the non-treatment controls [Table 1, Table 2].

The assessment of marital satisfaction, assessed with the Maudsley Marital Questionnaire [MMQ] (5), also indicated that there were no differences between the groups [Table 3].

Because there were no significant differences between the groups prior to and after treatment, the data of the follow-up assessment are not of interest and, therefore, are not presented.

As expected there was no reduction of pain or other physical complaints.

DISCUSSION

These results have led to the conclusion that this program of psycho-motor therapy combined with marital counselling was not sufficient to enhance significant and durable changes in fibromyalgia patients. The fairly positive evaluation could be the result of social desirability or maybe our assessment material is not sensitive enough to measure these changes.

At this moment we are modifying our treatment program. The new approach is based on cognitive behavioral therapy which offers more structure to the patients. A previous study, published in the *Journal of Rheumatology* (6), indicated that psycho-social aspects of fibromyalgia were very similar to other chronic pain syndromes. Therefore, the new treatment program corresponds with treatment programs which have been useful in other chronic pain syndromes. Our current program is based on the stress-inoculation therapy as developed by Meichenbaum and Turk (7). That therapy program is divided in 3 phases, an education phase, a training phase and an application phase.

Table 1. SCL-90R; comparison of experimental and control group pre- and post treatment.

	T=1 exp. n=50 (Mean ± SD)	Significance of t Value	T=1 con. n=50 (Mean ± SD)	T=2 exp. n=28 (Mean ± SD)	T=2 con. n=49 (Mean ± SD)	Significance of t Value
Anxiety	17.8 ± 6.4	NS	18.1 ± 6.5	18.3 ± 7.1	16.7 ± 5.3	NS
Agoraphobia	9.3 ± 2.8	NS	10.6 ± 5.0	10.1 ± 5.5	9.2 ± 4.3	NS
Depression	29.2 ± 10.5	NS	29.9 ± 11.0	29.4 ± 11.8	27.8 ± 8.3	NS
Somatization	29.4 ± 7.6	NS	31.6 ± 7.9	30.5 ± 7.8	29.4 ± 6.8	NS
Insufficiency	19.6 ± 5.7	NS	18.9 ± 4.5	20.3 ± 6.7	18.5 ± 4.8	NS
Sensitivity	28.3 ± 9.5	NS	28.3 ± 9.9	29.6 ± 10.0	27.6 ± 7.9	NS
Hostility	7.6 ± 2.1	NS	8.7 ± 9.9	8.2 ± 2.1	7.9 ± 1.9	NS
Sleep	8.4 ± 3.6	NS	9.5 ± 3.9	8.3 ± 4.1	8.4 ± 3.6	NS

p < 0.006, NS = not significant.

Table 2. UCL; comparison of experimental and control group pre-and post treatment.

| | T=1 | | | T=2 | | |
	exp. n=50 (Mean ± SD)	con. n=50 (Mean ± SD)	Significance of t Value	exp. n=27 (Mean ± SD)	con. n=47 (Mean ± SD)	Significance of t Value
active approach	17.4 ± 3.2	17.7 ± 3.2	NS	17.2 ± 3.4	17.2 ± 3.5	NS
palliative	18.8 ± 3.3	21.3 ± 10.9	NS	18.3 ± 3.7	19.1 ± 3.5	NS
avoidance reaction	16.2 ± 3.1	16.7 ± 3.9	NS	15.0 ± 2.7	15.5 ± 2.9	NS
social comfort	11.9 ± 3.3	12.7 ± 4.3	NS	12.2 ± 4.2	11.9 ± 3.4	NS
depressive	12.2 ± 3.2	13.1 ± 6.1	NS	12.0 ± 3.9	11.7 ± 2.8	NS
emotional/angry	5.4 ± 1.3	7.6 ± 11.9	NS	5.6 ± 1.6	5.5 ± 1.3	NS
comforting thoughts	13.5 ± 2.7	14.7 ± 8.6	NS	12.7 ± 2.9	13.2 ± 2.9	NS

p < 0.007, NS = not significant.

Table 3. MMQ; comparison of experimental and control group pre- and post treatment.

	T=1			T=2		
	exp. n=44 (Mean ± SD)	con. n=40 (Mean ± SD)	Significance of t value	exp. n=24 (Mean ± SD)	con. n=41 (Mean ± SD)	Significance of t value
Marital satisfaction	12.9 ± 10.3	13.6 ± 10.2	NS	16.4 ± 12.7	14.5 ± 12.2	NS
Sexual satisfaction	9.6 ± 8.2	13.1 ± 14.9	NS	12.5 ± 9.4	11.6 ± 8.3	NS
General Life satisfaction	12.5 ± 5.4	13.1 ± 8.0	NS	11.5 ± 4.3	12.4 ± 6.4	NS

$p < 0.02$, NS = not significant.

REFERENCES

1. Nijdam B, van Buuren H: Statistiek voor de sociale wetenschappen. Alphen aan de Rijn, Samson, 1980.

2. Myers JL: Fundamentals of Experimental Design. 3rd ed. Boston: Allyn and Bacon, 1979.

3. Arrindell WA, Ettema JHM: SCL-90R; handleiding bij een multidimensionele psychopathologie indicator. Swets en Zeitlinger, Lisse, The Netherlands, 1985.

4. Schreurs PJG, van de Willige G, Tellegen B, Brosschot JF: De Utrechtse copinglijst; UCL-handleiding. Vakgroep Klinische Psychologie, Rijksuniversiteit Utrecht, The Netherlands, 1986.

5. Arrindell WA, Boelens W, Lambert H: On the psychometric properties of the Maudsley Marital Questionnaire (MMQ): evaluation of self-ratings in distressedand 'normal' volunteer couples based on the dutch version. Person individ Diff 4: 293-306, 1983.

6. Birnie DJ, Knipping AA, van Rijswijk MH, de Blecourt AC, de Voogd JN: Psychological aspects of fibromyalgia compared with chronic and nonchronic pain. Journal of Rheumatology 18:12, 1845-1848, 1991.

7. Meichenbaum D, Turk D: The cognitive-behavioral management of anxiety, depression and pain. In P.O. Davidson (Ed.), the behavioral management of anxiety, depression and pain. New York: Brunner/Mazel, 1976.

Cervicobrachial Syndrome: Neck Muscle Function and Effects of Training

Allan Jordan
Jesper Mehlsen

SUMMARY. Objectives: Our study evaluated the neck function in a group of patients with chronic cervicobrachial syndrome [CBS] and a group of healthy controls. A second objective was to study the effect of neck muscle training on CBS patients.

Methods: We measured range of movement [ROM], maximum voluntary contraction [MVC] and isometric endurance at 60% of MVC [IE]. Measurements were made during dorsal, ventral and lateral flexion. ROM was measured with an electronic goniometer, and MVC was measured by a strain gauge dynamometer. A visual analog scale [VAS] was used to monitor pain perception.

Results: In healthy subjects, ROM, MVC and IE attained the highest values during dorsal flexion, whereas values obtained during ventral and lateral flexion were of comparable magnitude. Patients with CBS showed a decrease in ROM during dorsal flexion, a decrease in MVC in all directions and a decrease in IE during dorsal and lateral flexion. Two months of intensive neck muscle training improved both MVC- and VAS-values.

Allan Jordan, DC, and Jesper Mehlsen, MD, are both affiliated with the Department of Clinical Physiology, Frederiksberg Hospital, Frederiksberg, Denmark.

Address correspondence to: Jesper Mehlsen, MD, FACA, Assistant Professor, Department of Clinical Physiology, Frederiksberg Hospital, DK-2000 Frederiksberg, Denmark.

[Haworth co-indexing entry note]: "Cervicobrachial Syndrome: Neck Muscle Function and Effects of Training." Jordan, Allan, and Jesper Mehlsen. Co-published simultaneously in the *Journal of Musculoskeletal Pain* (The Haworth Press, Inc.) Vol. 1, No. 3/4, 1993, pp. 283-288; and: *Musculoskeletal Pain, Myofascial Pain Syndrome, and the Fibromyalgia Syndrome* (ed: Søren Jacobsen, Bente Danneskiold-Samsøe, and Birger Lund) The Haworth Press, Inc., 1993, pp. 283-288. Multiple copies of this article/chapter may be purchased from the Haworth Document Delivery Center [1-800-3-HAWORTH; 9:00 a.m. - 5:00 p.m. (EST)].

Conclusions: Our results are in accordance with findings in studies of the trunk musculature. The reestablishment of muscular strength and agonist/antagonist ratios appears to be of therapeutic value in CBS, as has been the case with chronic low back rehabilitation.

KEYWORDS. Neck muscle function, neck tension syndrome, dynamic training

INTRODUCTION

Ramazzini was the first to report on occupational/overuse syndromes among clerks and scribes in 1713 (1). He surmised that the aches and pains of his subjects were due to repetitive movements, constrained postures, and mental stress. These premises are still accepted though the underlying pathophysiological mechanisms remain poorly understood (2). Studies of shoulder musculature are abundant (3), but those of the neck musculature are rare.

This paper reports on the function of neck muscles for a group of patients suffering from CBS and a group of healthy subjects with comparable work conditions. We furthermore report on the effects of dynamic training in a small group of patients with CBS.

SUBJECTS AND METHODS

The study included 18 healthy subjects [41 years [28-55]] and 18 subjects [41 years [28-55]] with chronic cervicobrachial syndrome [duration: 12 years [5-20]] defined according to a standardized Nordic questionnaire for neck/shoulder pain (4).

Both groups had similar work conditions and were of comparable height [171 cm [162-183] vs. 169 cm [163-178] and weight [67.0 kg [55.0-80.0] vs. 64.0 kg [50.0-76.0]].

The function of the neck muscles was tested during lateral, ventral, and dorsal flexion in random order. The axis of rotation was centered at a level between the seventh cervical and the first thoracic vertebra, and was made of range of movement [ROM], maximum voluntary contraction [MVC] and isometric endurance [IE] at 60% of MVC. Tests of MVC were performed in a dynamometer with a starting position of 15° flexion in all directions. ROM was tested as the maximal deflexion in each direction by use of an electronic goniometer.

Ten patients participated in a two month training program with sessions twice a week, each session lasting one hour and comprising warm-up for 5 min on a bicycle ergonometer, dynamic exercises with 36 repetitions in each of the four directions [ventral, lateral and dorsal flexion] at 50 per cent of MVC and stretching of the involved muscle groups. The load was increased with five per cent of MVC each second week. Before onset of training the patients filled out a visual analog scale [VAS] in order to quantify the subjective symptoms of pain in the neck shoulder region. The VAS was used again after one month of training and at the end of the training program, at which time the measurements of MVC also were repeated. Data are given as median values with ranges in brackets. Comparisons between groups were made with unpaired rank sum test and comparisons within the groups were made with paired rank sum test. A two-sided significance level of 0.01 was used in order to reduce the inherent problem in multiple comparisons.

RESULTS

Measurements of lateral flexion in healthy subjects showed a high degree of symmetry between the left and right side for all variables, and the mean values of the two sides were thus used for further calculations.

Values obtained in testing the range of movement [ROM], maximal voluntary contraction [MVC], and isometric endurance [IE] are shown in Table 1. ROM was found to be significantly reduced in the patients during dorsal flexion and a similar non-significant tendency was seen with respect to lateral flexion. MVC was found to be significantly reduced in the patients during all types of movement. IE was found to be significantly reduced in the patients during lateral and dorsal flexion.

Training gave rise to increased values of MVC [Figure 1] and corresponding decreases in symptoms of neck pain [Figure 2].

DISCUSSION

This study has shown that a group of patients suffering from chronic cervicobrachial syndrome [CBS] differs from a group of healthy subjects with respect to several parameters characterizing the neck function. It has furthermore been shown that dynamic and specific training of the neck muscles may improve the clinical condition of patients with CBS.

Tabel 1: Neck muscle function in cervicobrachial syndrome compared to healthy subjects.

	Range of Movement (°)		Maximal Voluntary Contraction (kp)		Isometric Endurance (s)	
	Controls	CBS	Controls	CBS	Controls	CBS
Ventral Flexion	59 (44 - 75)	59 (34 - 69)	11 (9 - 18)	8 (4 - 19)*	47 (29 - 70)	32 (18 - 145)
Lateral Flexion	52 (37 - 64)	48 (32 - 64)	11 (8 - 19)	8 (5 - 20)*	62 (26 - 220)	34 (18 - 184)*
Dorsal Flexion	76 (41 - 92)	59 (30 - 94)*	16 (12 - 32)	12 (7 - 30)*	71 (32 - 149)	36 (24 - 138)*

Range of movement in healthy controls and patients with chronic cervicobrachial syndrome (CBS) was tested by an electronical goniometer. Maximum voluntary contraction (MVC) was tested by a strain gauge dynamometer. The axis of rotation was at the level of C_7/Th_1. Isometric endurance was tested at 60 per cent of MVC. Median values are given with ranges in brackets. Results were compared with the two-sample rank sum test (* p< 0.01).

FIGURE 1. Median values of neck muscle action during lateral, ventral and dorsal flexion in patients with chronic cervicobrachial syndrome. Measurements were made twice before [*solid bars*] and after two months of dynamic training [*hatched bars*].

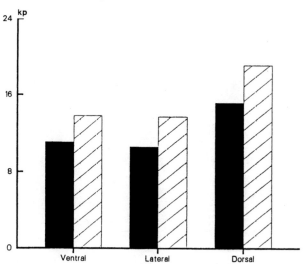

ROM was decreased in patients with CBS only during dorsal flexion and this deficiency may be due to facet joint arthrosis or to increased tone of antagonistic muscles. MVC was reduced in all directions in patients with CBS, and the reduction was more pronounced during dorsal flexion than during the other types of movement. Pain-induced increases of basal tone in antagonistic muscles may reduce the ability to generate force in the agonist and thus decrease MVC. IE was reduced in patients with CBS during dorsal and lateral flexion even though the loads used were smaller in this group. With reduced endurance levels, patients with CBS would be more prone to develop sustained pain from the neck musculature, when required to maintain static postures over longer periods of time

In conclusion, our study has shown that patients with chronic cervicobrachial syndrome [CBS] have deficiencies in several parameters of neck muscle function especially during dorsal flexion. These findings are in accordance with findings in studies of the trunk musculature, and reestab-

FIGURE 2. Median values of subjective pain rating from a visual analog scale. Measurements were made twice before training [*before I and II*] and after one [*during*] and two months [*after*] of dynamic training.

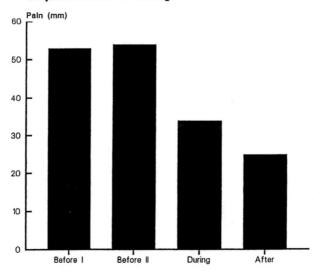

Chronic Cervicobrachial Syndrome

Subjective effect of training

lishing muscular strength seems to be of therapeutic value in CBS, as has been the case with chronic low back rehabilitation (5).

REFERENCES

1. Ramazzini B: Disease of Workers (English translation by Wright W.C.). New York: Hafner, 1940.

2. Edwards RHT: Hypothesis of peripheral and central mechanisms underlying occupational muscle pain and injury. Eur J Appl Physiol 57: 275-81, 1988.

3. Hagberg S, Kvarnström S: Muscular endurance and EMG in myofascial shoulder pain. Arch Phys Med Rehab 65: 522-5, 1984.

4. Kuorinka I, Johnsson B, Kilbom A, Vinterberg H, Biering-Sørensen F et al.: Standardized Nordic questionnaire for analysis of musculoskeletal symptoms. Appl Ergonom 18: 233-37, 1987.

5. Mannicke C, Hesselsøe G: Clinical trial of intensive muscle training for chronic low back pain. Lancet 11: 1473-6, 1988.

Injection Therapy for Treatment of Chronic Myofascial Pain: A Double-Blind Study Comparing Corticosteroid versus Diclofenac Injections

Asbjørn Mohr Drewes
Arne Andreasen
Lone Hvidtfelt Poulsen

SUMMARY. Objectives: The aim of this study was to compare prednisolone [P] and diclofenac [D] injections in treatment of chronic myofascial pain.

Methods: Patients with localized myofascial pain lasting between 1 and 7 months were included in a double blind study using either P or D injections. Patients and physicians evaluated the treatment during a 2 week period.

Results: Thirty-eight patients completed the study and 84% improved from the injection therapy. No difference between the treat-

Asbjørn Mohr Drewes, MD, is affiliated with the Department of Rheumatology, Aalborg Hospital, Denmark, and Department of Rheumatology, Viborg Hospital, Denmark.

Arne Andreasen, MD, and Lone Hvidtfelt Poulsen, MD, are affiliated with the Department of Rheumatology, Viborg Hospital, Denmark.

Address correspondence and reprint requests to: Asbjørn Mohr Drewes, MD, Department of Rheumatology, Aalborg Hospital, DK-9000 Aalborg, Denmark.

This study was supported by Ciba-Geigy A/S.

[Haworth co-indexing entry note]: "Injection Therapy for Treatment of Chronic Myofascial Pain: A Double-Blind Study Comparing Corticosteroid versus Diclofenac Injections." Drewes, Asbjørn Mohr, Arne Andreasen, and Lone Hvidtfelt Poulsen. Co-published simultaneously in the *Journal of Musculoskeletal Pain* (The Haworth Press, Inc.) Vol. 1, No. 3/4, 1993, pp. 289-294; and: *Musculoskeletal Pain, Myofascial Pain Syndrome, and the Fibromyalgia Syndrome* (ed: Søren Jacobsen, Bente Danneskiold-Samsøe, and Birger Lund) The Haworth Press, Inc., 1993, pp. 289-294. Multiple copies of this article/chapter may be purchased from The Haworth Document Delivery Center [1-800-3-HAWORTH; 9:00 a.m. - 5:00 p.m. (EST)].

ments was found at the clinical evaluations or in the patient question-naires.

Conclusion: Diclofenac injections might be an alternative in the treatment of myofascial pain.

KEYWORDS. Myofascial pain syndrome, trigger point, intramuscular injections

INTRODUCTION

As a treatment of myofascial pain syndromes, infiltration in the trigger-point [TP] with local anaesthetics or corticosteroid have been recommended (1). As preliminary reports (2) have shown good results using diclofenac sodium in aqueous solution, we conducted a double-blind study comparing corticosteroid and diclofenac injections.

MATERIAL AND METHODS

Patients with *localized* myofascial pain lasting for 1 to 7 months were included. The pain must have been felt in a specific area with a palpable TP in the muscle and palpation should elicit typical referred pain. In order to ensure a comparable distribution of the injections, patients were divided into 4 groups. In this way patients with TP in the 1. neck, 2. around the shoulder girdle, 3. in the back, and 4. in the gluteal region were randomized to one of the 2 treatments:

[P] = 1 ml 0.9% saline solution + 1 ml soluble prednisolone injectable [25 mg/ml, Delcortol[R], Leo] or

[D] = 2 ml diclofenac sodium injectable [25 mg/ml, Voltaren[R], Ciba-Geigy].

After randomization, the nurse prepared 2 syringes. The physician was given the first syringe containing either 1 ml 0.9% saline or 1 ml diclofenac, both clear fluids. After an attempt of aspiration, the agent was injected into the TP. The needle was left in the tissue and the physician injected the content of a new, but opaque, blinded syringe containing either 1 ml prednisolone or 1 ml diclofenac. Patients were seen again after 2 and 4 days. At this time, the injection procedure was repeated if pain was still present. Fourteen days after the first consultation a follow-up was performed. As analgesic paracetamol 1-3 g daily was permitted. At each consultation the physician evaluated the patient's pain during movements and at palpation at TP, and made a statement regarding the improvement during therapy compared to base-line [5 point verbal scales]. At the final consultation a global evaluation was made [patient and physicians general opinion of the treatment]. The patients filled out a pain-questionnaire [1-5 verbal scales] every day. Furthermore, side effects and paracetamol consumption were registered.

The statistical analysis were chi-square tests with Yates correction and non-parametric methods were used for description of the data.

RESULTS

Thirty-eight patients completed the study. Data from the study group appears from Table 1 and 2. Results from the clinical evaluation at the endpoint [day No. 14] are given in Table 3. No differences between the two treatment groups were found regarding "pain at palpation" or "pain at movements" [P = 0.56, P = 0.59, chi-square]. Eighty-four percent improved during therapy and 47% [Table 4] recovered completely, again no differences were observed between the groups [P = 0.39, P = 0.70, chi-square]. None of the patients had a worsening of the pain. There was a consistent improvement during the treatment period. In total 61% were satisfied with the treatment ["global evaluation"]. Results from the patients' self-evaluation at the endpoint visit appear from Table 5. Four patients in each group complained of pain at the injection site after the first injection, and two steroid treated patients had pain after the second and third injection.

TABLE I

Anatomical region	N	Male/female	Age, median and [range]	Duration in days, median and [range]
I	8	3:5	51.0 [37–68]	120 [30–165]
II	14	3:11	44.5 [35–57]	135 [31–180]
III	4	2:2	49.5 [24–63]	90 [45– 90]
IV	12	8:4	53.0 [35–69]	60 [31–150]
Total	38	16:22	50.0 [24–69]	90 [30–180]

Patient distribution by group. I: neck region, II: around shoulder girdle, III: back, IV: gluteal region.

TABLE 2

Treatment group	N	Male/female	Age, median and [range]	Duration in days, median and [range]
Prednisolone	22	10:12	54 [35-69]	90 [21-180]
Diclofenac	16	5:11	48 [24-60]	60 [37-150]

Patient distribution by treatment.

TABLE 3

Treatment group	No pain during movements	No pain at triggerpoint	Improvement of therapy
Prednisolone	15 [68%]	9 [41%]	18 [81%]
Diclofenac	8 [50%]	5 [31%]	14 [88%]
Total	23 [61%]	14 [37%]	32 [84%]

End point clinical evaluation by the physician [day No. 14].

TABLE 4

Treatment group	Day No.3	Day No.5	Day No.14
Prednisolone	2 [9%]	8 [36%]	11 [50%]
Diclofenac	3 [19%]	6 [38%]	7 [44%]
Total	5 [13%]	14 [38%]	18 [47%]

Distribution of patients assessed "cured" by the physician at the visits [day No. 3, 5 and 14].

Analgesic consumption and the number of injections given were equal in the two groups. Two thirds of the patients needed 3 injections.

DISCUSSION

Most localized myofascial pain disappears without specific treatment, but when the condition persists, TP injection is preferred by many authors (3,4). Exercises and massage might be more useful when the pain is

TABLE 5

Treatment group	No pain at rest	No pain at movements	No pain at self-palpation
Prednisolone	10 [46%]	7 [32%]	9 [41%]
Diclofenac	7 [44%]	6 [38%]	6 [38%]
Total	17 [45%]	13 [34%]	15 [40%]

Patients self-evaluations at the final evaluation [day No. 14].

diffuse and widespread. Eighty-four percent of our patients improved and 47% were totally cured despite symptoms for approximately 90 days, thus we recommend the injection therapy for long lasting symptoms. Studies of local injection therapy have demonstrated an effect of dry needling, pure saline, local anaesthetics, corticosteroids as well as diclofenac (2,4,5), but most studies were either open or semi-blind and in some of them treatment started rather early, thereby introducing bias. As even pure saline injections cannot be regarded placebo treatment, we omitted a "placebo" group. The design was made using 2 antiinflammatory agents as some studies have demonstrated slight inflammatory changes in the muscles. During the study, it was difficult to find patients who fulfilled the criteria of only one TP. Nevertheless the exclusion of all patients with diffuse pain or multiple TP was necessary as the evaluation of treatment otherwise might be ambiguous.

The injection therapy in general proved to be valuable. Local prednisolone treatment is mostly harmless as no vital systemic effect is expected, but injection near subcutaneous tissue can produce pitting of the skin and depigmentation, and steroid injections into muscle might give fiber damage (1). Diclofenac, however, may also produce skin necrosis, particularly in case of superficial injections. The side-effects observed in this study were few, therefore we conclude that injected diclofenac, although not an officially approved indication, may be an alternative in the treatment of myofascial pain.

REFERENCES

1. Travell JG, Simons DG: Myofascial Pain and Dysfunction: The Trigger Point Manual. Williams and Wilkins, Baltimore, 1983, Chapter 3.

2. Frost FA: Diclofenac compared with lignocaine in injection treatment of myofascial pain. Ugeskr Laeg 148:1077-78, 1986. [Summary in English].

3. Cooper AL: Trigger-point injections: Its place in physical medicine. Arch Phys Med Rehabil 42:702-9, 1961.

4. Bourne IHJ: Treatment of chronic back pain. Comparing corticosteroid-lignocaine injections with lignocaine alone. The practitioner 228:333-8, 1984.

5. Lewit K: The needle effect in the relief of myofascial pain. Pain 6:83-90, 1979.

CONSENSUS DOCUMENT ON FIBROMYALGIA: THE COPENHAGEN DECLARATION

INTRODUCTION

A consensus conference on fibromyalgia took place in Copenhagen on August 20, 1992 as part of the Second World Congress on Myofascial Pain and Fibromyalgia. This is the report from the consensus conference.

The consensus conference addressed the following questions:

1. What is fibromyalgia?
2. How do we diagnose fibromyalgia?
3. What causes fibromyalgia?
4. What is the frequency of fibromyalgia in the population?
5. How does fibromyalgia affect the individual?
6. What is the impact on society of fibromyalgia?
7. What sort of treatment is effective?
8. What research challenges must be met in the future?

The consensus conference consisted of two panels, an expert panel and a consensus panel.

The members of the two panels were

Finalized at the Consensus Conference at the Second World Congress on Myofascial Pain and Fibromyalgia, MYOPAIN '92, August 17-20, 1992, Copenhagen, Denmark.

[Haworth co-indexing entry note]: *"CONSENSUS DOCUMENT ON FIBROMYALGIA: THE CO-PENHAGEN DECLARATION."* Co-published simultaneously in the *Journal of Musculoskeletal Pain* (The Haworth Press, Inc.) Vol. 1, No. 3/4, 1993, pp. 295-312; and: *Musculoskeletal Pain, Myofascial Pain Syndrome, and the Fibromyalgia Syndrome* (ed: Søren Jacobsen, Bente Danneskiold-Samsøe, and Birger Lund) The Haworth Press, Inc., 1993, pp. 295-312. Multiple copies of this article/chapter may be purchased from The Haworth Document Delivery Center [1-800-3-HAWORTH; 9:00 a.m. - 5:00 p.m. (EST)].

EXPERT PANEL: Robert Bennett (Chairman), USA
Anders Bjelle, Sweden
Ann Bengtsson, Sweden
Carol S. Burckhardt, USA
Don Goldenberg, USA
Karl G. Henriksson, Sweden
Søren Jacobsen, Denmark
Marijke van Santen Hoeufft, The Netherlands
Henning Værøy, Norway
Frederick Wolfe, USA

CONSENSUS PANEL: Finn Kamper-Jørgensen [Chairman], Denmark
Liv Anne Andreassen, Consumer representative, Norway
Dag Bruusgaard, General practitioner, Norway
Bente Danneskiold-Samsøe, M.D., Denmark
Alfonse T. Masi, Epidemiologist/rheumatologist, USA
Janine Morgall, Sociologist, Denmark
[Robert Bennett, Chairman of expert panel, USA]

Appendix 1 compares an ordinary consensus conference with the modified *MYOPAIN '92* consensus conference. Appendix 2 presents a timetable and the addresses of panel members.

MUSCULO-SKELETAL DISEASES AND CHRONIC WIDESPREAD PAIN

Pain and discomfort from the musculo-skeletal system are common in the general adult population. Health surveys in industrialized countries have shown that 40-50% of the population report such symptoms within any two week period and about 20% regard the problem as serious.

Studies have shown that musculo-skeletal disorders when compared to other disease groups give rise to:

- most premature pensions
- most cases of longstanding or prolonged illness
- most limitation of activity in the population
- most lost good years of life
- most visits to general practitioners

Thus musculo-skeletal disorders have important socio-economic implications and should be considered a disease group that may endanger social welfare.

Defining the syndrome fibromyalgia in the early 1980's stimulated increasing interest in the scientific and clinical aspects of chronic muscular pain.

Recent population studies indicate that 10-20% suffer from chronic widespread pain. The fibromyalgia syndrome accounts for an important subset of these patients.

WHY DEFINE A NEW DIAGNOSIS?

Now and then new diagnoses in medicine are established. Medical diagnoses are social conventions/constructions conveying medical experience between doctors and between generations, and hence have both scientific as well as social implications.

The rationale for grouping patients and establishing a new diagnosis may vary. Criteria for grouping and diagnosis are for example based on common etiology [a bacteria], common patho-anatomic characteristics [ulcer, infarct], prognosis [AIDS], dysfunction of an organ [senile dementia], response to treatment [polymyalgia rheumatica], distinctive clinical appearance [fibromyalgia].

Ideally, the act of diagnosing identifies a homogenous group of patients. However, clinical experience usually shows large variations in clinical appearance, and prognosis among patients with the same diagnosis.

Fibromyalgia is a syndrome, i.e., a condition based on a set of characteristic symptoms. Experienced clinicians have found it useful to create the fibromyalgia concept in order to promote research, evaluate treatment programmes and improve patient management.

The World Health Organization in developing the International Classification of Disease [ICD] has incorporated fibromyalgia in the 10th revision of ICD; Fibromyalgia is number M 79.0.

WHAT IS FIBROMYALGIA?

Fibromyalgia is a painful, non-articular condition predominantly involving muscles; it is the commonest cause of chronic, widespread musculoskeletal pain. It is typically associated with persistent fatigue, non-refreshing sleep and generalized stiffness. Women are affected some 10-20 times more often than men.

Fibromyalgia is often part of a wider syndrome encompassing: headaches, irritable bowels, irritable bladder, dysmenorrhoea, cold sensitivity, Raynaud's phenomenon, restless legs, atypical patterns of numbness and tingling, exercise intolerance and complaints of weakness.

A varying proportion [20-50%] of fibromyalgia patients experience significant depression or anxiety which may contribute to the severity of the symptoms or result from having chronic pain.

Most fibromyalgia patients experience both diurnal and seasonal variations in symptoms. Typically, symptoms are worse during periods of cold damp weather, at the beginning and end of the day, and during periods of emotional stress.

HOW DO WE DIAGNOSE FIBROMYALGIA?

Fibromyalgia is a distinctive syndrome which can be diagnosed with clinical precision. It may occur in the absence [primary fibromyalgia] or presence of other conditions such as rheumatoid arthritis or systemic lupus erythematosus [concomitant fibromyalgia]. It is very rarely secondary to another disease, in the sense that alleviation of the associated disease also cures the fibromyalgia. It may be confidently diagnosed in patients with widespread musculo-skeletal pain [see Table 1] and multiple tender points.

TABLE 1. The American College of Rheumatology 1990 Criteria for the classification of fibromyalgia (Wolfe et al. 1990).

History of widespread pain.
> *Definition.* Pain is considered widespread when all of the following are present: pain in both sides of the body, pain above and below the waist. In addition, axial skeletal pain (cervical spine, anterior chest, thoracic spine or low back) must be present. Low back pain is considered lower segment pain.

Pain in 11 of 18 tender point sites on digital palpation.
> *Definition.* Pain, on digital palpation, must be present in at least 11 of the following 18 tender point sites:
>> *Occiput*: at the suboccipital muscle insertions.
>> *Low cervical*: at the anterior aspects of the intertransverse spaces at C5–C7.
>> *Trapezius*: at the midpoint of the upper border.
>> *Supraspinatus*: at origins, above the scapula spine near the medial border.
>> *Second rib*: upper lateral aspects of the second costochondral junction.
>> *Lateral epicondyle*: 2 cm distal to the epicondyles.
>> *Gluteal*: in upper outer quadrants of buttocks in anterior fold of muscle.
>> *Greater trochanter*: posterior to the trochanteric prominence.
>> *Knee*: at the medial fat pad proximal to the joint line.

Digital palpation should be performed with an approximate force of 4 kg. A tender point has to be painful at palpation not just "tender".

The tender point is defined as a discrete area of soft tissue which is painful to digital palpation at an approximate force of 4 kg. The patient should be instructed to indicate the presence of pain; tenderness without pain does not qualify. Tender points are found in characteristic locations as defined by the 1990 criteria of the American College of Rheumatology [see Table 1]. For the purposes of standardizing *research* protocols fibromyalgia is strictly defined in terms of widespread pain plus 11 or more out of 18 specified tender points [see Table 1].

From a *pragmatic* perspective in dealing with the individual patient, the diagnosis is commonly entertained in the presence of unexplained widespread pain or aching, persistent fatigue, generalized stiffness, non-refreshing sleep and multiple tender points. Most patients with these symptoms have 11 or more tender points, but a variable proportion of otherwise typical patients may have less than 11 tender points at the time of examination.

A potential cause of confusion is regional myofascial pain syndrome. These patients have a localized pain distribution and a limited number of tender points. They are usually responsive to specific myofascial therapy. Such patients seldom have the typical fibromyalgia profile of persistent fatigue, widespread stiffness and non-restorative sleep. In a minority of patients a regional myofascial pain syndrome may develop into a typical picture of fibromyalgia.

Few conditions mimic fibromyalgia; some, for example, include: hypothyroidism, widespread malignancy, polymyalgia rheumatica, osteomalacia, generalized osteoarthritis, early Parkinson's disease and the initial stages of a connective tissue disease. The presence of fibromyalgia symptoms in some patients with chronic fatigue syndrome and vice versa has been noted in several studies. The significance of these observations is not known as there is no clear definition of the chronic fatigue syndrome.

WHAT CAUSES FIBROMYALGIA?

The etiology and pathogenesis of fibromyalgia is not presently known. Contemporary studies provide some support for the following statements:

Psychological Factors

Although fibromyalgia patients often suffer from depression and other psychological problems it is not thought that pain and tenderness are caused primarily by emotional distress. However, the quality of life is often adversely affected by concomitant psychological distress.

Sleep Disturbance

Fibromyalgia patients invariably wake up feeling unrefreshed. Physiologically this sleep disturbance has been correlated with an electroencephalogram abnormality called alpha-delta sleep. This is a disturbance of the deeper stages of sleep characterized by an arousal pattern. Alpha-delta sleep is probably the cause of non-refreshing sleep symptoms. The relationship between the sleep anomaly and the other features of fibromyalgia is not understood. The possibility that alpha-delta sleep may interfere with the circadian secretion of some pituitary hormones is a subject of contemporary research.

Muscle Studies

Muscle biopsy studies in fibromyalgia patients have failed to reveal any changes that are characteristic or diagnostic of the condition. The morphological changes that have been described such as ragged red fibres, z-band smearing and reduced levels of high energy phosphates appear to have a focal distribution. Similar findings have been described in patients with work-related myalgia, suggesting that the muscle pain component of these two conditions may have a final common pathway. Serum levels of muscle enzymes, electromyography studies, exercise testing, and nuclear magnetic resonance have failed to show any *global* defect of muscle metabolism in fibromyalgia patients.

Pain

There is increasing evidence that fibromyalgia patients have a centrally enhanced perception of pain. One study has reported elevated cerebrospinal fluid levels of substance P, Metenkephalin Arg-Phe and dynorphin-A. Two studies have reported low levels of a tryptophan metabolite–namely 5 hydroxy indole acid. Cerebrospinal fluid levels of beta endorphins have been reported as normal. The relevance of these changes in cerebrospinal fluid neuropeptides to an enhanced central perception of pain has not yet been elucidated.

Increased Sympathetic Activity

Most fibromyalgia patients complain of cold sensitivity, some 20 to 40% have the primary form of Raynaud's phenomenon. Other complaints suggestive of increased sympathetic activity are dry eyes, dry mouth, fluid retention, and bladder irritability. Patients with Raynaud's phenomenon have been shown to have an up regulation of alpha-2 adrenergic receptors on platelets. This would make them more sensitive to their own endogenous production of catacholamines. One study has indicated that stellate ganglion blockade reduces both the overall feeling of pain and a number of tender points on the side of sympathetic block. Studies of serum catecholamine levels in fibromyalgia patients have not shown any changes. It would therefore appear that some fibromyalgia patients have an increase in sympathetic activity as a result of an enhanced responsiveness to physiologically normal stimulation of their sympathetic system.

WHAT IS THE FREQUENCY OF FIBROMYALGIA?

Health surveys in various countries point to a prevalence of 0.7-3.2% in the general adult population. Nearly all cases were found in women, yielding a female prevalence of at least 1.3% to 6% or more.

Onset of symptoms is most frequent from the age 20-40 years, but has been reported to occur at all ages, even in childhood.

Reported frequencies of fibromyalgia patients among adult males and females combined in primary health care has been 2-6% and in some rheumatology practices up to almost 20%. The fibromyalgia syndrome is often underdiagnosed when it follows an inflammatory or degenerative rheumatic disease. This may lead to inappropriate treatment.

Few data are available on the natural history of fibromyalgia. Existing follow up studies support the idea of fibromyalgia being a chronic condition with a poor social prognosis.

It was recommended that the American College of Rheumatology [ACR] criteria be used in future studies in order to provide comparable research.

As yet, there is no incidence data available and little is known about risk factors from population data.

HOW DOES FIBROMYALGIA AFFECT THE INDIVIDUAL AND THEIR LIVES?

Muscle Pain

Fibromyalgia may begin as localised muscle pain. The pain involves the whole body when the syndrome is fully developed. Most fibromyalgia patients also have subjective joint pain without evidence of arthritis. Muscle and joint stiffness is seen in 90% of the patients, worst in the morning and often lasting for 2-4 hours. The pain influences the individual as described below.

Functional Disability

Fibromyalgia patients have problems with mobility, arm function, grip strength, and household tasks that are comparable to rheumatoid arthritis patients.

Ergonomic assessment of functional work tests has shown that fibromyalgia patients have as much disability as rheumatoid arthritis patients and perform at only 60% of normal capacity. Their reduced work capacity is usually due to pain which limits movement. Functional disability tends to remain stable over time.

Poor Physical Fitness

Most individuals with fibromyalgia exercise very little. They also have low levels of physical fitness when compared to age-matched healthy subjects. Patients often complain of muscle weakness. On the average, maximum muscle strength is lower in fibromyalgia patients than in matched controls.

Work Disability

Many patients feel unable to cope with housework. Many have quit work outside the home, changed jobs, or work only part-time as a consequence of their fibromyalgia. There is a strong negative impact of fibromyalgia on work performance. When employed, individuals with fibromyalgia have a higher number of sick days, have more difficulty performing work accurately and completing work tasks efficiently compared to individuals with rheumatoid arthritis. They also report the need for more frequent rest periods and within-job modifications. Overall, having fibromyalgia makes it difficult for patients to be *competitively* employed.

In some countries, fibromyalgia accounts for a considerable amount of work disability payments.

Psychological Distress

There is no "fibromyalgia personality." Persons with fibromyalgia respond in very individualized ways and cannot be stereotyped.

Between 20 and 70% of individuals with fibromyalgia are depressed or have a history of depression. Other common psychiatric problems are generalized anxiety and phobia. Whether individuals with fibromyalgia have higher rates of psychiatric disorders than individuals with rheumatoid arthritis is unclear.

Psychological distress, in particular anxiety and worry about illness, is often more a consequence of pain, the uncertainty regarding the fibromyalgia diagnosis and non-ineffective treatment rather than a specific trait of the individual. Individuals with fibromyalgia have higher levels of stress as measured by daily "hassles." As with other chronic diseases patients with fibromyalgia have a high prevalence (20-70%) of anxiety and depression. This compounds their distress, but is not the primary cause of most of their symptoms. The pain associated with fibromyalgia may have the greatest effect on psychological state.

Decreased Quality of Life

Persons with fibromyalgia perceive their quality of life to be significantly lower than healthy persons or those with rheumatic diseases such as rheumatoid arthritis or systemic lupus erythematosus. Spheres of life with which they are particularly dissatisfied include health, relationships, and ability to engage in recreation.

Relationship Problems

Fibromyalgia patients perceive less support and understanding from family members and friends.

WHAT IS THE IMPACT ON SOCIETY OF FIBROMYALGIA?

Studies documenting societal impact hardly exist. Some ongoing studies have been identified. Rising disability pensions as the major part of indirect costs are of major concern.

WHAT SORTS OF TREATMENTS ARE AVAILABLE?

As long as we do not know the etiology of fibromyalgia no cure is available. Individualized multidisciplinary treatment programmes are of importance because fibromyalgia affects the patient physically, psychologically and socially.

The symptoms of fibromyalgia patients must be accepted by the doctor. Doctors need to explain to the patients that fibromyalgia is a chronic disorder and that long term treatment is required.

Physical Therapy

Very few studies of this kind have been carried out. Controlled trials are difficult because the option of placebo treatment is limited. It is therefore difficult to compare the effects of different treatments. Overall, the best results have been reported from a gentle physical training programme combined with psychological intervention. The idea behind physical training programmes for fibromyalgia patients is to avoid the effects of inactivity on muscle, to increase endorphin secretion and to provide an increased locus of control.

Education and Cognitive Restructuring

It is apparent that many fibromyalgia patients have been misinformed regarding their diagnosis. An increased understanding is likely to decrease anxiety and to lead to better treatment compliance. Many fibromyalgia patients have problems dealing with stress, and there is increasing evidence that cognitive restructuring techniques may be a useful addition to a treatment programme.

Drug Treatment

Few studies have been done on the effects of non-steroidal anti-inflammatory drugs, acetylsalicylic acid and paracetamol on fibromyalgia patients, although these treatments are frequently given. At most, such medications take the "edge" off the pain. The use of stronger painkillers needs to be restricted due to the development of dependence and minimization of exercise and other non-pharmacologic interventions.

Anti-depressive drugs have a well-documented effect on fibromyalgia patients. The typical dosage is only 1/10 of that which is administered to treat depression and the effect is much quicker than that seen in the treatment of depression. The long-term results of this medication are at present unknown. These drugs potentiate the effects of serotonin in the central nervous system and this is believed to modulate sleep and pain.

S-adenosylmethionine occurs naturally in the body and is involved in certain metabolic processes. Two studies show that S-adenosylmethionine seems both to reduce pain and increase physical strength in fibromyalgia patients.

Local injections of corticosteroids and anaesthetics are only of value in fibromyalgia treatment when an acute and localised worsening of pain occurs. (Systemic corticosteroids have no place in fibromyalgia treatment.)

In Conclusion

The most promising results for treatment of fibromyalgia seem to be an individualized multidisciplinary long-term approach to treatment. Several groups are now assessing multidisciplinary treatment programmes which employ a combination of approaches using modalities such as education, low dose anti-depressive drugs, aerobic conditioning, cognitive restructuring and myofascial therapy.

WHAT RESEARCH CHALLENGES MUST BE MET IN THE FUTURE?

It was agreed upon that research efforts be intensified and look at all aspects of fibromyalgia. Some priorities are described below.

Epidemiology

Many more women suffer from fibromyalgia than men. Studies of more precise common characteristics are needed. Also socioeconomic data are needed which look at variables such as civil status; economic status; occupational status, etc. Studies of incidence and prevalence should be conducted and efforts made to initiate cross-national studies. Subclassifications of fibromyalgia in epidemiologic studies are needed in order to increase comparability of studies. Criteria for subclassification may include, for example, levels of severity (mild, moderate, severe) as well as patients with significant physical predispositions (marked hypermobility, significant deconditioning or overuse/overload circumstances) and psychologic distress.

Longitudinal Studies of Early Disease

Controlled risk factor studies as well as longitudinal course of illness research on fibromyalgia patients starting in the earliest available stage of disease is essential in order to determine factors that may contribute to onset and prognosis versus those which result from the pain and dysfunction of this chronic condition.

Causal Modelling of Fibromyalgia

The continued search for causes of fibromyalgia should be developed. Biomedical etiologic models have been launched at the MYOPAIN World Congress 1992. Also broader models including living conditions, ecologic factors and lifestyle have been proposed as a conceptual starting point for a broader research strategy. When a better understanding of the causes of fibromyalgia are known prevention should be a research priority.

Muscle Research

Biopsies. Microscopic changes have been described in tender fibromyalgia muscle. These changes, however, are not specific to fibromyalgia. Future muscle research in fibromyalgia needs to answer the following questions:

1. Are the changes quantitatively different in fibromyalgia patients compared to normal individuals and are they sufficient in themselves to explain myopain?
2. Are the changes in fibromyalgia muscle biopsies primary or secondary to disuse?
3. Are the reported changes due to alterations in microcirculation and/ or mechanic microtrauma?
4. What are the relations of the reported muscle changes to pain?

Muscle function. Muscle function in fibromyalgia patients is reported to be impaired. The role of peripheral causes is still unclear. There is a need to evaluate muscle function in controlled studies using standardized procedures that can critically evaluate:

1. muscle strength
2. muscle endurance
3. perception of effort and pain
4. degree of relaxation at voluntary rest
5. focal muscle metabolism, e.g., by nuclear magnetic resonance studies.

Pain Research

An unresolved problem is the origin of myopain. Most likely there are both peripheral and central factors. The research on neurotransmitters should be expanded as well as studies of the sympathetic nervous system.

Psychological/Psychiatric Research

Psychological and psychiatric abnormalities are present in some patients. Studies comparing fibromyalgia patients with patients who suffer from other chronic pain-related diseases could clarify the role of psychological distress in fibromyalgia. The development of a psychological test which takes the pain factors into account would help with both prognosis studies and choice of treatment for fibromyalgia patients. The role of psychosocial stress in initiating sleep disturbance and the resulting neuroendocrine changes need to be studied in greater detail.

Clinical Therapy Trials

Future controlled therapy trials should more critically focus on indicators of the effectiveness of the various treatments, e.g., tricyclic antidepressive drugs, aerobic conditioning, cognitive behavioural therapy, education, triggerpoint injection therapy, non-steroidal anti-inflammatory drugs, etc. Studies to date have suggested that only a certain number of patients respond partially to any single therapeutic intervention. Future research should try to identify any subgroups which respond more effectively to a particular intervention or combinations of therapies.

Anthropological and Social Studies

It was suggested that the social and cultural aspects of fibromyalgia patients be explored using qualitative research methods. For example, by using in-depth interviews future research might look at cultural perceptions of pain, perceived control in the work situation, perceived control of one's personal life, etc.

Health Services Research

Little is known about how health services handle fibromyalgia patients. The utilization pattern and health economic aspects should be studied [cost effectiveness and quality of life]. Future research should include consumer studies such as patients' perceptions of and satisfaction with health services.

Long-Term Outcome Studies

Demonstrated effective therapies from individual and multidisciplinary programmes should be critically analyzed to determine improvements in outcome functioning and quality of life including return to work, vocational and non-vocational pursuits.

APPENDIX 1. MYOPAIN CONSENSUS CONFERENCE PROCESS

The modified consensus conference process was created by the organizers of MYOPAIN under the leadership of Finn Kamper-Jørgensen. As seen from the table below the MYOPAIN conference differs from the ordinary consensus conference. The MYOPAIN time-table only allowed the conference to last 4 hours.

A preliminary consensus document–made available to the panels about one month prior to the congress and to all congress participants at the beginning of the congress–was drafted by Søren Jacobsen, Bente Danneskiold-Samsøe, Robert Bennett, Else Bartels and Finn Kamper-Jørgensen.

The final document was able to consider not only the results of the consensus conference, but also all the presentations from the world congress.

Appendix 2 shows the timetable and the panels.

The final document was written immediately after the consensus conference by the consensus panel. The chairman of the expert panel was included in the consensus panel. The process lasted twelve hours.

CONSENSUS CONFERENCES		
	Usual consensus conference	MYOPAIN consensus conference
Time available	2–3 days	3–4 hours
Conference questions formulated before conference	Yes	Yes
Document available before conference?	No. Is written during conference	Yes. Preliminary version distributed to all congress participants
Responsible for consensus document?	Consensus panel	Consensus panel and chairman of expert panel
Role of experts	Present knowledge 10–20 min. related to a particular question	Defend or criticize the relevant section of the preliminary consensus document
Questions from consensus panel to expert panel – and discussion?	Yes	Yes
Possibility for interventions from the audience?	Yes	Yes

APPENDIX 2

FIBROMYALGIA CONSENSUS CONFERENCE
August 20, 1992 9.00 a.m. – 1.00 p.m.
Chairman: Finn Kamper-Jørgensen

TIMETABLE

9.00 – 9.55	**Presentation of highlights from seminars with particular reference to the fibromyalgia consensus document**
9.00 – 9.05	**Introduction** : Finn Kamper-Jørgensen
9.05 – 9.15	**Seminar I** : Frederick Wolfe
9.15 – 9.25	**Seminar II** : Robert M. Bennett
9.25 – 9.35	**Seminar III** : Ann Bengtsson
9.35 – 9.45	**Seminar IV** : Odd Kogstad
9.45 – 9.55	Possibility of one minute statements from other chairmen: Bente Danneskiold–Samsøe, Anders Bjelle, Jens Halkjær Kristensen, Søren Jacobsen, Henning Værøy, Gisela Sjøgaard, Don L. Goldenberg, Valur Johansson, Allan Wiik, Muhammad B. Yunus, Thorsten Ingemann Hansen
9.55 – 10.00	Preparing for panels.
10.00 – 10.15	What is a consensus conference? Introducing the questions, the panels and playing rules: Finn Kamper–Jørgensen
10.15 – 10.25	Introduction, overview by chairman of expert panel: Robert Bennett
10.25 – 10.30	**Question 1:** What is fibromyalgia? Robert Bennett
10.30 – 10.35	**Question 2:** How do we diagnose fibromyalgia? Frederick Wolfe
10.35 – 10.40	**Question 3:** What causes fibromyalgia? Karl G. Henriksson
10.40 – 11.00	Questions from consensus panel. Discussion
11.00 – 11.30	**COFFEE BREAK**
11.30 – 11.35	**Question 4:** What is the frequency of fibromyalgia in the population? Anders Bjelle
11.35 – 11.40	**Question 5:** How does fibromyalgia affect the individual? Carol S. Burckhardt

APPENDIX 2 (continued)

11.40 – 11.45	**Question 6:** What is the impact on society of fibromyalgia? Marijke van Santen–Hoeufft
11.45 – 11.50	**Question 7:** What sort of treatment is effective? Don L. Goldenberg
11.50 – 11.55	**Question 8:** What research challenges must be met in the future? Ann Bengtsson, Søren Jacobsen
11.55 – 12.20	Questions from the consensus panel. Discussion
12.20 – 12.45	Questions and comments from congress participants (max. 3 min per person)
12.45 – 13.00	Discussion between panels.
13.00	**CLOSURE OF CONSENSUS CONFERENCE**

MEMBERS OF PANELS

Expert Panel

Robert M. Bennett, M.D., FRCP, Professor, Chairman of panel
Department of Medicine
Oregon Health Sciences University
School of Medicine, Division of Arthritis
3181 S.W. Sam Jackson Park Rd. (L329A)
Portland, Oregon 97201-3098
USA

Ann Bengtsson, M.D., Ph.D., Assoc. Professor
Rheumatology Unit
University Hospital
581 85 Linköping
Sweden

Anders Bjelle, M.D., Ph.D., Professor
Sahlgren University Hospital
Department of Rheumatology
413 45 Göteborg
Sweden

Carol S. Burckhardt, Ph.D., RN, Assoc. Professor
Oregon Health Sciences University
3181 S.W. Sam Jackson Park Rd. (L329A)
Portland, Oregon 97201-3098
USA

Don L. Goldenberg, M.D., Professor
Tufts University, School of Medicine
Newton-Wellesley Hospital
2114 Washington Street
Newton, Massachusetts 02162
USA

Karl G. Henriksson, M.D., Ph.D.
University Hospital
Department of Clinical Neurophysiology
and Neuromuscular Unit
581 85 Linköping
Sweden

Søren Jacobsen, M.D.
Department of Rheumatology
Hvidovre Hospital
Kettegård Alle 30
DK-2650 Hvidovre
Denmark

Marijke Van Santen-Hoeufft, M.D., Ass. Professor
University Hospital Maastricht
Department of Internal Medicine
Division of Rheumatology
P.O. Box 5800, NL 6202 AZ Maastricht
Holland

Henning Værøy, M.D., Ph.D.
Oppland Regional Psychiatric Hospital
Presteseter
2840 Reinsvoll
Norway

Frederick Wolfe, M.D., Professor
School of Medicine, Arthritis Center
1035 N. Emporia, 230
Wichita, Kansas 67214
USA

Consensus Panel

Finn Kamper-Jørgensen, M.D., Ph.D., Director, Chairman of Consensus
    Conference
The Danish Institute for Clinical Epidemiology (DIKE)
Svanemøllevej 25
DK-2100 Copenhagen
Denmark

Liv Anne Andreassen
Norwegian Fibromyalgia Association
Postboks 6313, Etterstad
N-0604 Oslo
Norway

Dag Bruusgaard, M.D., Ph.D., Professor
Institute of General Practice
Frederik Stangsgate 11-13
0264 Oslo
Norway

Bente Danneskiold-Samsøe, M.D., Ph.D.
Head of Department of Rheumatology
Frederiksberg Hospital
Ndr. Fasanvej 57
DK-2000 Frederiksberg
Denmark

Alfonse T. Masi, M.D., DR.P.H., Professor
Department of Medicine
University of Illinois
College of Medicine at Peoria
One Illini Drive, P.O. Box 1649
Peoria, Illinois 62656
USA

Janine Marie Morgall, Ph.D., Sociologist
The Royal Danish School of Pharmacy
Department of Social Pharmacy
Universitetsparken 2
DK-2100 Copenhagen
Denmark

LISTING OF SCIENTIFIC PRESENTATIONS DURING THE SECOND WORLD CONGRESS ON MYOFASCIAL PAIN AND FIBROMYALGIA, AUGUST 17-20, 1992, COPENHAGEN, DENMARK

Scientific presentations including review lectures, oral presentations, guided posters and posters listed according to the programme topics and in alphabetic order of the first author.

Abstracts from the Second World Congress on Myofascial Pain and Fibromyalgia are published in: MYOPAIN '92. Scandinavian Journal of Rheumatology; Supplement 94, 1992.

REVIEW LECTURES ON MYOFASCIAL PAIN SYNDROMES AND FIBROMYALGIA

R. M. Bennett, The Origin of Myopain: An integrated Hypothesis of Focal Muscle changes and Sleep Disturbance.

J. R. Fricton, Myofascial Pain: Clinical Features and Diagnostic Criteria

R. D. Gerwin, Myofascial Pain Syndrome: Treatment Programme

D. L. Goldenberg, Fibromyalgia: Treatment programs

K. G. Henriksson, Chronic Muscular Pain–Etiology and Pathogenesis

H. Merskey, Chronic Muscular Pain–A Life Stress Syndrome?

H. Moldofsky, Seasonality of Pain, Mood, Energy and Sleep in Fibromyalgia vs. Rheumatoid Arthritis

O. M. Sejersted, Acute Localized Muscle Pain–Etiology and Pathogenesis

F. Wolfe, Fibromyalgia–Clinical Features and Diagnostic Criteria

SEMINAR 1
EPIDEMIOLOGY AND NATURAL HISTORY
OF MYOFASCIAL PAIN AND FIBROMYALGIA

Oral Presentations

A. Bengtsson, E. Bäckman, Long-term Follow up of Fibromyalgia Patients

P. Croft, J. Schollum, A. S. Rigby, R. F. Boswell, A. J. Silman, Chronic Widespread Pain in the General Population

C. Lyddell, O. L. Meyers, The Prevalence of Fibromyalgia in a Southern African Community

A. T. Masi, Aspects on the Epidemiology and Criteria of Myofascial Pain and Fibromyalgia

J. Nørregaard, P. Bülow, E. Prescott, S. Jacobsen, B. Danneskiold-Samsøe, A 4 year Follow-up Study in Fibromyalgia. Relationship to Chronic Fatigue Syndrome.

E. Prescott, S. Jacobsen, M. Kjøller, P. Bülow, B. Danneskiold-Samsøe, F. Kamper-Jørgensen, Prevalence of Fibromyalgia in the Adult Danish Population

H. Raspe, Ch. Baumgartner, The Epidemiology of the Fibromyalgia Syndrome (FMS) in a German Town

F. Wolfe, Fibromyalgia and Myofascial Pain: Lessons from the Clinic and the Community

Guided Posters

J. H. Andersen, O. Gaardboe, Myofascial Pain among Sewing-machine Operators

C. S. Burckhardt, C. A. O'Reilly, A. N. Wiens, S. R. Clark, S. M. Campbell, R. M. Bennett, Psychological Status of Women with Fibromyalgia

C. W. Chan, S. Goldman, D. Ilstrup, A. Kunselman, P. O'Neill, The Pain Drawing, Waddell's Non-organic Physical Signs and Low Back Pain

G. F. Ferraccioli, F. Salaffi, W. T. Rioda, M. Carotti, C. Cervini, Disability in Fibromyalgia, Rheumatoid Arthritis and Osteoarthritis

R. D. Gerwin, Myofascial Pain in Polio Survivors

D. J. Hawley, F. Wolfe, Depression in Fibromyalgia: A Comparative Study of 1522 Rheumatic Disease Patients

A. A. Knipping, J. N. de Voogd, A. C. E. de Blécourt, M. H. van Rijswijk, Psychological Aspects in Fibromyalgia

T. J. Romano, Coexistence of Fibromyalgia Syndrome and Systemic Lupus Erythematosus

T. J. Romano, Presence of Fibromyalgia Syndrome in Osteoarthritis Patients

T. J. Romano, Incidence of Fibromyalgia Syndrome in Rheumatoid Arthritis Patients in a General Rheumatology Practice

I. J. Russell, S. J. Russell, R. E. Cuevas, J. E. Michalek, Early Life Traumas and Confiding in Fibromyalgia Syndrome (FS)

J. Schollum, P. Croft, Symptoms Associated with Tender Points Counts in the General Population

L. Szczepanski, W. Walewski, Unclassified Generalized Pain and Fibromyalgia Syndrome

W. Walewski, L. Szczepanski, Epidemiological Studies of Fibromyalgia Syndrome Morbidity

Posters

P. Bolwijn, M. van Santen-Hoeufft, H. Baars, S. van der Linden, Social Network Characteristics in Patients with Primary Fibromyalgia and Rheumatoid Arthritis: A Pilot Study

S. Jacobsen, S. R. Bredkjær, Selfreported Diffuse Chronic Musculo-skeletal Pain in the Danish Population

R. Jensen, B. K. Rasmussen, J. Olesen, Muscle Tenderness and Pressure Pain Threshold in an Epidemiological Study of Tension-Type Headache

O. L. Meyers, The Epidemiology of Various Soft Tissue Rheumatic Syndromes in a Small Urban Community

P. A. Reilly, G. O. Littlejohn, Sleep Disturbance and Lumbar Hyperlordosis and their Relationship to Fibromyalgia Syndrome (FS)

N. B. Rosen, Toward a More Rational and Uniform Classification of Muscle Pain Disorders

W. Samborski, T. Stratz, W. Kretzman, P. Mennet, W. Müller, The Comparison of Incidence the Vegetative and Functional Symptoms in Patients with Fibromyalgia and Chronic Low Back Pain Syndrome.

M. Sinaki, P. Limburg, J. Rogers, P. Murtaugh, Trunk Muscle Strength in Children

SEMINAR 2
PERIPHERAL AND CENTRAL MECHANISMS IN MUSCLE PAIN

Oral Presentations

S. R. Clark, C. S. Burckhardt, S. M. Campbell, R. M. Bennett, Physical Fitness Characteristics of 94 Women with Fibromyalgia

A. M. Drewes, A. Andreasen, H. D. Schrøder, B. Høgsaa, P. Jennum, Muscle Biopsy in Fibromyalgia

G. Granges, G. O. Littlejohn, R. D. Helme, S. Gibson, Cerebral Event-related Responses Induced by Co 2 Laser Stimulation in Subjects with Fibromyalgia Syndrome

E. Houvenagel, G. Forzy, B. Cortet, G. Vincent, J. L. Dhondt, 5 Hydroxy Indol Acetic Acid in Cerebro Spinal Fluid in Fibromyalgia

R. Lindman, M. Hagberg, A. Bengtsson, K. G. Henriksson, L.-E. Thornell, Ultrastructural Changes in the Trapezius Muscle in Work-related Myalgia and Fibromyalgia

E. Saugen, A. M. Mengshoel, Ø. Førre, N. K. Vøllestad, Muscle Fatigue in Fibromyalgia patients

R. W. Simms, S. H. Roy, M. Hrovat, J. J. Anderson, G. S. Skrinar, S. R. LePoole, C. F. Zerbini, C. DeLuca, F. Jolesz, Fibromyalgia Syndrome is not Associated with Abnormalities in Muscle Energy Metabolism

K. Söderlund, E. Hultman, A. Bengtsson, Is a Reduced Energy Store or Energy Production Rate a Cause for Fibromyalgia?

M. Wærsted, T. Eken, R. H. Westgaard, Prolonged Psychogenic Activity in Single Motor Units: A Possible Mechanism for Muscle Injury?

Guided Posters

P. E. Baldry, Neurophysiological Basis for Superficial Dry Needling in the Deactivation of Myofascial Trigger Points

L. A. Bradley, G. S. Alarcón, J. E. Haile, I. C. Scarinci, Pain Perception and Psychological Distress Among Patients and Non-Patients with Fibromyalgia (FM)

W. Brückle, M. Sückfüll, W. Fleckenstein, W. Müller, Tissue-pO_2 Measurement in Tender Muscle (M.Erector Spinae)

A. C. E. de Blécourt, R. F. Wolf, M. H. van Rijswijk, R. L. Kamman, A. A. Knipping, E. L. Mooyaart, In Vivo 31P-MR Spectroscopy of Tender Points in Patients with Fibromyalgia

S. W. G. Derbyshire, A. K. P. Jones, W. D. Brown, P. Devani, K. J. Friston, L. Y. Qi, R. S. J. Frackowiak, Cortical and Subcortical Responses to Pain in Male and Female Volunteers Measured by Positron Emission Tomography

C.-Z. Hong, Y. Torigoe, D. G. Simons, Failure of Local Twitch Responses in Rabbit Skeletal Muscles with Repetitive Needling

C.-Z. Hong, D. G. Simons, Remote Inactivation of Myofascial Trigger Points by Injection of Trigger Points in Another Muscle

C. Jensen, K. Nilsen, K. Hansen, R. H. Westgaard, Shoulder-neck Complaints and Muscle Activity in Workers with Static Loads.

B. R. Jensen, K. Jørgensen, G. Sjøgaard, Muscle Fluid Balance During Submaximal Isometric Contractions

A. K. P. Jones, S. W. G. Derbyshire, P. Devani, K. J. Friston, L. Y. Qi, C. Feinmann, M. Harris, R. S. J. Frackowiak, Cerebral Responses to Pain in Patients with Atypical Facial Pain Measured by Positron Emission Tomography

E. Joos, N. Barette, K. De Meirleir, W. Buyens, P. Neirinck, K. Vandenborne, F. Dewitte, M. Osteaux, 31 P Magnetic Resonance Spectroscopy as a Diagnostic Tool in Patients with Fibromyalgia

M. W. W. Krapf, S. Müller, P. Mennet, T. Stratz, W. Müller, The Investigation of pH in the Musculus Erector Spinae by Patients with Low Back Pain and Fibromyalgia using vivo 31p Nuclear Magnetic Resonance (31p NMR)

P. Kröling, P. Schoeps, A. Beyer, C. Wonnerth, E. Senn, Pressure Pain Threshold (PPT) of Fibromyalgia Patients is Reduced at Typical Tender Points and Non Tender Points. A Patient Controlled Automatic PPT Device Improves Measurement Accuracy

M. Lindh, G. Johansson, G. Grimby, M. Hedberg, Muscle Function in Patients with Fibromyalgia

P. A. Reilly, Z. Khalil, R. D. Helme, G. O. Littlejohn, Axon Reflex Flare Responses in Patients with Fibromyalgia Syndrome (FS)

K. B. Veiersted, R. H. Westgaard, Do short Gaps in Myoelectrical Activity during Repetitive Manual Work Prevent Trapezius Myalgia?

S. H. Wigers, J. Aasly, G. Timm, P. Rinck, 31 Phosphorus Magnetic Resonance Spectroscopy of Leg Muscle in Patients with Fibromyalgia

Posters

J. Elert, S. Rantapää-Dahlqvist, B. Almay, M. Eisemann, Muscle Endurance, Muscle Tension and Personality Traits in Patients with Muscle or Joint Pain. A Pilot Study

G. Granges, G. O. Littlejohn, Monfas: An Activity Score for Fibromyalgia and Regional Pain Syndromes

A. Hietaharju, J. Kemppi, H. Pitkänen, P. J. Pöntinen, The Role of Thermography, Isokinetic Movement Analysis and Pain Threshold Measurements for Differentiation of Reflex Sympathetic Dystrophy (RSD) and Myofascial Pain Syndrome (MPS)–A Preliminary Report

S. Jacobsen, B. Holm, Muscle Strenght and Endurance Compared to Aerobic Capacity in Fibromyalgia

R. Lindman, A. Eriksson, L.-E. Thornell, A Morphological Approach to Chronic Trapezius Myalgia

B. Nickel, L. Nagymajtenyi, I. Desi, I. Szelenyi, Flupirtine a Centrally Acting Analgesic with Muscle Relaxing Activity

E. Prescott, J. Nørregaard, P. Rotbøl, L. Pedersen, B. Danneskiold-Samsøe, P. Bülow, Red Blood Cell Magnesium and Fibromyalgia

G. S. Skrinar, R. W. Simms, S. H. Roy, J. J. Anderson, C. F. Zerbini, C. DeLuca, How do Fibromyalgia Patients Rate Levels of Exertion? A Comparative Study with Sedentary Controls.

H. Sprott, C. Kovac, K. Birck, M. Lobisch, P. Mennet, N. Merz, T. Stratz, W. Müller, A New Method to Show Myotonolytic Effects in Man

P. Thoumie, F. Audisio, M. F. Kahn, M. Bedoiseau, Postural Control Evaluation in Fibromyalgia

SEMINAR 3
CLINICAL STUDIES IN MYOFASCIAL PAIN AND FIBROMYALGIA

Oral Presentation

J. E. Bachman, R. S. Roth, A. M. de Rosayro, A. McLoughlin, V. Mullin, Pain Experience, Psychological Functioning and Selfreported Disability in Chronic Pain of Myofascial Versus Fibromyalgia Origin

R. M. Bennett, S. R. Clark, S. M. Campbell, C. S. Burckhardt, Low Levels of Somatomedin-C in Fibromyalgia: A Neuro-endocrine Defect Involving the Sleep Related Secretion of Growth Hormone

C. S. Burckhardt, B. Archenholtz, K. Mannerkorpi, A. Bjelle, Quality of Life of Swedish Women with Fibromyalgia (FMS), Rheumatoid Arthritis (RA) or Systemic Lupus Erythematosus (SLE)

A. M. Drewes, K. D. Nielsen, P. Jennum, A. Andreasen, Alpha Intrusion of

Deeper Sleep Stages in Fibromyalgia–a Study based on Quantitative Frequency Analysis

E. N. Griep, J. W. Boersma, E. R. de Kloet, Evidence for Neuro Endocrine Disturbance following Physical Exercise in the Primary Fibromyalgia Syndrome (PFS)

V. Johannsson, Does it exist a Fibromyalgia Personality?

P. A. Reilly, G. O. Littlejohn, Diurnal Variation in the Symptoms and Signs of the Fibromyalgia Syndrome (FS)

G. Schuessler, J. Konermann, W. Mau, Psychosomatic Aspects of Primary Fibromyalgia Syndrome (PFS)

J. H. Mason, S. L. Silverman, A. L. Weaver, R. W. Simms, The Impact of Fibromyalgia on Multiple Aspects of Health Status

Guided Posters

J. Berlin, E. David, H. Schwendner, C. Naumann, W. Erdmann, M. Traub, Psychosomatic Aspects and Therapy of Fibromyalgia

A. M. Drewes, A. Andreasen, K. D. Nielsen, P. Jennum, A. Sjøl, Epidemiology of Sleep Related Complaints in Fibromyalgia and Rheumatoid Arthritis

B. Ellertsen, H. Værøy, MMPI Profiles and Duration of Disease in Fibromyalgia

W. Grassi, P. Core, G. Carlino, F. Salaffi, C. Cervini, Nailfold Capillary Permeability in Fibromyalgia Syndrome

C. Henriksson, Fibromyalgia–Changes in Psycho-social Consequences during a Five-year Period

W. Mau, H. Dans-Neeff, M. Bornmann, H. Weber, General Decrease of Pressure Pain Treshold in Fibromyalgia

Posters

O. Airaksinen, J. Ylinen, P. J. Pöntinen, Reliability and Repeatability of Handhold Tissue Compliance Meter

A. Bezzi, S. Canazza, D. Chiarini, R. La Corte, F. Trotta, Transcutaneous Electrical Nerv Stimulation (TENS) in Primary Fibromyalgia: An Evaluation with McGill Pain Questionnaire

M. Bornmann, H. Weber, S. Kallenberger, W. Mau, Aspects of Pain and Illness Behaviour in Fibromyalgia and Rheumatoid Arthritis

J. C. Branco, R. Santos, T. Paiva, Sleep Studies in Fibromyalgia

J. C. Branco, I. Abreu, R. Humbel, V. Tavares, M. Caetano, Inflammatory Protein Profile in Patients with Fibromyalgia

E. Cantelli, P. Cicogna, M. Ercolani, Psychological and Sleep Disorders in Primary Fibromyalgia Syndrome

G. A. Cassisi, S. Todesco, A. Ianniello, F. Ceccherelli, G. P. Giron, Pain in Fibromyalgic Syndrome (FS): Evaluation of Pain Threshold and Psychological State

A. M. Drewes, A. Andreasen, L. H. Poulsen, A Cross Frontiers Comparison of Pain in Fibromyalgia and Rheumatoid Arthritis

A. Gam, S. Jacobsen, C. Egsmose, M. Olsen, B. Danneskiold-Samsøe, G. F. Jensen, Bone Mass and Turnover in Fibromyalgia

D. M. Heath, B. M. Sucher, Myofascial & Somatic Dysfunction in Biceps Tendonitis

S. Jacobsen, K. Main, B. Danneskiold-Samsøe, N. E. Skakkebæk, Urinary Excretion of Growth Hormone in Fibromyalgia

S. Jacobsen, I. S. Petersen, Relationship of Clinical Features with Chronic Muscle Pain–with Reference to Fibromyalgia

A. Jordan, J. Mehlsen, Deficiency of Neck Muscles in Cervico-brachial Syndrome

J. Lautenschläger, J. Seglias, W. Brückle, W. Müller, Comparisons of Spontaneous Pain and Tenderness in Patients with Primary Fibromyalgia

G. Neeck, W. Riedel, Thyroid Function in Patients with Fibromyalgia Syndrome (FMS)

U. Nordenskiöld, Grip Force Involves Pain in Women with Fibromyalgia and Rheumatoid Arthritis

G. Pestelli, R. M. Rossi, A. Serra, P. Maltoni, A. Zoli, Fibromyalgia : What the best for?

P. J. Pöntinen, L. Vuoto, Pressure Algometry in Low Back Pain Patients and Healthy Controls

N. B. Rosen, Overuse Syndromes Versus Overload Syndromes: Part of the Spectrum of Myofascial Pain and Dysfunction?

N. B. Rosen, Myoedematous Response in Patients with Fibromyalgia and/or Myofascial Pain

S. H. Roy, R. W. Simms, S. R. LePoole, J. J. Anderson, M. Hrovat, C. F. Zerbini, G. S. Skrinar, C. J. De Luca, F. Jolesz, Surface EMG Measurement of Fatigue in Fibromyalgia Syndrome (FMS)

R. Saggini, M. A. Giamberardino, L. Dragani, L. Vecchiet, Myofascial Pain Syndrome of the Peroneus Longus: Biomechanical Approach

B. M. Sucher, Myofascial Release of Carpal Tunnel Syndrome–A Four Case Report

B. M. Sucher, D. M. Heath, S. Andrews, R. N. Hinrichs, Myofascial & Somatic Dysfunction in Repetitive Strain Syndrome

E. de Klerk, S. van der Linden, M. van Santen-Hoeufft, P. Bolwijn, Concordance of Self-assessment and Observed Functional Capacity in Fibromyalgia and Rheumatoid Arthritis

S. H. Wigers, T. C. Stiles, A. Holst, T. Moen, HLA-antigens in the Primary Fibromyalgia Syndrome

A. Zizzo, F. Casamassima, M. Ercolani, Personality Assessment of 10 Fibromyalgic Patients by Means of the Rorschach Test

SEMINAR 4
TREATMENT OF MYOFASCIAL PAIN AND FIBROMYALGIA

Oral Presentation

C. S. Burckhardt, K. Mannerkorpi, A. Bjelle, A Randomized, Controlled Trial of Education and Physical Therapy for Women with Fibromyalgia Syndrome (FMS)

S. R. Clark, C. S. Burckhardt, S. M. Campbell, C. A. O'Reilly, R. M. Bennett, Prescribing Exercise for Patients with Fibromyalgia

J. N. de Voogd, A. A. Knipping, A. C. E. de Blécourt, M. H. van Rijswijk, Treatment of Fibromyalgia Syndrome with Psycho-motor Therapy and Marital Counselling

A. M. Drewes, A. Andreasen, L. H. Poulsen, Injection Therapy for Treatment of Chronic Myofascial Pain

D. L. Goldenberg, K. H. Kaplan, M. G. Nadeau, A Prospective Study of Stress Reduction, Relaxation Response (SRRR) Therapy in fibromyalgia

R. Isomeri, M. Mikkelson, P. Latikka, Effects of Amitriptyline and Cardiovascular Fitness Training on the Pain of Fibromyalgia Patients

A. Jordan, J. Mehlsen, Cervicobrachial Syndrome: Neck Muscle Function and Effects of Training

O. Kogstad, F. Hintringer, Y. M. Jonsson, Patients with Fibromyalgia in Pain Schools

A. M. Mengshoel, H. B. Komnæs, Ø. Førre, Physical Fitness Training in Female Patients with Fibromyalgia

Guided Posters

C. S. Burckhardt, S. R. Clark, S. M. Campbell, C. A. O'Reilly, A. N. Wiens, R. M. Bennett, Multidisciplinary Treatment of Fibromyalgia

J. R. Fricton, D. D. Arancio, Comparison of Rehabilitation Treatment of Myofascial Pain with no Treatment

E. Gerecz-Simon, W. F. Kean, W. W. Buchanan, J.-A. Heale, Statistical Correlative Study of Outcome Measures in Fibromyalgia: Evidence that Anxiolytic Therapy has no Therapeutic Benefit

M. Ghirardini, L. Betelemme, F. Fatti, The Use of Trazodone AC 150 for Primary Fibromyalgia (P.F.). An Open Study Concerning 167 Patients

H. Himmelstrup, S. Jacobsen, J. Mehlsen, Vacusac Treatment in Primary Fibromyalgia

O. Høydalsmo, I. Johannsen, H. Harstad, S. Jacobsen, P. Kryger, Effects of a Multidisciplinary Training Programme in Fibromyalgia

T. Ingemann-Hansen, L. B. Andersen, K. Grunnet, K. Høgh, Muscular Endurance Training for Neck/Shoulder and Relaxation Exercises in Sewing-machine Operators

Posters

O. Airaksinen, K. Tiittola, P. J. Pöntinen, Tension Neck Patients Unresponsive to Neck School

M. Avalle, Treatment of Myofascial Pain with High Voltage Stimulation (HVGS)

M. Ercolani, G. Fornasari, E. Montanari, D. Pasotti, E. Zetti, A. Zizzo, S. Ferri, Clinical Approach to Fibromyalgia Syndrome: Comparative Evaluation of Various Therapeutic Methods

J. B. Eyskens, Provisional Report Concerning the Standardization of Physical Therapy Treatment Plans for Musculo-Skeletal Pain Syndromes

M. Ghirardini, L. Betelemme, F. Fatti, Study on the Therapy of Primary Fibromyalgia in Pediatric Age with 5 Hydroxy-L-Tryptophan

I. Krajnc, M. Siftar, Z. Turk, J. Barovic, T. Nikolic, The Effect of Balneotherapy on the Low-back Pain Disease at the Moravci Spa and the Department of Physiotherapy and Rheumatology–Maribor Teaching Hospital

F. Maccabruni, M. Ghirardini, L. Betelemme, F. Fatti, Treatment of Primary Fibromyalgia with Peridural Sacral Therapy

D. Mihajlovic, V. Bosnjakovic, S. Bozilov, Balneotherapy in Myofascial Pain

E. T. Morris, Cryotherapeutic Treatment of Myofascial Pain Syndrome

B. M. Salim, Myofascial Pain–Trigger Point Injections VS Transcutaneous Electrical Stimulation

W. Samborski, T. Stratz, M. Sobieska, P. Mennet, W. Müller, J. S. Mönting, The

Intraindividual Comparison of Effectiveness of Total-body Cold Therapy and Hot Packs Therapy in the Patients with Generalised Tendomyopathy (Fibromyalgia)

V. Ulzibat, S. Shishov, Operative Treatment of Primary Fibromyalgia (Myofibrillosis)

A. Zizzo, R. Zanelli, M. Ercolani, R. Chattat, An Experience of Group Psychotherapy Body-oriented in Fibromyalgic Syndrome (FS)

MISCELLANEOUS POSTERS ON MYOFASCIAL PAIN SYNDROMES, FIBROMYALGIA AND OTHER RHEUMATIC CONDITIONS

Guided Posters

L. Janssens, Trigger Points and Fibromyalgia in the Dog: Symptoms, Anatomy and Treatment Results

D. Kaunaite, Pathogenesis of Chest Muscular Pain Syndrome in Patients with Coronary Heart Disease

K. H. Njoo, E. Does, Trigger Points in Aspecific Low Back Pain Patients–A Critical Perspective on the Diagnostic Criteria

G. Skylv, Muscular Imbalance Found in Examination of Posture in Torture Victims

G. Skylv, L. Olsen, K. Christensen, L. Tived, B. Carstensen, Late Sequels After Falanga Torture

G. Skylv, A Medical Model for Rehabilitation of Torture Victims

Posters

E. M. Bartels, J. Nørregaard, M. Harreby, S. Amris, B. Danneskiold-Samsøe, Single Cell Morphology in Fibromyalgia

J. C. Branco, I. Abreu, R. Humbel, V. Tavares, M. Caetano, Is the Immunopathology Component Important in Some Patients with Fibromyalgia

R. B. Buckingham, Temporomandibular Joint Dysfunction Syndrome: A Close Association with Systemic Joint Laxity (the Hypermobile Joint Syndrome)

L. Caparoski, I. Dejanov, T. Caparoska, The Heterogenous Nature of Fibromyalgia

P. Cardemil, M. Correa, C. Pino, M. T. Almarza, Team Work: A Need

P. Cardemil, Dealing with Pain

M. Carrabba, E. Paresce, G. La Maida, G. Ceravolo, S. Spinelli, D. S. Pedemonti, A. Galanti, An Uncommon Case of Isolated ACTH Deficiency Associated with a Stiff-Man Syndrome

G. S. Chakhunashvili, I. M. Kvachadze, D. O. Tabutsadze, Muscular Hypothrophy in Children with Articular-and-Visceral form of Rheumatic Arthritis Depending on the Process Activity

H. Göbel, M. Dworschak, D. Soyka, Cortical Magnetical Stimulation Induced Interoceptive Suppression in Patients with Tension-Type Headache

L. G. Schoen, B. J. Eason, A. L. Hinkle, Multidisciplinary Treatment of Chronic Pain: Outcome and Maintenance

H. Jensen, R. M. Mikkelsen, E. T. Paulsen, Therapeutic Riding for Bechterew Patients

J. Kemppi, A. Hietaharju, P. J. Pöntinen, Circulatory Effects of Two Isometric Loading Tests

S. Luigi, Neuro-Myo-Fascial Pain

S. Morris, S. Benjamin, R. Gray, J. Heath, A. Quayle, D. Bennett, Psychiatric Diagnoses and Illness Behaviours in Patients with Temporomandibular Joint Pain Dysfunction Syndrome (TMJPDS)

V. Moshchich, Z. Volobuyeva, V. Shevchenko, The Evaluation of the Efficacy of the Rheumatoid Arthritis Local Therapy

I. Narycheva, Myopain and Hypermobility Syndrome of Joints

T. Päi, Rehabilitation of Patients with Various Kinds of Painful Conditions due to Rheumatoid Diseases with Whole Body Extreme Cold Exposure and Exercises

T. Richter, Prevalence of Joint Dysfunctions of the Lumbar-Pelvic-Region

M. Sander, Physiotherapie of Patients with Myofascial Pain

G. Skylv, The Social Construction of Fibromyalgia–A "New" Disease

J. Tarrant, C. Pedley, A Five-year Study on the Interdisciplinary Treatment for Chronic Somatic Pain

D. R. Trotter, M. L. Taylor, M. E. Csuka, The Incidence of Physical-sexual Abuse in Women with Primary Fibromyalgia

Z. Turk, J. Barovic, F. Vajd, Lumbal Spondylolysthesis Conservative Treatment with Magnetic Field Therapy

Z. Turk, J. Barovic, M. Kramberger, M. Siftar, Postoperative Rehabilitation following Arthroscopic Operations of the Shoulder Joint in Impingement Syndrome Therapy

V. Ulzibat, The Myopain–What is it?

Index

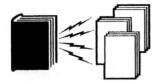

Haworth
DOCUMENT DELIVERY
SERVICE
and Local Photocopying Royalty Payment Form

This new service provides (a) a single-article order form for any article from a Haworth journal and (b) a convenient royalty payment form for local photocopying (not applicable to photocopies intended for resale).

- *Time Saving:* No running around from library to library to find a specific article.
- *Cost Effective:* All costs are kept down to a minimum.
- *Fast Delivery:* Choose from several options, including same-day FAX.
- *No Copyright Hassles:* You will be supplied by the original publisher.
- *Easy Payment:* Choose from several easy payment methods.

Open Accounts Welcome for . . .
- Library Interlibrary Loan Departments
- Library Network/Consortia Wishing to Provide Single-Article Services
- Indexing/Abstracting Services with Single Article Provision Services
- Document Provision Brokers and Freelance Information Service Providers

MAIL or *FAX* THIS ENTIRE ORDER FORM TO:

Attn: **Marianne Arnold**
Haworth Document Delivery Service
The Haworth Press, Inc.
10 Alice Street
Binghamton, NY 13904-1580

or **FAX:** (607) 722-1424
or **CALL:** 1-800-3-HAWORTH
(1-800-342-9678; 9am-5pm EST)

PLEASE SEND ME PHOTOCOPIES OF THE FOLLOWING SINGLE ARTICLES:
1) Journal Title: _____
   Vol/Issue/Year:_____Starting & Ending Pages:_____
Article Title:_____

2) Journal Title: _____
   Vol/Issue/Year:_____Starting & Ending Pages:_____
Article Title:_____

3) Journal Title: _____
   Vol/Issue/Year:_____Starting & Ending Pages:_____
Article Title:_____

4) Journal Title: _____
   Vol/Issue/Year:_____Starting & Ending Pages:_____
Article Title:_____

(See other side for Costs and Payment Information)

COSTS: Please figure your cost to order quality copies of an article.

1. Set-up charge per article: $8.00
   ($8.00 × number of separate articles) _____

2. Photocopying charge for each article:
   1-10 pages: $1.00 _____
   11-19 pages: $3.00 _____
   20-29 pages: $5.00 _____
   30+ pages: $2.00/10 pages _____

3. Flexicover (optional): $2.00/article _____

4. Postage & Handling: US: $1.00 for the first article/
   $.50 each additional article _____
   Federal Express: $25.00 _____
   Outside US: $2.00 for first article/
   $.50 each additional article _____

5. Same-day FAX service: $.35 per page _____

6. Local Photocopying Royalty Payment: should you wish to copy the article yourself. Not intended for photocopies made for resale. $1.50 per article per copy (i.e. 10 articles x $1.50 each = $15.00) _____

GRAND TOTAL: _____

METHOD OF PAYMENT: (please check one)

❑ Check enclosed ❑ Please ship and bill. PO # _____
(sorry we can ship and bill to bookstores only! All others must pre-pay)

❑ Charge to my credit card: ❑ Visa; ❑ MasterCard; ❑ American Express;

Account Number: _____ Expiration date: _____

Signature: X _____ Name: _____

Institution: _____ Address: _____

City: _____ State: _____ Zip: _____

Phone Number: _____ FAX Number: _____

MAIL or *FAX* THIS ENTIRE ORDER FORM TO:

Attn: **Marianne Arnold**
Haworth Document Delivery Service
The Haworth Press, Inc.
10 Alice Street
Binghamton, NY 13904-1580

or FAX: (607) 722-1424
or CALL: 1-800-3-HAWORTH
(1-800-342-9678; 9am-5pm EST)